Handbook of Research on Informatics in Healthcare and Biomedicine

Athina A. Lazakidou
University of Piraeus, Greece

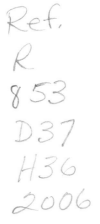
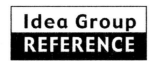

IDEA GROUP REFERENCE
Hershey · London · Melbourne · Singapore

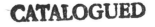

Acquisitions Editor: Michelle Potter
Development Editor: Kristin Roth
Senior Managing Editor: Amanda Appicello
Managing Editor: Jennifer Neidig
Copy Editor: Shanelle Ramelb
Typesetter: Diane Huskinson
Cover Design: Lisa Tosheff
Printed at: Yurchak Printing Inc.

Published in the United States of America by
    Idea Group Reference (an imprint of Idea Group Inc.)
    701 E. Chocolate Avenue, Suite 200
    Hershey PA 17033
    Tel: 717-533-8845
    Fax: 717-533-8661
    E-mail: cust@idea-group.com
    Web site: http://www.idea-group-ref.com

and in the United Kingdom by
    Idea Group Reference (an imprint of Idea Group Inc.)
    3 Henrietta Street
    Covent Garden
    London WC2E 8LU
    Tel: 44 20 7240 0856
    Fax: 44 20 7379 3313
    Web site: http://www.eurospan.co.uk

Library of Congress Cataloging-in-Publication Data

Handbook of research on informatics in healthcare & biomedicine / Athina Lazakidou, editor.
    p. cm.
    Summary: "This collection describes and analyzes recent breakthroughs in healthcare and biomedicine providing comprehensive coverage and definitions of important issues, concepts, new trends and advanced technologies"--Provided by publisher.
    Includes bibliographical references and index.
    ISBN 1-59140-982-9 (hardcover) -- ISBN 1-59140-983-7 (ebook)
    1. Medical informatics. 2. Bioinformatics. I. Lazakidou, Athina, 1975-
    R853.D37H36 2006
    610'.285--dc22
                        2006009481

British Cataloguing in Publication Data
A Cataloguing in Publication record for this book is available from the British Library.

Editorial Advisory Board

List of Contributors

Table of Contents

Section I
Medical Data and Health Information Systems

Section II
Standardization and Classification Systems in Medicine

Section IX
Image Processing and Archiving Systems

Section X
Signal Proessing Techniques

Section XI
Use of New Technologies in Biomedicine

Section XII
Ergonomic and Safety Issues in Computerized Medical Equipment

Section XIII
Health Economics and Health Services Research

Detailed Table of Contents

Section I
Medical Data and Health Information Systems

Paper-based health records have a number of significant disadvantages. The implementation of electronic health records systems is not simple; it concerns not a single system but a collection of interlocking systems that are tied to a series of complex clinical and administrative work flows.

Chapter II

In this chapter the authors explain how exactly the information flow takes place in medical systems, and they identify which mechanisms are usually being used to prevent violence of those systems. Finally, they present some examples of security deficiency and what impacts have been recorded.

Chapter III

Between 2001 and 2003, a project conducted in Croatia aimed to establish and develop a health information system based on the latest technologies. Extraordinary results in the trial run give the authors the ground to recommend such an approach to all transitional post communist countries. The development of such systems is feasible in transitional countries because most of them are still having one main insurer.

This chapter has reviewed the regulatory requirements definitions of FDA, AFSSAPS, EC and how computer systems can be validated with a relevant approach. By directing validation activities into a clear action plan, first, we need to analyze the specific organizational need according to the priorities and impacts to construct the required validation plan which can fulfill the requirements. The aim of the authors is to focus on a general approach to validation that can support several needs without addressing the technical aspects.

Chapter V

In many countries organizations of primary care services have been established at local or district levels. In Australia, divisions of general practice have played a key role in supporting general practices to provide more systematic care through disseminating evidence-based guidelines, educating GPs and consumers, supporting shared-care and self-management education, providing allied health services, and coordinating local registers for recall and audit. The authors have been involved in one widely implemented computer-based register system which has demonstrated improvements in the quality of care.

Section II
Standardization and Classification Systems in Medicine

Chapter VI

Standards in health and medical informatics are a means of enabling better healthcare. Healthcare is supposed to be better if healthcare providers can access data from patient health records, read records, or add new data that other healthcare providers taking care of the patient can access. There are a variety of organizations and groups developing standards, cooperating with ISO and CEN, or acting as administers and coordinators in standardization. For example, there are Health Level 7 (HL7); Digital Imaging and Communications in Medicine (DICOM); American National Standards Institute (ANSI), a non-profit organization that administers and coordinates the U.S. voluntary standardization and conformity assessment system; and others.

Chapter VII

Since the introduction of information systems in health, the demand for coding systems has been great. Medical coding systems are fundamental to medical record keeping as well as to gathering and communicating public health statistics. They are used for a variety of purposes: recording causes of death, coding diseases and procedures, and physician billing and reimbursement.

Section III
Virtual Reality Applications in Medicine

Chapter VIII

This chapter explores the technological quest of virtual reality within the field of medicine. Although the author does not intend to provide an exhaustive review of the various health informatics applications of VR over the past 15 years of its development, he presents some of the major technological breakthroughs and their impact in the provision of healthcare services to the point-of-need, (i.e. the patient).

Chapter IX

Computer simulation of biological processes is a convenient tool for biomedical research that is easy to handle with various applications. The complexity of biological systems imposes limits in their usage; most often the results are limited to a small number of variables and cover just certain relations while always neglecting others. However, the programs will become more complex, covering more variables, trying to get closer to the great challenge in this field in the (near) future—to simulate an entire cell.

Chapter X

Virtual reality today is an important part of modern scientific methodology and research, using the modern high speed computers of the most recently designed technologies for research and simulation in various scientific fields such as ergo physiology and bio kinetics. This is a new field in contemporary science and methodology of the experimentation, and it will continue with great success. An important field using this new way of research is the simulation of the human movement in ergo physiology and applied bio kinetics science.

Section IV
Virtual Learning Environments in Healthcare and Biomedicine

Chapter XI

In this chapter the authors report on their experiences in education of both students of healthcare engineering at Graz University of Applied Sciences and students of medicine at the Medical University Graz, which were gained during the winter term of 2004. Care2x is an open source Web-based integrated healthcare environment (IHE). It allows the integration of data, information, functions, and workflows in one environment. The system is currently consisting of four major components, which can also function independently: hospital information system (HIS), practice management (PM), a central data server (CDS), and a health exchange protocol (HXP). Although the components are under heavy development, the HIS has reached a degree of stability, where one can use it at least for educational purposes.

Chapter XII

Learning objects (LO) are theoretically based on granular, reusable chunks of information. In this chapter the authors argue that LOs should consist of more than just content, (i.e., they should include pre-knowledge questions on the basis of the concept of the advanced organizer), self-evaluation questions (assessment), and appropriate metadata. The used metadata concept must be based on accepted standards, such as learning object metadata (LOM) and the shareable object reference model (SCORM). A best practice example of the realization of these concepts is the Virtual Medical Campus Graz (VMC-Graz), which actually is the realization of an information system to make a new curriculum digitally accessible.

Chapter XIII

Motivating and teaching healthcare students to use information and communication technologies represent a challenge. For successful integration of healthcare and technology, it must be invested in organization, but particularly in people. Motivation and a lot of practical work are mandatory for teaching informatics in healthcare. Practical knowledge of informatics is an investment for healthcare students which can improve the quality of study, work efficiency, and their everyday life. In this chapter, four examples of connecting their jobs with informatics are presented. Connecting their work and everyday life with lecturers is an efficient way of motivating healthcare students to use information and communication technologies.

E-learning is developing rapidly worldwide. The volume of the information, which e-learning systems render, grows too. Nowadays, the critical issue is to acquire more knowledge in less time and effort. The chaotic volumes of information provided must be elaborated and transformed into knowledge. Contemporary e-Learning systems, although they embody up-to-date technology, AI techniques, and pedagogical methods, they address to a flat spectrum of users. The user agents deal with this weakness. Also, the wide and manifold spectrum of the health and social sector parties will definitely benefit from the architecture proposed, as most e-learning systems lack this feature.

E-learning has the potential to transform learning for healthcare and social care, supporting the aims of the NHS Plan and raising standards of care for patients and service users across health and social care. This chapter sets out a vision of healthcare and social care services in the 21st century, and a strategy for making it a reality. The authors present and discuss here the basic principles and benefits of e-learning for healthcare professionals, medical students, and patient education.

Chapter XVI

Information technology is an increasingly important tool for accessing and managing medical information—both patient-specific and more general scientific knowledge. Medical educators are aware of the need for all medical students to learn to use information technology effectively. Computer-based learning has been developed for the beginning medical student and the experienced practitioner, for the lay person and the medical expert. In this chapter, the authors present examples of actual programs that are being used to support medical education for each of these categories of learners.

Clinically, it is currently used in the diagnosis of disease and the assessment of disease progression, and for preoperative surgical planning in functional neurosurgery, which is a rapidly advancing field that offers minimally invasive and highly effective treatment options for many difficult neurological disorders. Recent technological advances in neuroimaging techniques, the development of larger sensor arrays, the use of sophisticated computer hardware and superior graphics, and the development of new mathematical tools for modeling the head and the intracranial sources underlying the externally recorded neurophysiological signals, gradually make more apparent the relevance of this technique, by providing answers to complex questions about the structural and functional connectivity of the brain, and the way it represents and processes information.

Chapter XVIII

The authors present a general review of electrocardiogram (ECG) diagnosis using decision support systems. Computerized ECG processing can be divided into several stages. The most important ones are the analysis and the diagnosis. The variety of the systems developed in order to address the automation of these two tasks shows the great interest for this scientific area and its clinical importance. The developed methods differ in terms of accuracy, but each one of them has unique advantages. Proper combination of the above techniques can improve the results of ECG analysis and diagnosis.

Information seeking is one of the most important aspects of information processing. While the different types of information processing strategies used by people when making decisions have been extensively studied, the role of the decision context has only recently received some attention. Information processing is modified significantly by the decision-making context and decision task characteristics. Knowledge of clinical decision-making is therefore becoming increasingly important when designing an intervention that will produce sustained behavioral change. An exploration of the context and information seeking aspects of prescribing is emerging as a first step towards building the concept of task-specific decision support design.

Data mining techniques have been used as a recent trend for gaining diagnostics results especially in medical fields such as kidney dialysis, skin cancer and breast cancer detection, and also biological sequence classification. The primary problem for urological dysfunction is acute and chronic renal failure which can be treated through dialysis. This chapter describes the data mining techniques for predicting the life span of kidney dialysis patient.

Model fit in data mining requires the attention of at least 3 aspects: the data, the model to be fitted, and the optimization criterion. Spline fitting means the calculation of the parameters of the chosen spline function from the given data. The data, the class of the functions, and the optimization criterion determine the calculation method for the parameters of the spline function.

Statistical parameter estimation is a standard task in most data mining procedures. It is presupposed that the data are a sample of the interesting random variable. Parameter estimation procedures are developed following special principles and considering the distribution of the random variables. They should fulfill quality requirements. The chapter describes all aspects of parameter estimation.

Model fit is a general task in data mining. It is a basic component of general problems like optimization, statistical data evaluation, data imaging, and so forth. The method of least squares is a widely used principle to fit a model to given data and has geometric character. Many data related optimization criteria are extensions of the classic least squares method. Statistical parameter estimation and the method of least squares are closely connected in linear statistical models (e.g., the Gauss-Markov theorem in mathematical statistics). The method of least squares is explained in examples presented within the chapter. In addition, difficulties are demonstrated occurring in the model linearization.

Section VII
Current Aspects of Knowledge Management in Medicine

Health informatics is still an emerging and rapidly expanding academic discipline located at the intersection of information and communications technology (ICT) and the many areas of healthcare. Its growth is a direct consequence of the dramatic expansion of ICT across the health service over the last two decades. The heterogeneous nature of the discipline means that it finds itself enmeshed in the many methodological and epistemological issues involved in the practice of healthcare. Indeed, even health informatics' most basic formula—the generation and transformation of data to information and knowledge—invites divergent opinions about the assumptions that underpin its claims.

The knowledge management (KM) model constitutes a hopeful innovation in the health sector with more possibilities and uses. It's about time for a qualitative upgrade of health services provision to take place. The KM is a tool that helps healthcare professionals to implement the best practices while considering the special needs of each patient and sometimes to innovate. Information technology in knowledge management is just the "enabler"; the idea is for people to start sharing experiences and ideas with a common aim.

Chapter XXVI

This chapter presents the basic principles and theoretical aspects of use of knowledge management (KM) in medicine. KM is a basic tool for all those working in the health field and for hospitals. It helps in sending the right information, to the right part, to the right person, at the right time, so that the right decisions can be made, depending on the existing problems. It is certain that with the help of knowledge management, the effectiveness in the health field will be increased through unified systems, processes and methods, the cultivation of exchanging knowledge, and the promotion of the effective use of available information.

Chapter XXVII

Organizations all over the world are adapting to rapid changes in many ways, and an approach that has made significant contributions to resurrection of post-war Japanese industry is the Deming's philosophy of total quality management (TQM). Deming's TQM is indeed applicable to the management of Internet businesses and eminently suitable for telemedicine and data mining projects in life sciences. The purpose of this chapter is to highlight the capability of Deming's total quality management to provide the directions and impetus to establish a framework for data mining in life sciences and to demonstrate through a simple application the different ways to apply Deming's 14 charter points in actual practice. The future possibilities are varied and some thoughts will be shared towards creating an International Consortium for Research and Development of Telemedicine Applications.

Section VIII
Telemedicine and E-Health Services

Chapter XXVIII

The development of information systems technology had led us to an increased number of telemonitoring applications to help with patient healthcare. These applications enable health professionals carry-out home health visits (virtual visit). Such applications/systems complete the management of data collection and reinforce their analysis. Telemedicine services can be shared among patients and several regional hospitals and health and other specialized centers. The authors present here new telemedicine systems and devices for patient monitoring.

Chapter XXIX

Rapidly emerging information and communication technologies (ICT) have spurred the recent escalation of various telehealth applications. There is an enormous interest in finding new ways to apply telehealth as much as telemedicine as a special part of telehealth. This chapter has along with providing a better understanding of what telehealth is, investigated the ways in which such an avant-garde, advancing, and newly emerging technology could be used in order to be available in an upper-healthcare level.

Chapter XXX

The healthcare industry is experiencing a substantial shift to care delivery away from the traditional nursing areas due to the convergence of several technology areas. Increasingly, capable health monitoring systems are moving the point of care closer to the patient, whereas the patient, better informed and aware now, undertakes an active role to self care and/or prevention. Emerging ICT technologies in conjunction with the medical device industry development (intelligent devices, biosensors, novel software, etc.) demonstrate the personalized healthcare delivery potential without geographical limitations.

Chapter XXXI

In pathology, the sample subject of analysis by the doctor is most often a biological tissue specimen cut in very thin sections, disposed over a glass slide, and colored with suitable stainings in order to make morphological structures and biochemical components visually apparent. In particular, telepathology has been traditionally constituted by the set of techniques for remotely transmitting images acquired from a glass slide through a microscope. This chapter provides a brief overview on telepathology and digital pathology techniques and applications.

Chapter XXXII

It is easily understood why chronically ill children and adults feel more comfortable receiving care at home rather than having to visit a healthcare facility. The medical professional needs to work in close cooperation with a variety of health specialists and the patient's family for obtaining best care. For this reason, a great variety of homecare systems and services have been developed. The related legal and ethical implications or constraints that concern homecare systems and medical procedures are taken into account, so as to ensure that all the appropriate technological and operational measures are delivered.

Chapter XXXIII

Electronic solutions are more and more common in the healthcare sector (e.g., electronic prescription), and it may be useful to submit pharmaceutical products electronically. This chapter gives a closer look at the opportunities of the electronic way of submission concerning process, time, and costs.

Chapter XXXIV

The Semantic Web provides a mechanism for adding meaning to data, essential in healthcare where the same clinical information can have many different representations. Combining the Semantic Web and Web services in relation to the healthcare domain results in Semantic Web services for healthcare, which will ultimately enable automated interpretation of clinical data. Semantic Web services for healthcare open new possibilities in knowledge management, clinical decision support, and application integration. Semantic Web services have the potential to support an advanced health care environment, offering new applications and services to health networks. Primary issues of concern are data security and confidentiality.

Section IX
Image Processing and Archiving Systems

New developments are continually making the technology faster, more powerful, less invasive, and less expensive. Imaging technology was primarily used in medical diagnosis initially, but it is being increasingly used in pure neuroscience, psychological research and in many other fields such as biomedicine and bioengineering.

Compression of medical images is an area of discussion among the medical community due to the fact that compressing an image could lead to vital diagnostic information being lost. In telemedicine applications, compression of medical images plays a paramount role in reducing the image file size, thereby, reducing the bandwidth for transmission over a network. The main objective of this work is to evaluate different integer wavelets on the basis of their lossy and lossless compression performance for various medical images.

Three-dimensional image elaboration is a very strong tool in medical diagnostics. Many of the diseases with tissue and microscopic interest are able to have an early diagnosis and therefore to be cured. Especially benefited are the fields of research medicine, pharmacology, and genetics, where the elaboration and depiction of three-dimensional models is extremely crucial for their development. The appearance of more and more evolved depiction devices and the growth of more powerful and more complete software of digital graphic elaboration predispose for even bigger steps of evolvement in the near future.

Magnetoencephalography (MEG) is a relatively new medical imaging modality for monitoring and imaging of human brain function. While spatial resolution is significantly lower than that of PET and fMRI, the ability to monitor neuronal activation at the millisecond time scale makes this modality, together with EEG, a unique window on the human brain. Recent developments in instrumentation have lead to the manufacture of whole head MEG arrays in excess of 300 magnetometers. Coupled with new data analysis tools for mapping brain function from MEG data, these systems will lead to important new insights into the workings of the human brain with applications in both clinical and cognitive neuroscience.

One of the main aims in medical image processing is to extract important features from the radiological image data, called region(s) of interest, for accurate diagnostic analysis, interpretation, and better patient treatment. Coding the region(s) of interest (ROI coding) is significant for easy, rapid transmission and also for efficient storage. This is useful in the applications areas of tele-radiology, picture archiving and communication systems (PACS), hospital information systems (HIS). ROI coding is a very significant and promising research area that can benefit many medical computing applications. Generic scaling and maxshift methods are popular among image processing communities and are well established. This chapter is an introduction for the curious developer.

The purpose of this chapter is to revisit the assessment of the perfusion CT imaging in many clinical applications, to suggest new clinical fields (e.g., brain death diagnosis) for possible future application of perfusion CT, and to emphasize the pitfalls of the method suggesting a new distributed-parameter (DP) kinetic model for generating more accurate perfusion parametric maps.

Section X
Signal Proessing Techniques

Chapter XLI

The aim of the present study is to compare nonlinear techniques' effectiveness to identify significant variations in electroencephalography (EEG), which reflect alterations in cerebral function induced by hypoxia. Cerebral hypoxia is caused by failure of the human body's systems to deliver adequate oxygen to the brain, and it is a crucial clinical condition especially in intensive care units.

Section XI
Use of New Technologies in Biomedicine

Chapter XLII

Devices of the future will incorporate information technology, nanotechnology, and biosciences. In the near future, a convergence between engineering and biology is expected. Medical technology should develop new skills in molecular and cell biology in order to correspond to the demands of medical science. As industry trends move toward smaller, lower-power, sensor-driven devices, new sciences such as protein-based therapies present new targets and new opportunities.

This chapter introduces the field of artificial intelligence in medicine, a new research area that combines sophisticated representational and computing techniques with the insights of expert physicians to produce tools for improving healthcare. This introductory chapter describes the historical and technical foundations of the work and provides an overview of the current state of the art and research directions. The authors describe prototype computer programs that tackle difficult clinical problems in a manner similar to that of an expert physician.

Dental researchers collaborating with bioinformaticians have achieved advances in oral health research by actualizing the impact of genetics in oral health. With the help of bioinformatics, a spectrum of questions in dentistry can be addressed. Comparative genomics approaches are used to identify the functional domains of a protein and suggest similarities for assigning 3D structures by homology modeling. Three-dimensional structure predictions developed by modeling of conserved domains of proteins supports a key role for specific residues in processes like mineralization.

Chapter XLV

Recently developed bioinformatics algorithms and tools exploit such relevant information within heterogeneous and widely distributed databases of the biomolecular databanks accessible through Web servers to extract a list of the most significant genes as a cause of disease and to gather and evaluate the relevance of the gene annotations related. Genomic databanks and bioinformatic databank-based tools are useful to highlight significant biological characteristics and to support a global approach in order to improve the understanding of complex cellular mechanisms and patophisiological knowledge.

The proper and harmonious expression of a large number of genes is a critical component of normal growth and development and the maintenance of proper health. Disruptions or changes in gene expression are responsible for many diseases. Using traditional methods to assay gene expression, researchers were able to survey a relatively small number of genes at a time. The emergence of new tools enables researchers to address previously intractable problems and to uncover novel potential targets for therapies. Microarrays allow scientists to analyze expression of many genes in a single experiment quickly and efficiently.

The analysis of the frequency distribution of biological data facilitates a diagnostic insight into the control systems of the organism to be gained easily. The regulatory type can be classified and quantified. With chaotic or rigid inclination go both conditions and illnesses. In this study the authors demonstrate that these results can be used to recognize the genetic disposition and the heritability. The presented analysis has not only an objective character and an evidence basis, but also it can give the therapist information about the existing risks and possible illnesses in the future for the individual and the descendants.

Chapter XLVIII

Several standardized models (questionnaires) exist for the measurement of health-status for population concerning the quality of life (health-related quality of life-HRQOL). These tools produce a depicted plan of prosperity, and portray changes of levels of natural and mental health before and after a patient's introduction to the health system.

Section XII
Ergonomic and Safety Issues in Computerized Medical Equipment

Chapter XLIX

In the case of medical equipment, the design can impact enormously on its successful use. In particular, errors in operating such equipment are often caused, at least in part, by the design of the user interface. Such errors can not only hamper patient care, but in some cases can even lead to injury or death. It is obviously important that medical equipment be designed with special consideration given to the impact of design on safe operation.

Chapter L

Computers are now increasingly being introduced into safety-critical systems like nuclear power plants and aircraft and, as a consequence, have occasionally been involved in deadly mishaps. As the cost of microcomputer technology continues to drop, computers also now are being used increasingly in medical systems and equipment such as ventilators or pacemakers, sometimes with safety-critical results. This note illustrates some of the special concerns that arise when computer technology is introduced into medical equipment, using two case studies as examples. Also discussed are some of the regulations that have been proposed by the (American) Food and Drug Administration (FDA) to help tackle the special problems that can arise when developing software-based medical equipment.

Chapter LI

Alarms are frequently employed in safety critical environments such as in aviation and nuclear power plants. Now that microcomputer technology has revolutionized the design of patient monitors for use in modern hospital operating rooms (ORs) and intensive care units (ICUs), alarms are used in countless medical products ranging from infusion pumps to ventilators. This is especially true in anesthesia/surgical and critical care environments. In this brief chapter the authors examine the use of alarms in the acute care clinical environment, focusing on their strengths and limitations in the setting of patient monitoring equipment.

Section XIII
Health Economics and Health Services Research

Chapter LII

There is a general recognition that numerous organizational factors will influence the success of an informatics intervention. This is supported by a body of evidence from multi-disciplinary and health-specific research. Organizational factors are highly interrelated and the exact nature and contribution of each to the success of an intervention is not clear. A health-specific understanding and recognition of these factors is necessary if informatics applications are to reach their potential in healthcare settings.

Chapter LIII

The big growth of sciences and technology in the last decades of the 20th century has resulted in the rapid development of medical science and also the models of demand of health services. These developments, which influenced all the professions of health and helped benefit health services, are carried out henceforth in the frames of completely organized systems of health. It is exceptionally critical to for professionals, or the future professionals of health, to understand not only the sectors of their professions, but also the nature, the organization, and the operation of systems in which they make their professions. It is also critical for citizens to understand how important it is to evaluate the health sector and economic output.

Chapter LIV

This chapter is an attempt to use a rather new economic framework in order to define the value and the placement of ICT within the healthcare sector—the way that it transforms the previous healthcare delivery into a co-produced activity. This effort might be proven helpful to facilitate implementation issues and to diffuse telemedicine in each healthcare system.

Chapter LV

Advances in information technology and telecommunications may offer many potential benefits to Australia's under-served communities by reducing the barriers of distance and space that disadvantage rural areas; this can only happen where projects enable the participation of all groups in the community. Improvements in the knowledge and use of such technologies have been identified as being beneficial in improving health literacy in rural communities and will continue to be an area of attention to reduce health inequities in Australia.

Preface

Advances in information and communication technologies (ICT) have provided the tools and the environment to study, analyze, and better understand complex medical problems. This technological development has enabled researchers to provide increasingly advanced services, including computer-assisted radiology, telemedicine, robotized tele-operating systems, and so forth.

In recent years, research in computer applications applied to healthcare and biomedicine has dramatically intensified. The *Handbook of Research on Informatics in Healthcare and Biomedicine* aims to provide a platform for researchers to describe and analyze recent breakthroughs in these areas. This handbook will be most helpful as it provides comprehensive coverage and definitions of the most important issues, concepts, new trends and advanced technologies in healthcare and biomedicine. This important new handbook will be distributed worldwide among academic and professional institutions and will be instrumental in providing researchers, scholars, students, and professionals access to the latest knowledge related to information science and technology in the areas of healthcare and biomedicine.

This handbook provides a compendium of terms, definitions, and explanations of concepts, processes, and acronyms. Additionally, this volume features short chapters authored by leading experts offering an in-depth description of key terms and concepts related to different areas, issues, and trends in information science and technologies in hospitals and other organizations worldwide.

The *Handbook of Research on Informatics in Healthcare and Biomedicine* is an excellent source of comprehensive knowledge and literature on the topic of health and biomedical informatics.

The topics in this handbook cover useful areas of general knowledge including medical data and health information systems, standardization and classification systems in medicine, virtual reality applications in medicine, virtual learning environments in healthcare and biomedicine, computer-assisted diagnosis, data mining and medical decision making, current aspects of knowledge management in medicine, telemedicine and e-health services, image processing and archiving systems, signal processing techniques, use of new technologies in biomedicine, ergonomic and safety issues in computerized medical equipment, health economics, and health services research. Speicifically, these useful terms and key words have been included and analyzed in the concrete sections of this publication.

A healthcare provider's competitiveness, level of efficiency, and quality of care may be in direct relationship to the rate of progress toward a paperless system—with digital documentation of all clinical and administrative care processes. Each small step toward the electronic health record should be analyzed according to its benefits and costs. Hospitals and delivery networks must share secure health information and improve processes and efficiency in handling IT. The first section, "Medical Data and Health Information Systems", contains chapters related to the current status and future prospects of the electronic health record systems, the security in health information systems, and various applications in the area of health informatics.

For more than 130 years the systematic collection and record of medical information has been based on the use of traditional classifications, nomenclatures, and coding schemes of various kinds. Until relatively recently, such schemes were used mainly for recording causes of death and gathering minimal diagnostic information for statistical and epidemiological purposes. Despite their many limitations, schemes such as the international classification of diseases (ICD) have been successful in supporting the collation and comparison of national and international statistics on morbidity and mortality, and advancing our understanding of the distribution and causes of diseases. The second section, "Standardization and Classification Systems in Medicine", contains chapters related to standardization and classification systems in health.

Medicine will benefit from virtual reality. As recorded in the military, virtual reality can provide an excellent training mechanism when there is no room for mistakes. Doctors will be able to practice alone or in teams to fine tune their skills for highly sensitive operations without having to risk a human life. Virtual reality can improve the doctor's performance during operations by superimposing vital information on the patient during an operation. Superimposed images can increase the effectiveness of radiation treatment and reduce the scarring of a surgery. In the third section, "Virtual Reality Applications in Medicine", various virtual reality applications in (bio) medicine and their benefits are presented.

The application of computer technology to education often refers to computer-assisted learning (CAL), computer-based education (CBE), or computer-aided instruction (CAI). Computer-based learning has been developed for the beginning medical student and the experienced practitioner, for the lay person and the medical expert. In the fourth section, "Virtual Learning Environments in Healthcare and Biomedicine", examples of actual programs that are being used to support medical education for each of these categories of learners are presented.

Digital imaging still remains one of the key technologies for progress in healthcare. With further advances in processing, display, and communication of medical imaging it becomes the key to solve many problems in diagnosis and therapy. As well as computer-assisted diagnosis, computer-assisted surgery relies increasingly on some type of image management. Typical examples can be found in craniofacial surgery, neurosurgery, orthopaedic surgery of the hip and spine, plastic/reconstructive surgery, otolaryngology, and so forth. The fifth section, "Computer-Assisted Diagnosis", includes a large number of examples in the area of computer-assisted diagnosis.

The process of extracting useful information from a set of data is called "data mining". Data mining techniques have been used as a recent trend for gaining diagnostic results especially in medical fields such as kidney dialysis, skin cancer, and breast cancer detection and also biological sequence classification. Various "Data Mining and Medical Decision Making" are presented in the Section VI.

Knowledge management is a basic tool for all those who work in the health field and in hospitals. It helps sending the right information, to the right part, to the right person, at the right time, so that the right decisions can be made, depending on the existing problems. It is certain that with the help of knowledge management the effectiveness in the health field will be increased through unified systems, processes and methods, the cultivation of exchanging knowledge, and the promotion of the effective use of available information. In Section VII, basic principles and theoretical aspects of the use of knowledge management in medicine are clearly presented.

Rapidly emerging information and communication technologies (ICT) have spurred the recent escalation of various telehealth applications. It is true that there is an enormous interest in finding new ways to apply telehealth as much as telemedicine as a special part of telehealth. Section VIII, "Telemedicine and E-Health Services", has, along with providing a better understanding of what telehealth is, investigated the ways in which such an avant-garde, advancing, and newly emerging technology could be used in order to make an upper healthcare level to be available. This section aims to help someone to clarify confused terms such as telehealth and telemecine or even telecare and e-health.

The rapid progress in imaging technologies during the last decades has stimulated many developments and applications in medicine, biology, industry, aerospace, remote sensing, meteorology, oceanography, and environment. New developments are continually making the technology faster, more powerful, less invasive, and less expensive. Imaging technology was primarily used in medical diagnosis initially, but it is being increasingly used in pure neuroscience, psychological research, and in many other fields. The quantitative nature of data will be relevant to the effective diagnostic as well as therapeutic management of patients—

whatever disease they may have. In the ninth section, "Image Processing and Archiving Systems", various imaging technologies and their applications in Biomedicine are clearly presented.

In digital signal processing, numerous powerful algorithms, both linear and non-linear, have been developed during the past three decades. These have given rise to tremendous progress in speech and image processing. But digital signal processing is not restricted to communications and information processing. It also plays a leading role in such diverse fields as measurement, automatic control, robotics, medicine, biology, and geophysics to mention just the most important ones. New signal processing techniques for use in medicine are clearly presented in Section X.

Medical technology is a science discipline that has been rapidly growing over the last decades. It is characterized by a constant flow of innovations and a high level of research and development. Many technological achievements have dramatically changed the way that medicine diagnoses and treats human disease. Improved healthcare technology has presented many revolutionary medical devices that reduced mortality and morbidity. New various technologies applied in biomedicine are presented in Section XI.

As the cost of microcomputer technology continues to drop, computers are being used increasingly in medical systems and equipment such as ventilators or pacemakers, sometimes with safety-critical results. "Ergonomic and Safety Issues in Computerized Medical Equipment" are clearly presented and discussed in Section XII.

Health services research is research that seeks to improve the quality, organisation and financing of health services. Its concern extends from the care of individuals through health care organisations to national and international policies. Section XIII contains chapters related to health economics and health services research.

Athina A. Lazakidou, PhD
Editor

Acknowledgments

The editor expresses her deep gratitude to the chapter authors whose original contributions served as the foundation for this important handbook.

The editor also would like to acknowledge and express her appreciation to all members of the editorial board who generously allocated their time and expertise to reviewing the manuscripts which was a significant contribution to the overall quality of the publication. They include Professor George Vassilakopoulos, Health Informatics Laboratory, University of Piraeus, Greece, Dr. Andriani Daskalaki, Free University of Berlin, Germany, Dr. Melpomeni Lazakidou, General Hospital Salzburg, Austria, Dr. Konstantinos Konstantinidis, General Hospital Salzburg, Austria, Dr. Konstantinos Siassiakos, University of Piraeus, Greece), Dr. Iordanis Evangelou, National Institutes of Health, USA, and Dr. Sotirios Bisdas, Johann Wolfgang Goethe University, Frankfurt, Germany).

Michelle E. Potter, acquisitions/development editor, provided editorial assistance and guidance over the past six months, and Jan Travers, managing director, provided guidance and support over the year since the project began.

Special thanks to our publisher: Idea Group Inc. Without you, we could not have completed this undertaking.

This book is respectfully dedicated to my parents Apostolos and Paulina and to my sisters Georgia and Melina.

Athina A. Lazakidou, PhD
Editor

About the Editor

Dr. Athina A. Lazakidou currently works at the University of Piraeus as a teaching assistant and at the Hellenic Army Academy as a lecturer in informatics. Prior to that, she worked as a visiting lecturer at the Department of Computer Science at the University of Cyprus (2000-2002). She did her undergraduate studies at the Athens University of Economics and Business (Greece) and received her BSc in computer science in 1996. In 2000, she received her PhD in medical informatics from the Department of Medical Informatics, University Hospital Benjamin Franklin at the Free University of Berlin (Germany). She is also an internationally known expert in the field of computer applications in healthcare and biomedicine, with four books and numerous papers to her credit. Her research interests include health informatics, e-learning in medicine, software engineering, graphical user interfaces, (bio)medical databases, clinical decision-support systems, hospital and clinical information systems, electronic medical record systems, telematics, and other applications in medicine.

Section I
Medical Data and
Health Information Systems

A healthcare provider's competitiveness, level of efficiency, and quality of care may be directly related to his or her rate of progress toward a paperless system, with the digital documentation of all clinical and administrative care processes. Each small step toward the electronic health record should be analyzed according to its benefits and costs. Hospitals and delivery networks must share secure health information and improve processes and efficiency in handling IT.

Chapter I
Electronic Health Records

Olga Galani
National and Kapodistrian University of Athens, Greece

Ageliki Nikiforou
National and Kapodistrian University of Athens, Greece

ABSTRACT

The electronic health record is a means of organizing patient data making profound use of the advances in the field of information technology. Its purpose is to fulfill the various needs for information not only of patients and healthcare providers but also of other beneficiaries. The implementation of EHR systems in healthcare organizations is very complex and involves many parameters. This article is about the challenges faced by those undertaking such a task and about the potential benefits from a successful implementation.

INTRODUCTION

Advances in computer technology have the potential to solve some of the most persistent problems in healthcare. There is a consensus in healthcare that there is a need for creating information and communication systems that reduce cumbersome and outdated paperwork. Paper-based health records have been in use for centuries since they require relatively little investment to use and produce compared to more sophisticated supports, and they are familiar to users who do not have to acquire new skills or behaviors to use them properly. Despite all these, paper-based health records also have a number of significant disadvantages. First of all, paper is a very fragile medium that requires large storage facilities. In addition, paper-based health records require large human effort to keep the files and archives organized and updated, they are available only in one place at a time, and the aggregation of data for research is difficult. Furthermore, we are moving to a model where the patient is no longer a passive recipient of the services provided by nurses, physicians, and others, but is an active partner (a consumer or a client) with the healthcare practitioners. A successful partnership requires open access to the healthcare information. The creation and implementation

Figure 1. Creation of an electronic health record

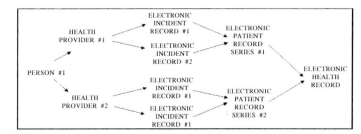

of electronic health record (EHR) systems is at the heart of addressing these needs (Daskalaki, Lazakidou, Philipp, Jacob, & Berlien, 2001; Mantas, 2002; Medical Records Institute, http://www.medrecinst.com/index.asp; Wang et al., 2003).

COMPONENT PARTS OF AN ELECTRONIC HEALTH RECORD

Figure 1 depicts an oversimplified view of how the EHR is created.

To gain a more accurate appreciation of the EHR's complexity and breadth of information, one must recognize the wide range of health information sources. Each time an individual visits a healthcare provider, data are generated. Figure 2 identifies some of the sources of data for an EHR as listed by the Institute of Medicine (Institute of Medicine, 1997).

The component parts of utmost importance of an EHR are the following:

- Patient's demographic details
- Family history
- Allergies and alerts
- Medical history
- Procedures
- A summary of services provided to an individual by:
  - Hospitals during admissions for treatment

- Outpatient and emergency departments
- Community and allied health
- General practice
- Dental clinics
- Diagnostic results (pathology and radiology)
- Documents such as assessments, discharge referrals, and letters
- Multidisciplinary and multiservice care plans

USE AND BENEFITS OF THE EHR

The primary purpose of the EHR is to provide a documented record of care that supports present and future care by the same or other

Figure 2. Sources of health-related data

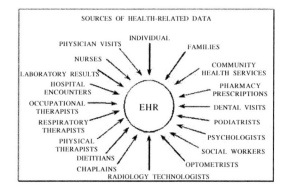

clinicians. This documentation provides a means of communication among clinicians contributing to the patient's care. The primary beneficiaries are the patient and the clinicians.

Any other purpose for which the medical record is used may be considered secondary as are any other beneficiaries. Much of the content of EHRs is currently defined by secondary users as the information collected for primary purposes was insufficient for purposes such as billing, policy and planning, statistical analysis, accreditation, and so forth.

Secondary uses of EHRs include the following:

- **Medico-Legal Uses:** Evidence of care provided, indication of compliance with legislation, reflection of the competence of clinicians
- **Quality Management:** Continuous quality-improvement studies, utilisation review, performance monitoring, benchmarking, accreditation
- **Education**
- **Research:** Development and evaluation of new diagnostic modalities, disease-prevention measures, epidemiological studies, population health analysis
- **Public and Population Health:** Access to quality information enables the effective management of real and potential public health risks
- **Policy Development:** Health-statistics analysis, trends analysis, casemix analysis
- **Health-Service Management:** Resource allocation and management, cost management
- **Billing, Finance, and Reimbursement:** Insurers, government agencies, funding bodies (Schloeffel & Jeselon, 2002)

The use of EHR can yield to a number of benefits, which can be described in terms of the following attributes.

Patients

- Integrated health services
- Improved healthcare and decreased risks (e.g., adverse drug reactions)
- Not having to repeat basic information, such as name and address
- Increased confidence knowing that all healthcare professionals have access to all relevant parts of one's medical history
- Access to their own health records helps patients to make informed decisions about their health
- Avoidance of duplicate, invasive, and/or expensive tests

Public

- Expanded reach of effective healthcare
- More secure information
- Access to information about how the healthcare system works

Health Professionals

- View of patient data
- Access to other related and integrated patient information
- Access through a portal to related health services
- Seamless care through the coordination of multiprofessional and multiagency care
- Development of decision-support systems

Health Administrators

- Increased patient care time
- Access to data to support clinical governance and local planning
- Reduced healthcare costs

Policy Makers

- Improved and effective health maintenance and education
- Support for medical and administrative decision-making processes
- Improved long-term planning

Researchers

- Access to timely, high-quality data for research
- Access to up-to-date research findings, and treatment and medication options
- Data aggregation
- Improved trend analysis

Governments

- Improved accountability
- Improved health-resource allocation (Upham, 2004)

THE EHR TODAY

The barrier to the adoption of the EHR that is probably the most difficult to overcome is the lack of easily apparent returns on investment (ROI). Many writers on the subject have noted that healthcare decision makers find it difficult to readily demonstrate ROI or justify the expenditure of dollars and time to undertake a comprehensive EHR system within their organizations, particularly while healthcare costs continue to spiral out of control and taking into consideration the fact that the initial investment on equipment can be quite expensive. Another factor that complicates the adoption of the EHR is the fact that data are heavily structured, being recorded in their allocated space. This implies a deep knowledge of the system to know where to record any piece of information

Figure 3. Clinical data repositories in use and planned for use within 1 to 4 years

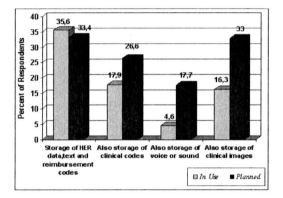

(which requires a period of time to learn), or searching for the appropriate location to record most pieces of information (which requires time to search). Training is an important issue as this is required by a large amount of the population. In addition, one should always keep in mind the fact that the population has different levels of computer literacy (Upham, 2004). All the above characteristics of the EHR have contributed to a slow increase in the adoption of such systems in many hospitals. One example of an important shift in the EHR market is seen in Figure 3, which includes responses to the survey question, "What functions or components of an EHR system do you have in use or are planned for implementation?" Of the 436 who responded to the question, 35.6% said they have already implemented the basic repository capabilities of storing data, text, and reimbursement codes. Combined with those planning to add these basic capabilities, the percentage is expected to grow to 67% in the next 4 years. On top of the fundamentals are plans to add storage for clinical codes, voice or sound, and clinical images.

The EHR survey also included an analysis by market segment with some interesting find-

Figure 4. Some barriers, by market segment, to implementing EHRs

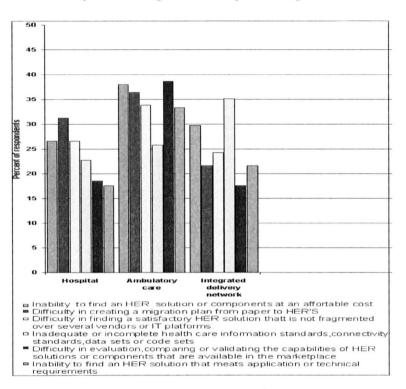

ings. Figure 4 shows some of the results from the 477 respondents to the question, "What are the major barriers to your plans for implementing an EHR?"

For example, respondents from ambulatory-care facilities indicated that they face more barriers in implementing EHRs than respondents from hospitals or integrated delivery networks. In particular, ambulatory-care respondents reported challenges in finding an affordable solution, creating a migration plan, finding a solution that is not fragmented among vendors, evaluating solutions, and finding a solution that meets their technical requirements (Blair, 2003).

THE EVOLUTION OF THE EHR

Although we should always expect a medical record to be populated with data about a specific patient, in the electronic implementation of such records, we may also expect to find data regarding populations of patients, integrated access to the biomedical literature, and interactive environments for offering clinical guidelines or frank consultative advice. We can envision a world in which the enterprise LAN (local area network) is seamlessly connected to the full Internet, with integrated access to a wide variety of information sources that are geographically distributed well beyond local institutions. Although such a concept raises important issues related to patient privacy and confidentiality, there are technical and policy measures that can be taken to help to assure that such virtual records are kept secure but also available at times of medical need.

Realizing the vision described above will depend on at least four factors.

- **An Enhanced Internet:** An Internet with much higher bandwidth and reliability, increased response time, and financial models that make the applications cost effective and practical is required. Major research efforts are underway to address some of these concerns, including the federal Next Generation Internet activity in the United States. All exploratory efforts that continue to push the state of the art in Internet technology have significant implications for the future of healthcare delivery in general and for computer-based health records in particular.

- **Better Education and Training for Healthcare Providers:** There is a difference between computer literacy (familiarity with computers and their routine uses in our society) and the knowledge of the role that computing and communications technology can and should play in our healthcare system. More medical-informatics training programs and the expansion of existing programs are needed. In addition, junior faculty in health-science schools who may wish to seek additional training in this area should be supported.

- **Changes in the Management and Organization of Healthcare Institutions:** Healthcare provides some of the most complex organizational structures in society, and it is simplistic to assume that off-the-shelf products will be smoothly introduced into a new institution without major analysis, redesign, and cooperative joint-development efforts.

- **Just Like the Healthcare Industry, Technology Cannot Stand Still:** Sys-tems must continue to evolve to meet the industry's changing needs. While today's imaging and work-flow applications are excellent for viewing and accessing information, healthcare institutions continue to push for more. Suppliers must keep developing greater intelligence within their systems to serve this dynamic industry.

Since the actual realization of EHRs requires full interoperability within and among healthcare enterprises, total industry adoption is not likely to be achieved within the near future (most predict it will be 5 to 10 years). Unlike EHRs, the continuity-of-care record (CCR) is designed to provide a snapshot of essential patient information that will enable a physician to understand a patient's context and provide appropriate care. Some of the core elements of the CCR are document-identifying information (to and from fields, date sent, purpose), patient-identifying information, patient insurance and financial information, advance directives, patient health-status information (may include conditions, diagnoses, problems, family medical history, adverse reactions and allergies, social history and health-risk factors, medications, immunizations, vital signs and physiological measurements, laboratory results and observations, procedures, and imaging), care documentations, care-plan recommendations, and a list of healthcare practitioners. The CCR is gaining momentum across the industry because it will achieve many of the immediate short-term goals and benefits envisioned by HL7 as we continue to define and develop the EHR: It may even provide the impetus needed to stimulate more rapid EHR development. It is increasingly being viewed as a practical, more immediately achievable solution while the industry continues to wait for a defined EHR (Carpenito, 2004; Golden, 2004; Shortliffe, 1999).

CONCLUSION

The implementation of EHR systems is not simple; it concerns not a single system but, rather, a collection of interlocking systems that are tied to a series of complex clinical and administrative work flows. This implementation will involve a long-term, highly coordinated commitment from a large number of stakeholders and a significant financial investment. The changes required are massive since the EHR-related initiative is trying to implement a total healthcare solutions. To this end, projects that address part of the puzzle are under way (i.e., pharmaceutical systems), others are developing application models (emergency health records) on which to base further development, and still other projects are using new technology models such as smart cards (Office of Health & Information Highway Health Canada, 2001).

REFERENCES

Blair, J. (2003). The EHR today. *Health care informatics online*. Retrieved from http://www.healthcare-informatics.com/index.htm

Carpenito, L. (2004). A report on the CCR. *Symantec enterprise solutions*. Retrieved from http://www.symantec.com

Committee of European Normalization, Technical Committee on Medical Informatics (CEN/TC 251). (n.d.). *Medical informatics vocabulary working document* (PT 011/N 300 V.1.00). Approved European Standard in Healthcare Informatics ENV 12017.

Daskalaki, A., Lazakidou, A., Philipp, C., Jacob, C., & Berlien, H. P. (2001). Introducing electronic health record into laser medicine. *Medical Informatics, 5*, 85-86.

Golden, R. (2004). *The evolving electronic patient record system.* Retrieved from http://www.infotivity.com

Institute of Medicine. (1997). *Computer-based patient records. A review of the environmental and technical changes in the healthcare industry in the United States.* Retrieved from http://www.iom.edu

Mantas, J. (2002). Electronic health record. In J. Mantas & A. Hasman (Eds.), *Textbook in health informatics: A nursing perspective* (pp. 250-257). Amsterdam: IOS Press.

Office of Health & Information Highway Health Canada. (2001). *Toward electronic health records.* Retrieved from http://www.hc-sc.gc.ca

Schloeffel, P., & Jeselon, P. (2002). *ISO/TC 215 ad hoc group report: Standards requirements for the electronic health record & discharge/referral plans.* Retrieved from http://www.iso.org

Shortliffe, E. (1999). The evolution of electronic medical records. *Academic Medicine, 74*(4), 414-419.

Upham, R. (2004). *The electronic health record: Will it become a reality?* Phoenix Health Systems. Retrieved from http://www.hipaadvisory.com

Wang, S., Middleton, B., Prosser, L., Bardon, C., Spurr, C., Carchidi, P., et al. (2003). *Academic publication proves that EMRs are cost effective:* A cost-benefit analysis of electronic medical records in primary care. *American Journal of Medicine, 114*(5), 397-403.

URL REFERENCES

Center for Health Information Technology: http://www.centerforhit.org

Medical Records Institute: http://www.medrecinst.com/index.asp

NSW Electronic Health Record: http://www.nsw.com

KEY TERMS

CCR: The continuity-of-care record is an emerging standard for communicating patient information electronically among providers. The CCR is intended to provide a snapshot of essential patient information, rather than a complete patient record, that will enable a physician to understand a patient's context and provide appropriate care. The format of the CCR allows it to be used universally to help to bridge the gaps between EHR systems and improve the portability of patient information.

Decision-Support System: Any computer-based support of medical, managerial, administrative, and financial decisions in health using knowledge bases and/or reference material.

EHR: A healthcare record in computer-readable format.

EHR System: Information system that manages and operates on the EHR.

Healthcare Record: Systematic record of the history of the health of a patient kept by a physician or other healthcare practitioner.

HL7: A specification for a health-data interchange standard designed to facilitate the transfer of health data resident on different and disparate computer systems in a healthcare setting.

LAN (Local Area Network): A system of connecting computers and computer equipment together with physical links that do not use a telecommunications network.

Smart Card: An integrated circuit card that incorporates a processor unit. The processor may be used for security algorithms, data access, or for other functions according to the nature and purpose of the card.

Chapter II
Security in Health
Information Systems

Christina Ilioudi
University of Piraeus, Greece

Athina A. Lazakidou
University of Piraeus, Greece

ABSTRACT

The development of Internet technology and Web-based applications made health information more accessible than ever before from many locations by multiple health providers and health plans. In this chapter, security in health information systems is put into perspective. The further penetration of information technology into healthcare is discussed, and it is concluded that information systems have already become a vital component, not only for the logistics of the healthcare institution but also for the rendering of care and cure.

INTRODUCTION

Before the computer age, healthcare information was typically stored in the physician's office. All information specific to a patient was generally kept in a medical record and filed in the office filing cabinet. The introduction of technology changed how physicians and other health organizations keep personal health information. Nowadays medical data are being kept in a computer, so we talk about an electronic patient record (EPR) and not about a printed medical record. Thus, health information systems rely upon a computerised infrastructure. The development of Internet technology and Web-based applications made health information more accessible than ever before from many locations by multiple health providers and health plans. In the near future, the Internet will probably be the platform of choice for processing health transactions and communicating information and data. But along with this acces-

Figure 1.

Very important
Important
Not important

Figure 2.

a	b	c	d
Data			

sibility come increased threats to the security of health information, and those who would steal, divert, alter, or misuse your information are becoming even more skilled at finding what they want and covering their tracks.

In healthcare, it is very important to develop secure systems because we want to ensure that the medical data that contain the personal information of patients will not be violated by anyone. Thus, what is under question is the availability of the right data to the right user at the right time (availability). Information technology deeply affects the confidential relationship between patient and doctor since it increasingly surrounds and mediates it. Hence, the protection of personal medical data (confidentiality) is a necessity without which medical treatment will hardly be successful. This will sometimes include the anonymity of a patient. In addition to the protection of data from unauthorized reading, data also have to be protected against unauthorized modification (integrity). Also, healthcare professionals are personally responsible and mostly liable for their decisions in favour of a particular action or against it. This raises the need for health information systems that are capable of providing an individual with undoubted proof that he or she took a certain action or did not (accountability). Below we will explain how exactly the information flow takes place in medical systems, which security model we used in the past, what the threats are, which mechanisms are usually being used to prevent the violence of those systems, and finally we will present some examples of security deficiency and what impacts have been recorded.

INFORMATION-FLOW CONTROL

In security engineering, there are two approaches to information-flow control. The first approach (Figure 1) is multilevel security (top-down approach), in which lower level information may move up in the hierarchy, but higher level information may not move down. The main representative of this approach is the Bell-LaPadula policy. The second approach (Figure 2) is multilateral security, in which information is prevented from flowing across departments. One representative of this approach is the BMA model developed by the British Medical Association to describe the information flows permitted by medical ethics. This kind of security applys very well in healthcare systems as it covers the use of techniques such as anonymity. However, we will not make further analysis of it here because this is not our goal.

THREATS TO HEALTH INFORMATION SYSTEMS

One question of vital importance for health information systems could be "What are the threats that could have a major impact on health information?" If we try to answer the question, we would count some of the potential threats. A threat can be an agent who either accidentally or intentionally gains unauthorized access to the protected IT systems. Threats may be physical or logical. Physical threats include the following:

- Employees (common threat)
- Ex-employees
- Hackers
- Terrorists
- Criminals
- Customers
- Visitors
- Destruction of physical storage devices
- Natural disasters

Protection against these threats comprises a variety of different methods and techniques.

Logical threats involve unauthorized logical access to information. They can result in the disclosure of confidential information, the illegal modification of data, or the destruction of stored data. The threats can be classified as follows:

- The disclosure of confidential information includes direct or indirect access to protected information.
- Illegal modification of data can be caused by improper, possibly accidental, data handling or intentional modifications by an illegal user (these threats are related to all attacks to data integrity).
- Denial of service can be caused by monopolizing system resources in such a way that other users cannot access them. This involves all attacks on availability.

SECURING HEALTH INFORMATION SYSTEMS

Healthcare information systems are secure if a protection mechanism enforces the security policy. A security policy must have appropriate security features. These features should be supported by a security mechanism. In the following, we specify those mechanisms.

- Protect health information. Healthcare systems will lose medical data unless they take reasonable steps to protect them. Operating computer networks should have firewalls, security monitoring, and effective password-protection mechanisms and policies, not allowing critical data to walk out of the door unprotected on laptops and PDAs (personal digital assistants).
- Protect against hackers and computer malice. Individuals (often ex-employees) can wreak havoc to a computer system by means of unauthorized access. We need authentication and authorization controls that ensure that only authorized users gain access to a system and to only those parts of the system necessary to perform his or her responsibilities. Appropriate authentication and access controls not only protect against unauthorized access, but also reduce the risk of systems being infected by malicious software.
- Avoid public-relations issues. Breaches in information security can be a source of embarrassment to an organization, especially one that relies on public trust.
- Avoid productivity issues. Lapses in information security can cause downtime and the corruption of data and systems, which in turn can cripple the operations of a company.
- It is important to develop strong cryptographic technologies end to end, where end points will range from patients' homes to large hospitals, and often may terminate in a mobile device such as a PDA or Internet-enabled cellular telephone. In addition, digital signatures should be used to verify that data, whether in transit or in a database, have not been modified by unauthorized parties. Digital signatures ensure that the accompanying data are

tamperproof and that signers cannot later deny access or use.

Apart from security measures and policies through computer technologies, there is another way to ensure security in health information systems. In particular, the Health Insurance Portability and Accountability Act of 1996 (HIPAA) has issued a detailed proposed regulation regarding security requirements for healthcare information. HIPAA includes requirements to protect the security, integrity, and confidentiality of this health-related information. To be HIPAA compliant, departments (especially hospitals that work with health information) must develop, implement, and enforce a comprehensive security program including administrative, technical, and physical safeguards as determined appropriate for the institution and data. In addition to developing their own safeguards, departments are responsible for taking steps to ensure that their affiliates and service providers safeguard customer information in their care.

EXAMPLES OF SECURITY-RISK IMPACTS

Below we mention the impact of threats in healthcare systems. We believe that this is a good way for those who are involved in healthcare to take the enforcement of security in such systems seriously.

The most common security problem within healthcare systems is the access of employees (threat from inside). Specifically, people who work in a hospital have the ability to view the protected health information (PHI) of anyone. This raises the probability for legal action, which causes major impacts. It is conceivable how important it is to enforce security policies. It is important to the introduction of security

policies that the people who have the authority to make decisions set boundaries under which the staff can operate.

Besides inside threats, it is possible for damage to occur in a healthcare system due to outside threats such as hackers. In this case, it is very important to develop mechanisms that minimize this risk. Therefore, we cannot allow an insecure Internet connection in the internal network of the healthcare system. Also, firewalls are another solution to minimize the impact of the threat.

DISCUSSION

Because of the rapid development of Internet technology and Web-based applications, it is obvious that in the near future, if we want to be more straightforward, our electronic medical records will contain personal health information about our parents or genetic information. For this reason, it is easy for everyone to understand how meaningfulness it is to find out security models or extend those that already exist. This is desirable because the most important thing for healthcare systems is to ensure our medical data.

The privacy, confidentiality, and security of health information will be achieved only when the following happen:

- Privacy and confidentiality protections are uniform and set the high standard throughout the country through federal laws that establish fair, reasonable, and uniform health-information practices, across all states. These laws should respect the rights of the individual and the public, and apply to the medium in which such information is stored, transferred, or accessed.
- An individual will have the right to access his or her health information in any setting

(with minimal limits), to have an understanding of his or her privacy rights and options, to be notified about all information practices concerning his or her information, to appropriately challenge the accuracy of his or her health information, and to opt in or authorize the collection or use of information beyond what is originally authorized by the individual or the law in certain electronic or Internet situations.

- The collection and use of health information will be permitted only for legitimate purposes and only as provided by law, and will be uniform across all jurisdictions and entities and for all individuals.
- Credentialed health-information management professionals, given their training and education in privacy and information-release and health-information management, are considered the primary custodians of health information and principal experts in maintaining the privacy, confidentiality, and security of information in the healthcare industry.
- Laws, practices, and technologies are put in place to provide protections required to maintain the appropriate privacy, confidentiality, security, and integrity of health information.

CONCLUSION

The information being transferred between hospitals or between departments that constitute a hospital is referred to as sensitive data because it concerns patients' private data. It is easy for everyone to understand how important it is to ensure security for healthcare environments. As we use computer networks and the Internet more often now than ever, when exchanging health information, the threats will become bigger. The only way to protect our

sensitive information is a systematic approach to security. The people and organizations that are involved with health information should document the steps they have taken to minimize the risk to security.

REFERENCES

Aderson, R. (n.d.). *Security engineering: A guide to building dependable distributed systems.*

Baraani-Dastjerdi, A., Pieprzyk, J., & Safavi-Naini, R. (n.d.). *Security in database: A survey study.* University of Wollongong, Department of Computer Science.

Bleumer, G. (n.d.). *Guidelines for a secure environment for information systems in medicine: SEISMED.* Hildesheim, Germany: Universität Hildesheim, Institut für Informatik Samelsonplatz.

Castano, S., Fugini, M., Martella, G., & Samarati, P. (1995). *Database security.* Addison-Wesley, ACM Press.

Clark, D. D., & Wilson, D. R. (1987). A comparison of commercial and military computer security policies. *Proceedings of IEEE Computer Society Symposium on Security and Privacy* (pp. 184-194).

Cyber Security Industry Alliance (CSIA). (n.d.). *Ten steps for securing electronic health care systems* (CSIA security briefing).

Iowa State University. (n.d.). *Health information privacy and security policy.*

Kang, M. H., Froscher, J. N., & Costich, O. (1992). A practical transaction model and untrusted transaction manager for multilevel-secure database systems. *Proceedings of 6th Annual IFIP WG11.3 Working Conference on Database Security* (pp. 289-310).

Kang, M. H., Froscher, J. N., & Moskowitz, I. S. (n.d.). *An architecture for multilevel security interoperability*. Center for High Assurance Computer Systems, Naval Research Laboratory.

National Health Policy Forum. (n.d.). *Protecting the confidentiality of health information*.

Workgroup for Electronic Data Interchange (WEDI). (2003-2004). *Strategic national implementation process (SNIP): Background to information security*.

Workgroup for Electronic Data Interchange (WEDI). (2004). *Strategic national implementation process (SNIP): Background to information security* (Final draft).

URL REFERENCES

http://www.healthcareedu.org/phs_page3c.cfm

http://www.hhs.gov/ocr/combinedregtext.pdf

http://www.hipaabasics.com/glossary.htm

http://www.hipaadvisory.com/

http://www.hutchlaw.com/resources/docs/104047-v3.doc

http://library.ahima.org/xpedio/groups/public/documents/ahima

http://www.ncipher.com/investors/glossary.php

http://www.public.iastate.edu/~health/documents/

http://security.uwmedicine.org/securitypolicies.asp

http://www.w3.org/TR/2002/WD-ws-gloss-20021114/#securitypolicy

KEY TERMS

Availability: Ensuring that authorized users have access to information and associated assets when required.

Confidentiality: The property that information is not made available or disclosed to unauthorized individuals, entities, or processes (ISO 7498-2 as cited in *HISB Draft Glossary of Terms Related to Information Security in Health Care Information Systems*).

Cryptography: The art and science of using mathematics to secure information and create a high degree of trust in the electronic realm. See also *public key*, *secret key*, *symmetric key*, and *threshold cryptography*.

Digital Signature: The encryption of a message with a private key.

ePHI (Electronic Protected Health Information): ePHI is any information specifically identifying a person that is stored electronically, or sent or shared electronically.

Hacker: A person who tries and/or succeeds at defeating computer security measures.

Healthcare: Care, services, or supplies related to the health of an individual. Healthcare includes, but is not limited to, the following: (a) preventive, diagnostic, therapeutic, rehabilitative, maintenance, or palliative care, and counseling, service, assessment, or procedure with respect to the physical or mental condition or functional status of an individual that affects the structure or function of the body, and (b) the sale or dispensing of a drug, device, equipment, or other item in accordance with a prescription.

Health Information: The term health information means any information, whether oral or recorded in any form or medium, that is created or received by a healthcare provider, health plan, public health authority, employer, life insurer, school or university, or healthcare clearinghouse. It can relate to the past, present, or future physical or mental health or condition of an individual, the provision of healthcare to an individual, or the past, present, or future payment for the provision of healthcare to an individual.

HIPAA: The Health Insurance Portability and Accountability Act of 1996.

Integrity: Safeguarding the accuracy, completeness, and control of information and processing methods.

Password: A character string used as a key to control access to files or to encrypt them.

Protected Health Information (PHI): Individually identifiable health information that is transmitted by, or maintained in, electronic media or any other form or medium. Protected health information excludes individually identifiable health information in (a) education records covered by the Family Educational Rights and Privacy Act (FERPA), and (b) employment records held by the University of New England in its role as employer.

Security Mechanism: A process (or a device incorporating such a process) that can be used in a system to implement a security service that is provided by or within the system.

Security Model: A schematic description of a set of entities and relationships by which a specified set of security services are provided by or within a system.

Security Policy: The framework within which an organization establishes needed levels of information security to achieve the desired confidentiality goals. A policy is a statement of information values, protection responsibilities, and organization commitment for a system (OTA, 1993). The American Health Information Management Association (AHIMA) recommends that security policies apply to all employees, medical staff members, volunteers, students, faculty, independent contractors, and agents (AHIMA as cited in *HISB Draft Glossary of Terms Related to Information Security in Health Care Information Systems*). It is part of the security-management process on the matrix.

Trojan (or Trojan Horse): Trojans are programs (often malicious) that install themselves or run surreptitiously on a victim's machine. They do not install or run automatically, but may entice users into installing or executing them by masquerading as another program altogether (such as a game or a patch), or they may be packaged with hacked legitimate programs that install the trojan when the host program is executed. Hence, a user thinks he or she is installing a new game found for free, but will actually be installing a nasty piece of software. While trojans are not capable of spreading by themselves, there have been several reports of worms that carry trojans, dropping them onto infected machines as they spread.

Worm: A worm is a self-contained program that spreads by creating multiple copies of itself. Unlike viruses, worms do not require a host file. Common modes of transmission used by worms include e-mail, IRC, peer-to-peer file sharing, and network drives.

Chapter III
Development of a Health Information System in a Post-Communist Country

Ranko Stevanovic
Croatian Institute of Public Health, Croatia

Ivan Pristas
Croatian Institute of Public Health, Croatia

Ana Ivicevic Uhernik
Croatian Institute of Public Health, Croatia

Arsen Stanic
Orthopaedic Clinic, Croatia

ABSTRACT

Between 2001 and 2003, a project conducted in Croatia aimed to establish and develop a health information system based on the latest technologies. Extraordinary results in the trial run give the authors the ground to recommend such an approach to all transitional post communist countries. The development of such systems is feasible in transitional countries because most of them are still having one main insurer.

INTRODUCTION

Between 2001 and 2003, a project conducted in Croatia aimed to establish and develop a health information system based on the latest technologies. The most important experience and idea applied in the Croatian project was based on the concepts developed by Professor Andrija Stampar. According to these, primary healthcare is a venue where the major health problems of a population are resolved, and a point at which outcomes of changes in the system are most significantly reflected. A central health information system should be established and developed in parallel with the primary healthcare activity. Extraordinary results in the trial run give us the ground to recommend such an approach to all transitional post-communist countries. The development of such systems is feasible in transitional countries because most of them still have one main insurer. In developed countries, however, developing these could be difficult for they have a number of insurance companies that do not find their business interest in the full integration of health information and data. Indeed, for countries with a single dominant, basic insurance company, the above is the only positive alternative. Subsequent linkups of supplemental, auxiliary, and other future insurers with the single information system on the national level will be much simpler to make.

At the beginning of 2004, that is, 6 months after software for primary healthcare was tested in Croatia, the European Public Health Alliance published a document titled *Communication from the Commission to the Council, the European Parliament, the European Economic and Social Committee and the Committee of the Regions. E-Health: Making Healthcare Better for European Citizens. An Action Plan for a European E-Health Area* (text with EEA relevance). As made clear in this document, European Union (EU) member states will start implementing in 2007 the solution Croatia reached in 2003. Establishing and developing this information system in transitional countries is one of the strategic projects for the coming years. Without rapid, reliable, and comprehensive information availability, developing, implementing, and monitoring any healthcare development strategy and system reform would be difficult. One would be unreasonable to expect a poor health system to keep and save enough money for "computerization to happen spontaneously." One should do exactly the opposite: Computerization should be installed in the system as a money keeping tool and implemented with the aim of exerting total control over the consumption as well as the rationalizing of it in order to save substantially more money than the cost of installing the information system.

In fact, the share of investment in information systems is directly proportional to the financial effectiveness of the system (e.g., banks and insurance systems spend 5 to 6% of their total budgets on the computerization of business operations). Whereas EU member states spend at least 2 to 3% of the health budget on computerization, in the United States, this share varies around 4 to 10% (Bates, Ebell, Gotlieb, Zapp, & Mullins, 2003). Among transitional countries, it is difficult to find one investing more than 0.2 to 0.5 % of its health budget. This raises the question of whether this might be the starting point for the vicious circle of ineffectiveness in transitional countries' health systems.

The elements of new organizations (new business rules) cannot be set, nor can the foundation of a redesign be made without investing in the computerization aligned with modern concepts (Stevanovic, 2002a, 2003), under which information (processed data) becomes a business resource (Krcmar, Stevanovic, Kovacic, & Merzel, 2001). At the same time, the information communication system for primary healthcare warrants the confidentiality of data on patients and the standardization of good practice for most common acute and chronic mass diseases (Stevanovic & Erceg, 2003). The system should provide the basic contents for the establishment of effective management.

GOALS AND IMPROVEMENTS

Ample help offered by computerization relates to the rapid retrieval of documents and insurees (Stevanovic, 2002b; Varga & Stevanovic, 2003), the replacement of manual data input, typing on typewriters, and the writing of recipes, referral notes, invoices, individual forms, and reports. The information system should give real time insight into the data and information, as well as enable prompt interventions within the system.

Improving the overall care of patients and insurees, more rapid diagnosis, and accuracy in prescribing a therapy are the major goals of such an approach. The system should enable better utilization of the capacities, shorter waiting times, and shorter stays in health institutions (Booth, 2003).

The project was the first to introduce electronic smart cards here for all physicians and nurses. Thus, at each medical checkup or hospital admission, the new information system also verifies both the insuree's and the physician's status and rights. Equally, as in banking or other card business, only a linkup between the magnetic card and the doctor's card makes the transaction possible.

Insurance-Provider Benefits

BI (business intelligence), or the utilization of accurate and comprehensive data and information required in health-insurance management, is one benefit. Data are standardized, and their input is independent of the wishes, ambitions, and interests of teams and institutions. This sets the insurer and physician free of worries about data collection and primary data processing because the information system takes care of these with standardized applications. Thus, doctors and insurers can devote all their energy to the execution of managerial and professional activities. Within the information system, per-formance monitoring accurately measures the effectiveness and outcomes, as well as teamwork coverage and contents.

Benefits for the Health Ministry and Public Health

The benefits include PHI (public health intelligence), the use of accurate and comprehensive data and information needed to run the public health system and public health initiatives. MI (management intelligence), the utilization of accurate and comprehensive data and information needed by the ministry of health, health managers, and decision makers for efficient guidance and running of the system, is another benefit. An integration tool will enable the full integration of the health system's information and data. Currently, data on more than 500 parameters are collected from the primary health service with the aim of extracting just a few pieces of information, that is, qualitative indicators (exclusively on the level of ratios or trends). The future system with a few standardizes characteristics will offer the possibility of analyzing a much greater number of indicators. Regarding the reporting of statistics, registering with public health registries (obligatory notifications of immunizations, infectious diseases, melanomas, psychotics, the disabled, etc.) will be carried out automatically, interactively, and proactively. Linkage makes the carrying out of coordinated and joint preventive and curative interventions feasible. The system guarantees the confidentiality and safety of personal information and of data on health and diseases (VPN, PKI [public-key infrastructure], encryption, smart cards, separate authentication servers, data servers, and data repositories). With an accident and catastrophe early-alert system, one can boot the whole system with all data and information in 24 hours.

Benefits for Physicians and Teams, and the Medical Chamber

The utilization of guidelines, instructions, and tools needed by physicians and insurees in order for standardized, quality care to be provided and for more rapid diagnosis setting and the selection of good and rational therapy in the treatment of disease is one benefit (healthcare intelligence). The dissemination and utilization of the knowledge necessary to provide good medical care is another (knowledge intelligence). Another benefit is still a linkage with other participants in the process of treatment and prevention of disease (online linkage of all care providers). Equally beneficial are the regulated and safe utilization of all data on the health and disease of an insuree in care, online consultations with networked experts, e consultations with specialists, telemedicine, and the direct engagement in scientific and technical public-health projects and programs. There is also the benefit of time and money savings in office, postal, and other expenditures.

Benefits for the Citizen, Patient, and Insuree

First, there is EI (equity intelligence), the equity or enabling of all who are in the same medical insurance (and market) position to avail themselves of the same conditions and quality. Then there is the continuity, irrevocability, and transferability of the safe storage of data on the care of an individual insuree. Next are the benefits of guaranteed confidentiality and the security of personal data. The final benefit is the communication option, that is, two way (or multiple) communication between a physician and the citizen, patient, or insuree (e-information, e-active-calling, e-instruction-sending).

Data Standards

For software applications and the central information system, use has been made of EU and certain other engineering standards in order for this system to be open from the outset and built for Croatia as an EU member state. It should support international and EU data standards and classifications, for example, HL7 (Health Level 7) Version 3, ICPC (International Classification of Primary Care, 2nd edition), ICD-10 (International Classification of Diseases, 10th revision), CEN TC 251 (European Committee for Standardization/TC251 Work Groups), and others.

Technical Elements and Standards for the System and Applications for Transitional Countries

Technical elements and standards should include the following: one common system with several licensed applications; an Internet infrastructure (to enable paperless operation); XML (extensible markup language) and HL7 standards; system safety standards like PKI; marking clinical and other documents with bar codes; electronic medical files; global registration and an insuree database; a global database on codebooks (Hofmans-Okkes & Lamberts, 1996; Lamberts & Hofmans-Okkes, 1996; Lamberts & Wood, 1987; Okkes, Oskam, & Lamberts, 1998; WONCA, 1998; World Health Organization [WHO], 1994); access to external databases; data integration into the primary health service's information system; direct linkage with the insurance administration, public health, and the ministry of health, e-recipes, e-referral-notes, e-business, and so forth; and the standardized, equitable, and measurable use of guidelines (Brage, Bensten, Bjerkedal, Nygard, & Tellnes, 1996; Lamberts, Wood, & Hofmans-Okkes, 1993).

CONCLUSION

- In transitional countries, an information system for primary healthcare is a strategic component of health reform. Its goal is to improve the quality of primary healthcare and rationalize its consumption.
- Investments in a primary-healthcare information system have no alternative. They are strategic and would yield a return of investment in 2 years.
- In transitional countries, health computerization projects should be defined (through measurable targets) in phases by priorities and conducted all the way down to their execution phase.
- New concepts and proven methodologies of project management should be used to guarantee the effectiveness of the project (investment).
- In countries in transition, the primary health service's information system should allow physicians and nurses to switch to a new, facilitated mode of operation that gives them more time for patients and practice-management improvement.
- A primary-healthcare information system grants access to data to all authorized staff needing it, as well as the proactive use of knowledge, standards, guidelines, procedures, and algorithms. It should enable direct IT communication between the citizen, wherever he or she may be, and hospitals, specialists, home-care services, home-visiting services, and diagnostic units, as well as all later linkages in the process of treatment.
- The system should permit the utilization of diagnostic and therapeutic guidelines, warrant equality in approaching the patients, and make the necessary knowledge available to the physician.
- The system should permit association with interest groups for special research projects, and business- and problem related linking and networking.

REFERENCES

Bates, D. W., Ebell, M., Gotlieb, E., Zapp, J., & Mullins, H. C. (2003). A proposal for electronic medical records in U.S. primary care. *JAMA, 10,* 1-10.

Booth, N. (2003). Sharing patient information electronically throughout the NHS, *BMJ, 327,* 114-115.

Brage, S., Bensten, B. G., Bjerkedal, T., Nygard, J. F., & Tellnes, G. (1996). ICPC as a standard classification in Norway. *Fam Pract, 13,* 391-396.

Hofmans-Okkes, I. M., & Lamberts, H. (1996). The international classification of primary care (ICPC): New applications in research and computer based patient records in family practice. *Fam Pract, 42,* 294-302.

Krcmar, N., Stevanovic, R., Kovacic, L., & Merzel, M. (2001). Health center, family medicine and community health care reform. *Seventh Congress on Family Medicine,* 219-227.

Lamberts, H., & Hofmans-Okkes, I. (1996). Episode of care: A core concept in family practice. *J Fam Pract, 42.*

Lamberts, H., & Wood, M. (Eds.). (1987). *ICPC: International classification of primary care.* Oxford: Oxford University Press.

Lamberts, H., Wood, M., & Hofmans-Okkes, I. (Eds.). (1993). *The international classification of primary care in the European community.* Oxford: Oxford University Press.

Okkes, I. M., Oskam, S. K., & Lamberts, H. (1998). *Van klacht naar diagnose* [From complaint to diagnosis]. Bossum, Coutinho.

Stevanovic, R. (2002a). Computer software for family medicine offices. *Med Fam Croat, 9,* 30-33.

Stevanovic, R. (2002b). ICT of the primary health care. *First Croatian Congress on Telemedicine with International Participation,* 86-87.

Stevanovic, R. (2003). Collection and managing of health data, the linkage of informatics systems and quality of health data. In D. Cvoriscec & V. Madaric (Eds.), *Quality management standards in hospital care* (pp. 100-109). Koprivnica, MOH.

Stevanovic, R., & Erceg, M. (2003). A proposal for national preventive medicine informatic & communication system. *First Croatian Congress on Preventive Medicine and Health Promotion with International Participation,* 308.

Varga, S., & Stevanovic, R. (2003). Health informatics system: Preventive benefits. *First Croatian Congress on Preventive Medicine and Health Promotion with International Participation,* 295.

WONCA. (1998). *International Classification Committee: The international classification of primary care* (2nd ed.). Oxford: Oxford University Press.

World Health Organization (WHO). (1994). *International statistical classification of diseases and related health problems: Vol. 3. Alphabetical index* (10th revision). Geneva, Switzerland: Author.

KEY TERMS

Business Intelligence (BI): The process of gathering information about a business or industry matter, or a broad range of applications and technologies for gathering, storing, analyzing, and providing access to data to help make business decisions.

European Committee for Standardization/TC251 Work Groups (CEN/TC251): Standardization in the field of health ICT to achieve compatibility and interoperability between independent systems and to enable modularity. This includes requirements on the health information structure to support clinical and administrative procedures, and technical methods to support interoperable systems, as well as requirements regarding safety, security, and quality.

Extensible Markup Language (XML): A simple, very flexible text format derived from SGML (ISO 8879). Originally designed to meet the challenges of large-scale electronic publishing, XML is also playing an increasingly important role in the exchange of a wide variety of data on the Web and elsewhere.

Health Level Seven (HL7): One of several departments of the American National Standards Institute (ANSI), whose mission is to provide standards for the exchange, management, and integration of data that support clinical patient care and the management, delivery, and evaluation of healthcare services.

International Classification of Diseases, 10th Revision (ICD-10): The international standard diagnostic classification for general epidemiology and many management purposes.

International Classification of Primary Care (ICPC): Instrument necessary to research general practice that was developed by the WONCA Classification Committee. It is available in more than 20 languages and has reached its second edition.

Public-Key Infrastructure (PKI): A system of digital certificates, certificate authorities, and other registration authorities that verify and authenticate the validity of each party involved in an Internet transaction.

Chapter IV
Computerized Systems Validation in the Pharmaceutical Industry

Kashif Hussain
University of Valenciennes, France

Shazia Yasin Mughal
University of Valenciennes, France

Sylvie Leleu-Merviel
University of Valenciennes, France

ABSTRACT

This chapter has reviewed the regulatory requirements definitions of FDA, AFSSAPS, EC and how computer systems can be validated with a relevant approach. By directing validation activities into a clear action plan, first, we need to analyze the specific organizational need according to the priorities and impacts to construct the required validation plan which can fulfill the requirements. The aim of the authors is to focus on a general approach to validation that can support several needs without addressing the technical aspects.

INTRODUCTION

The term validation appeared in the '60s, has become a topic of business concern today, and is considered to be one of the core issues in the pharmaceutical industries in terms of meeting regulatory requirements. In the recent past, an increase in the use of computerized-system validation (CSV) compelled quality and validation standards to be more precise to meet the industrial need. The utility of CSV has been an important catalyst in audits. Today, the pharmaceutical industry makes use of CSV for several purposes (services, computers, equipment, process verification, change management [CM], etc.), exploring the ways how validation ensures the system in use is compliant and how to decrease failure rates, risks, long-term costs, and so forth. Currently, official inspections concentrate more and more on the validation of computerized systems due to good manufacturing practices (GMPs; Hoffmann, Kähny-Simonius, Plattner, Schmidi-Vckovski, & Kronseder, 1998).

Worldwide regulatory authorities have issued rules, regulations, and guidelines that are aimed to ensure true and real practices in the pharmaceutical organizations concerning public health. These requirements to maintain quality processes are the way to ensure that final consumers receive only safe and effective medical products. These authorities verify the required compliance before approving the license to the manufacturer. These requirements are available in several forms like GxP (good [clinical, laboratory, manufacturing] practice) or BPF (bonne pratique de fabrication). Each country has its own interpretation of quality and compliance requirements for the development of systems and procedures to achieve quality; however, basic rules and principles remain the same and are universally applicable. These regulatory requirements are established to define uniform standards that emphasize public health and safety as a first concern. In all cases, these regulations give an overview of the minimum requirements and dictate what must be done and by whom without specifying how it is to be done. It is the responsibility of management with respective validation teams for identifying schedules, priorities, and resources required for the preparation to meet these standards.

Computerized System

Several definitions are available to define a computerized system. We start with the principle described by the European Parliament in Annex-11 (Computerized System), relating to medicinal products for human use and investigational medicinal products for human use:

The introduction of computerised systems into systems of manufacturing, including storage, distribution and quality control does not alter the need to observe the relevant principles given elsewhere in the Guide. Where a computerised system replaces a manual operation, there should be no resultant decrease in product quality or quality assurance. Consideration should be given to the risk of losing aspects of the previous system which could result from reducing the involvement of operators. (EC, 2003)

The Food and Drug Administration (FDA, 1987) defines a computerized system as "computer hardware, software, and associated documents (e.g., user manual) that create, modify, maintain, archive, retrieve, or transmit in digital form information related to the conduct of a clinical trial."

A computerized system may include data input, electronic processing, and the output of information to be used either for reporting or automatic control. It may include automated manufacturing equipment, process-control systems, automated laboratory equipment, laboratory-data capture systems, clinical or manufacturing database systems, and so forth. Our study provides an overview of CSV acceptance criteria in the pharmaceutical industry. To carry out our study, we used the regulations applicable via the European Union parliament for France, and for America, we use the FDA as the reference authority.

Validation is a process that requires dedicated attention, and we summarize a clear approach to validation that can be incorporated with quality to implement validation principles. We start with some general definitions of validation used by AFSSAPS (French Health Products Safety Agency), EC, FDA, and ISO (International Organization for Standardization). We go on to discuss a validation planning method that may be suitable in general in high-assurance disciplines, and then we link validation with quality. We conclude with some possible future research opportunities in computerized-system validation.

VALIDATION APPROACH

Validation remains one of the important issues in the pharmaceutical industry as it has for many years. Validation is an important aspect in the age of global competition and the rapidly changing technology environment not because of the regulatory requirements only, but also for an effective, true approach in the long run for the computer systems used in the industry. Validation is vital for organizational global competitiveness, growth, and compliance requirements. The basic aim is always to assure quality and that the process is capable to develop a product meeting the predefined conditions and respecting all the applicable norms. Validation teams are focusing on their role in the development of quality orientation validation plans by providing valuable insight and guidance in order to keep pace with the latest changing technology. The major objective behind a validation strategy is always to assure quality for all deliverables of a computer system and to verify compatibility with all compliance (functional, security, integrity, etc.) requirements. Valida-

tion is defined by AFSSAPS as the establishment of the proof that the implementation or the use of every process, procedure, material, raw material, product, activity, or system really makes it possible to reach the anticipated results and the fixed specifications (Ministry of Health & Social Protection, France, 2004).

The directives of 2003/94/EC describe the validation process:

The extent of validation necessary will depend on a number of factors including the use to which the system is to be put, whether the validation is to be prospective or retrospective and whether or not novel elements are incorporated. Validation should be considered as part of the complete life cycle of a computer system. This cycle includes the stages of planning, specification, programming, testing, commissioning, documentation, operation, monitoring and modifying. (EC, 2003)

The FDA (1987) defines validation as "[e]stablishing documented evidence that provides a high degree of assurance that a specific process will consistently produce a product meeting its predetermined specifications and quality attributes." The organization addresses the development of a proper validation plan that performs and documents validation tasks to assess software development.

Validation should be considered a part of the complete life cycle of a computerized system (Stokes, 1998). Validation basically concerns all steps in the production process that could affect the final quality of the product (Hoffmann et al., 1998). Thus, it is important to specify the compatibility and usefulness of the computer system, and to define specifications and quality dimensions of the computerized system under consideration before developing or purchasing. Therefore, the documentation of user requirements and the documentation of system specifications are equally essential (Ermer, 2001). The FDA in its guidance indicated the expectation of a risk-based approach to determining which systems should undergo validation. Most pharmaceutical and biotechnology professionals have experienced the qualitative difference between making high-risk and low-risk decisions. In low-risk situations, one is often willing to gamble and reach hasty, if not faulty, conclusions. In high-risk situations, one usually takes more time to gather and analyze all relevant information (Woodrum, 1998).

As defined in the ISO/IEC 17025 international standard, validation is the "confirmation by examination and the provision of objective evidence that the particular requirements for a specific intended use are fulfilled." So, for validation, both the procedures and systems components (hardware, software, etc.) that can affect the results of measurements need to be validated.

As the validation of computerized systems is a regulatory requirement for the FDA because of 21 CFR Part 11, validation can be treated as a proof of suitability that is linked to the whole system life cycle to ensure that the system meets the user requirements, ensures compliance expectations, and will be properly maintained to guarantee a secure environment with accurate, reliable, and traceable information throughout its life cycle. Validation is a process that begins with defining the requirements and ends with ensuring that the needs are being fulfilled consistently (Carter, 2005).

Numerous life-cycle models (waterfall method, enhanced waterfall method, spiral model, V model, CMM [capability maturity model], etc.) have been introduced in order to accomplish software validation. In general, software validation involves a series of activities and tasks that must be planned and executed at required stages depending on the life-cycle model used, the software used, the associated risks, and the scope of changes made as the project advances. This is based on the assumption that an organized approach, while using one, many, or a combination of these models, can result in fewer defects, thus, ultimately providing better results (Uzzaman, 2003). The documented collection of policies, processes, and procedures is equally important. We will not go into the details of these models as they are not in the primary objective of this chapter.

Validation of a Computerized System

The principles of good practices for the use of a computerized system via validation are now well established as the means by which quality is built into the development of these systems. Major phases of the validation of a computerized system producing documented evidence are described as follows.

- Network and infrastructure
- Validation master plan
- User-requirements specification (URS)
- Risk analysis
- Supplier audit and vendor selection
- Legal requirements
- Functional specification (FS)
- Validation strategy planning
- Design specification (DS)
- Implementation and testing
- Qualification phase
  - Installation qualification (IQ)
  - Operational qualification (OQ)
  - Performance qualification (PQ)
- Standard operating procedures (SOPs)
- Training
- Final validation report
- Change management
- Maintenance and regular review
- Decommissioning

Network and Infrastructure Tools

Infrastructure and network services including LAN (local area network), WAN (wide area network), intranet, security access, and so forth must provide reliable, trustworthy information, data, and delivery, and must be assured and maintained by detailed specification documentation (approved procedures) and change management.

Validation Master Plan

The master plan provides a complete documentation list for the computerized system to be validated according to the business and process priorities.

User-Requirements Specification

URS is a definition of the system requirements in terms of how the user perceives the system to operate in the intended use and environment. The URS should define what one wants to do or what the system is required to do for its users. It may identify integration with other existing systems, functional needs (e.g., data presentation, records, reports), regulatory requirements, working-environment constraints, system performance, the maintenance required, the documentation required, and so forth. The final user should be involved in this phase to ensure a good understanding of the system requirements and the functionalities required of the installed system. All URSs should be verified and assured before final confirmation.

Risk Analysis

One of the most important steps in validation is defining the risk areas. In order to guarantee as much security as possible during the routine utilisation of the system, critical functions have to be defined and certain numbers of test runs have to be done (FDA, 1987). Risk analysis includes a strategy and methodology, the risk associated with different parts of the system, and an action plan to minimize these risks. The analysis should result in solutions for all risks identified. What has been agreed upon during the supplier or vendor selection and specified during the continuous contact with the supplier might give additional advice to define critical functions and modules (Friedli, Kappeler, & Zimmermann, 1998). For validation of the software, risk analysis is affected module-wise (Arnold, 1998).

Supplier Audit and Vendor Selection

Pharmaceutical companies are held responsible for any inadequacy observed by the regulatory teams of their selected suppliers. A supplier audit is recommended and required to ensure the supplier is able to provide the services required with all necessary documentation. This audit includes the verification of a quality-management system, standards, tools, programming standards, working conditions, market repute, development methodology, customer support, change management, and so forth. The audit-report findings should be confirmed and verified. Depending on the audit results, the supplier or vendor may be asked to reply to the audit observations and findings.

Legal Requirements

Whenever external service providers are involved, legal contracts and service-level agreements (SLAs) should be incorporated and assured so that the regulatory requirements of the company are confirmed.

Functional Specification

The FS provides details about what the system should do to satisfy the user requirements. The functional specification, also termed preliminary functional design, identifies any constraints or potential deviations from the planned requirements. It should describe what the system should do and how it should do it. It explains how each feature of the system functions.

Validation Strategy Planning

Validation strategy planning is used to define the validation responsibilities, plan, strategy, and approach, and the acceptance criteria. However, for smaller systems, this phase can be replaced by the validation master plan. The final validation report is actually based on validation strategy planning.

Design Specification

The DS translates the requirements of the URS into a technical solution. Both developer and user involvement is required to facilitate this phase, and a detailed review during the project development phase is highly recommended to maintain the design methodology. The DS includes the functional, structural, and technical design depending upon the system size and complexity with detailed documentation. It explains how the system is intended to function or operate.

Implementation and Testing

The purpose of implementation and testing is to assure the suitable implementation of the system components (hardware, software, etc.) depending upon the size and complexity of the system. Proper documentation including that of development tools is required at this stage.

Testing is a sensitive issue, provoking failures and maximizing confidence, that involves certain limitations depending on the goals. Testing helps reliability and involves source-code review or peer review to identify any errors and to verify the codes with applicable coding standards. To evaluate the system performance against expectations, end users are required to perform user acceptance tests. A review of the user acceptance test results before system installation at the operation site should be done in order to satisfy the requirements. If executed test plans and test results are verified, organized, and documented, significant qualification workload can be reduced. Traceable records among URS, FS, DS, and testing should be maintained at this stage in order to move for effective qualification.

Qualification

Qualification covers several steps including installation qualification, operational qualification, and performance qualification; however, depending upon the size and complexity of the system, these steps can be carried out in single stage. Installation and operational qualification are usually based on system functionality.

Installation Qualification

IQ ensures that the system has been installed against the predetermined design criteria and has been specified and set up in compliance with the requirements of both parties (manufacturer and the user), and that complete documentation is available to prove this for the users. Usually, installation involves checking that all major system hardware, software, tools, peripherals, user manuals, and reference documents are readily accessible, and that a regular maintenance program along with backup is in place.

Operational Qualification

The IQ of the test system should be completed with complete SOPs and personal training before launching OQ. OQ is carried out as a documented verification to ensure that the system is in optimal working conditions and involves all functionalities and process operations, security access, and backup facilities according to the predefined specifications. OQ should be performed in a test environment when possible. After test execution, a review report with expected and achieved results, deviations found, and a conclusion must be approved to commence PQ.

Performance Qualification

PQ is documented verification to assure that the system operates throughout all operating ranges according to the requirements (stable system, operational documents in place, trained personnel) over a predefined period of time, and that the results are in accordance with the expectations in the system's actual use environment. System stability through continuous operation for a significant amount of time should be confirmed. This allows encountering a wide range of conditions to verify any error or fault in system that does not appear in normal activities.

Standard Operating Procedures

Approved SOPs must capture the details to standardize the validation-procedure performance. Departments charged with abiding by or following these SOPs must first be trained against them. SOPs may involve system operation, backup, restoration, security, data handling, change management, disaster recovery, training, and so forth.

Training

Training is one of the essential elements for any successful validation. All concerned members (users, developers, and persons involved in development, validation, maintenance, and so forth) of the validation project must be trained. Training records must be documented and maintained. Training should be performed in a test environment in order to avoid any effects on the system. Typically, training initiates within the validation group. It is essential that the lead validation resource for a given validation project initiate, facilitate, coordinate, and/or communicate the need for resource training (Neal, 2003).

Final Validation Report

A review of all activities is done after PQ to perform the final system release verification and data transfer plan, if any, to assure all deliverables identified in the validation plan and to sum up the completion of the validation cycle via a final validation report. Based on positive conclusions, the computer system can be released for use (Friedli, 1998).

Change Management

Any changes to the system must be thoroughly documented and managed by a change-management process. CM verifies all impacts of a proposed or planned change on the system before that change is done. CM defines the complete set of processes employed for tracking all changes on systems, applications, and environments defined by a respective pharmaceutical regulatory conformance standard, and manages systematically the effects of change. The changes are evaluated in order to decide the extent of validation required by the implementation of the change.

Maintenance and Regular Review

The purpose of this phase is to assure the optimal use of the system by properly maintaining the validation until the system is decommissioned. Periodic reviews should be performed and documented including reviews of SOPs, security, access, change management, backup files, training records, and so forth.

Decommissioning

Decommissioning is done to retire a system after the completion of its intended use and when it is no more required, using proper procedural methods and keeping in mind the impact on the rest of the system.

The CM process should be used to track all changes related to the system decommissioning to avoid any impact on other systems. An update of the disaster recovery plan (DRP) and the deactivation of SOPs if applicable are equally recommended. It is estimated that only 15% of organizations have attested to having an effective DRP plan (Snelham & Wingate, 2000).

Quality Approach

In general, quality can be specified as the ability of a product or service to fulfill the requirements and expectations defined by the customers. Quality is a dynamic issue that should lead toward continuous improvement. We believe that validation is directly linked with the quality of a system, and the use of quality tools can enhance the validation plan and assist in successful validation.

Various studies have considered validation as a part of a quality system (Randsell, 1996), quality assurance (Muller, Gempler, Schweie, & Zeugin, 1996), and total quality management (Christensen, Kristiansen, Hansen, & Nielsen, 1995), involving all resources (manpower, machines, knowledge, etc.) of a company to achieve customer satisfaction while allowing for the system to be considered safe and efficient by the legal authorities of the company.

DISCUSSION

Validation is highly dependent upon the effectiveness of the planning that goes into it. In many cases, validation may require considerable resources in terms of time, money, and specialized personnel, so getting it right and getting it done on time is crucial. Organized, well-planned validation increases the reliability of a computerized system, thereby decreasing compliance problems and increasing the company's confidence to fulfill the requirements of regulatory agencies. A better understanding of the validation of a computerized system is of high importance and will continue to play an important role in various aspects to minimize risk and enhance compliance, overall effectiveness, and efficiency. Obviously, achieving the validation of a computer system involves developing, maintaining, and releasing a computerized system throughout its life cycle and assures that the system consistently meets it specifications, thus, making it worthy for its intended use. The cost of validation is determined by the time spent on documentation, the development of protocols, SOPs, actual fieldwork, data collection, and analysis (Stocker, 1994). It is interesting to note that a good rule of thumb is that total validation costs may run from 4 to 8% of the total project cost for typical pharmaceutical-plant expansion projects (Gloystein, 1997). Some researchers have experienced system for which validation reduced maintenance-support costs by 75% (Wingate, 1997).

We are hopeful that advancement in technologies, standardization, and the harmonizing of the definitions of the required validation regulatory requirements will, in general, help any organization develop a standard, consistent, global approach for computerized systems. In the future, the key to mastering smart validation will lie in weighing the real risks that can affect the computerized system.

CONCLUSION

This chapter has reviewed the regulatory requirement definitions of the FDA, AFSSAPS, and EC, and how computer systems can be validated with a relevant approach. In directing validation activities into a clear action plan, we first need to analyze the specific organizational needs according to priorities and impacts to construct a required validation plan that can fulfill the requirements. Our aim is to focus on a general approach to validation that can support several needs without addressing the technical aspects. It must be recognized that the validation of a computerized system is highly important. A well-defined validation plan can formalize the validation process, the associated strategy, the responsibilities, and the acceptance criteria applicable to the computerized system, including risk analysis. The approach presented here can help to avoid some of the common pitfalls in the validation of computerized systems. The real challenge is in how a company plans for and documents the validation activities for the system in order to better implement these guidelines in the least possible time and with the least possible resources. We believe that the guidelines for validation can lead to a common approach and to establishing common procedures and vocabulary. Validation can further lead to the harmonization of audit inspections and the improvement of inspection systems, thus improving the chances for successful inspection. Together with the general rules of validation applicable worldwide, it is clear that the validation process

outline here encompasses the entire pharmaceutical business environment. Validation should be regarded as part of an integrated concept to ensure the quality, safety, and efficacy of pharmaceuticals (Ermer, 2001).

REFERENCES

Arnold, L. (1998). Software assessment under consideration of validation aspects: PPS and PMS systems. *Pharmaceutica Acta Helvetiae, 72*, 327-332.

Carter, E. R. (2005). Systems validation: Application to statistical programs. *BMC Medical Research Methodology, 5*, 3.

Christensen, J. M., Kristiansen, J., Hansen, A. M., & Nielsen, J. L. (1995). Method validation: An essential tool in total quality management. *The Proceedings of Sixth International Symposium on the Harmonization of the Role of Laboratory Quality Assurance in Relation to TQM* (pp. 46-54).

EC. (2003). Directive of 2003/94/EC of 8 October 2003: Laying down the principles and guidelines of good manufacturing practice in respect of medicinal products for human use and investigational medicinal products for human use. In *Annex 11: Computerised system: Vol. 4. Medicinal products for human and veterinary use: Good manufacturing practice* (p. 11). Retrieved April 13, 2005, from http://pharmacos.eudra.org/F2/eudralex/vol-4/home.htm

Ermer, J. (2001). Validation in pharmaceutical analysis: Part 1. An integrated approach. *Journal of Pharmaceutical and Biomedical Analysis, 24*, 755-767.

Food and Drug Administration (FDA). (1987). *Guidelines on general principles of process validation.* Retrieved April 14, 2005, from http://www.fda.gov/cder/guidance/pv.htm

Friedli, D., Kappeler, W., & Zimmermann, S. (1998). Validation of computer systems: Practical testing of a standard LIMS. *Pharmaceutica Acta Helvetiae, 72*, 343-348.

Gloystein, L. (1997). Protocol structure and IQ/OQ costs. *Journal of Validation Technology, 3*(2), 140.

Hoffmann, A., Kähny-Simonius, J., Plattner, M., Schmidi-Vckovski, V., & Kronseder, C. (1998). Computer system validation: An overview of official requirements and standards. *Pharmaceutica Acta Helvetiae, 72*, 317-325.

Ministry of Health & Social Protection, France. (2004). Décrets, arrêtés, circulaires. *Journal Officiel de la République française, 23*(95). Retrieved May 10, 2005, from http://agmed.sante.gouv.fr/htm/3/pta/ptaa1_190804.pdf

Muller, K. M., Gempler, M. R., Schweie, M.-W., & Zeugin, B. T. (1996). Quality assurance for biopharmaceuticals: An overview about regulations methods and problems. *Pharmaceutica Acta Helvetiae, 71*, 421-438.

Neal, C. (2003). Prerequisites for successful validation. *Journal of Validation Technology, 9*(3), 240-245.

Randsell, T. E. (1996). The cost of validation. *Journal of Validation Technology, 3*(2), 142-143.

Snelham, M., & Wingate, G. (2000). Validation laboratory information management systems. *Journal of Validation Technology, 6*(4), 740-748.

Stocker, A. C. (1994). Why does validation cost so much and take so long? And what we can do about it. *Journal of Validation Technology, 1*(1), 5-8.

Stokes, T. (1998). *The survive and thrive guide to computer validation.* Buffalo Grove, II: InterPharm Press.

Uzzaman, S. (2003). Computer systems validation: A system engineering approach. *Pharmaceutical Engineering, 23*(3), 52-66.

Wingate, G. A. S. (1997). *Validating automated manufacturing and laboratory application: Putting principles into practices.* InterPharm Press.

Woodrum, D. T. (1998). Computer system validation: Value added activities meeting regulatory imperatives. *Drug Information Journal, 32*, 941-945.

KEY TERMS

21 CFR Part 11: FDA code of U.S. Federal Regulations, Title 21, Part 11: Electronic Records. Electronic signatures that define parameters by which pharmaceutical companies can author, approve, store, and distribute records electronically.

AFSSAPS: The French Health Products Safety Agency is the French authority for all safety decisions taken concerning health products from their manufacturing to their marketing, that is, medicinal products; raw materials for pharmaceutical use; organs, tissues, and cells, and products of human and animal origins, and so forth.

Bonne Practique de Fabrication (BPF): Stands for bonne pratique de fabrication and is the equivalent of GMP.

Change Management: The complete set of processes employed for tracking all changes in existing and new systems, applications, and environments defined by a respective pharmaceutical regulatory conformance to mange systematically the effects of change.

Capability Maturity Model (CMM): The capability maturity model is a method for evaluating and measuring the maturity of the software-development process of organizations on a scale of 1 to 5. The Software Engineering Institute (SEI) at Carnegie Mellon University in Pittsburgh, USA, developed the CMM.

Computerized System: A system that includes software, hardware, application software, operating-system software, supporting documentation, and so forth, for example, automated laboratory systems; control systems; manufacturing-, clinical-, or compliance-monitoring database systems; and so forth.

Current Good Manufacturing Practice (cGMP): Current good manufacturing practice is an international set of quality regulations and guidelines applicable to the manufacture, testing, and distribution of drugs, medical devices, diagnostic products, biological products for human or veterinary use, and so forth. The FDA ensures product quality applicable to GMP via the 21 CFR Part 210 and 211 regulations.

Disaster Recovery Plan (DRP): A disaster recovery plan is the plan for business continuity in the event of a disaster that destroys business resources. The goal of DRP is to recover the technical infrastructure that supports business continuity in the event of a serious incident in the least possible time.

Food and Drug Administration (FDA): The Food and Drug Administration is the branch of the U.S. federal government that approves new drugs for sale and is responsible for ensuring the safety and effectiveness of all drugs, biologics, vaccines, and medical devices, including those used in diagnosis, treatment, regulation, and so forth for the USA.

Good Clinical Practice (GCP): Good clinical practice is an international set of quality regulations and guidelines for the design, conduct, monitoring, recording, auditing, analysis, and reporting of studies applicable to clinical or human studies in the evaluation of drugs, medical devices, biological products, and so forth. The FDA ensures product quality applicable to GCP via 21 CFR Parts 50, 54, and 56.

Good Laboratory Practice (GLP): Good laboratory practice embodies an international set of quality regulations and guidelines applicable to nonclinical studies in the evaluation of drugs, medical devices, biological products, and so forth. GLP provides a framework within which the FDA ensures laboratory studies are planned, performed, monitored, recorded, reported, and archived under 21 CFR Part 58.

GxP: GxP is the generalization of any quality guidelines used in the pharmaceutical industry that groups together the following compliance practices: cGMP, GLP, and GCP.

International Organization for Standardization (ISO): The International Organization for Standardization is responsible for a wide range of standards for a large number of industries. ISO provides a means of verifying that a proposed standard has met certain requirements for due process, consensus, and other criteria by those developing the standard.

Life-Cycle Model: A life-cycle model is the order in which a series of processes are performed to create or update a product or service. Examples include the waterfall, incremental-build, and evolutionary-build approaches.

Service-Level Agreement (SLA): Provides the predefined and standard level of services available in the organization.

Spiral Model: Also known as the spiral life-cycle model, it is a systems-development method used in information technology. This model of development combines the features of the prototyping model and the waterfall model.

The spiral model is favored for large, expensive, and complicated projects.

Standard Operating Procedure (SOP): A standard operating procedure is a written document that describes in detail how a particular procedure or method is executed for repetitive use. It is generally intended to standardize the procedure performance.

Validation: Documented evidence providing a high degree of assurance that a specific process under consideration does what it purposes to do. Validation deals with the entire system life cycle to ensure a system satisfies user requirements, meets compliance expectations, and is adequately maintained to provide a secure environment with accurate, reliable, and traceable information from conception to retirement. The term is also used to describe the overall validation approach including qualification. Validation includes but is not limited to manufacturing processes, equipment, computerized systems, and so forth.

V Model: The V model is a software-development model that describes the activities and results that have to be produced during software development.

Waterfall Model: Introduced in 1970, the waterfall model is a software-development model describing the theoretical approach to software development in which development is seen as flowing steadily through the phases of requirements analysis, design, implementation, testing (validation), integration, and maintenance. It is the basis for the V model used in the pharmaceutical industry.

Chapter V
Chronic Disease Registers in Primary Healthcare

M. F. Harris
University of New South Wales, Australia

D. Penn
University of New South Wales, Australia

J. Taggart
University of New South Wales, Australia

Andrew Georgiou
University of New South Wales, Australia

J. Burns
University of New South Wales, Australia

G. Powell Davies
University of New South Wales, Australia

ABSTRACT

Systematic care of patients with chronic diseases needs to be underpinned by information systems such as disease registers. Their primary function is to facilitate structured care of patients attending services—supporting identification of patients at risk, structured preventive care and provision of care according to guidelines, and supporting recall of patients for planned visits. In Australia general practitioners using division-based diabetes registers are more likely to provide patient care that adhered to evidence-based guidelines. Critical data issues include privacy, ownership, compatability, and capture as part of normal clinical care and quality.

INTRODUCTION

Chronic diseases account for over 70% of the burden of disease in countries such as Australia (Mathers, Vos, & Stevenson, 1999), and more than one in four problems managed by general practitioners relate to one or more of these chronic conditions (Australian Institute of Health and Welfare [AIHW], 2002). Systematic team care of patients with chronic diseases such as diabetes and cardiovascular disease is associated with improved health outcomes (Dunn & Pickering, 1998; Wagner, 1998; World Health Organization [WHO], 2001). This needs to be underpinned by information systems that assist with recall and audit according to evidence-based guidelines.

In many countries, organizations of primary-care services have been established at local or district levels. In Australia, the Divisions of General Practice have played a key role in supporting general practices to provide more systematic care through disseminating evidence-based guidelines, educating general practitioners and consumers, supporting shared care and self-management education, providing allied health services, and coordinating local registers for recall and audit. The authors have been involved in one widely implemented computer-based register system that has demonstrated improvements in the quality of care.

BACKGROUND

Functions

Disease registers have a variety of purposes ranging from facilitating longitudinal research to providing epidemiological surveillance. Their primary function in primary healthcare is to facilitate the structured care of patients attending services: supporting the identification of patients at risk, structured preventive care, the provision of care according to guidelines, and the recall of patients for planned visits.

Location

Registers may be located at the service (e.g., within a general practice) or at the healthcare organization level (e.g., a diabetes centre or the Division of General Practice). Registers within practices or services have the advantage of ease of data capture, avoiding problems of data transfer. Registers at the district or regional level held by a specialized service or primary-healthcare organization have greater capacity for analysis and are able to monitor the care provided by a multidisciplinary team across different services.

Data

Registers contain individual-identifying information, such as basic demographic profiles for recall purposes, together with information about the process and outcomes of care. This information needs to be standardized to allow comparison using nationally accepted units of measurement and frequencies for routine testing and recall. In Australia, standardized minimum data sets have been developed based on evidence-based guidelines for the management of diabetes or cardiovascular disease (National Health Data Committee, 2003a, 2003b), overseen by committees representative of primary-care providers, nongovernment organizations (NGOs), specialist providers, government agencies, and consumers.

Data Capture

Patient data may be recorded and captured in a variety of ways. Historically, data have been recorded on forms or copies of patient-held records,

Figure 1. Sources of data capture for chronic disease registers in Australian general practice

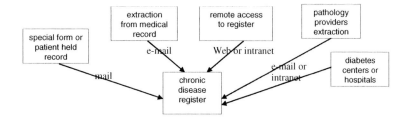

which are subsequently entered from paper format into a computer database either at the practice or division level. Increasingly, data are either extracted from electronic health records (EHRs) and sent to a register or entered directly into a Web-based register. HL7 (Health Level 7) message specifications and agreed standard EHRs allow register and recall developers to design systems that feature seamless interoperability for the communication of clinical data.

Reporting

Reports facilitate the functions of the register, principally providing prompts and audit reports against standards or other peer services (see Table 1).

Implementation

In countries where patients are required to register with general practices, establishing such registers may be an integral part of the patient registration system. In the United Kingdom, case ascertainment via an electronic-record linkage method showed high concordance between general-practice registers and data collated from various sources (Morris et al., 1997).

In Australia, registers may be held within general practices, at a Division of General Practice, at a specialist centre, or at a hospital. A survey of 81 Divisions of General Practice in 2002 revealed that 31 had an electronic-register recall system for diabetes and 8 had one for CVD. The number has steadily increased since 1993 (Georgiou, Burns, Penn, Infante, & Harris, 2004; Penn, Burns, Georgiou, Powell Davies, & Harris, 2004). The National Integrated Diabetes Program established by the Australian government in 2001 introduced incentive payments for practices having a disease register to help support best-practice care and for the completion of an annual cycle of care for diabetes.

Table 1. Types of reports generated from chronic disease registers

Function	Reports
Recall	Lists or recall notices for patients who are overdue for aspects of care
Audit	Frequency of visits or assessments Behavioural or physiological risk factors Intermediate health outcomes Complications, hospitalizations, and death Management: prescribing and referral
Follow-Up	Lists of patients with poor control for interventions (e.g., referral)
Accountability	Lists of patients for financial reporting or claims
Service Management	Health-service attendance, workload, and population coverage

Effectiveness

Register-recall systems are important facilitators to structured evidence-based care for the improved quality of clinical care (Weingarten et al., 2002). Research in Australia has shown that general practitioners using division-based diabetes registers were more likely to provide patient care that adhered to evidence-based guidelines (Harris, Priddin, Ruscoe, Infante, & O'Tool, 2002). This has also been demonstrated for the secondary prevention of coronary artery disease (Moher et al., 2001).

Recall or reminders for patients have been shown to improve adherence with planned or preventive care (Pirkis et al., 1998). However, it is important to ensure that such reminders are culturally appropriate, are personalized, and address financial barriers to attending the service (Hunt et al., 1998).

Registers in Australian Divisions of General Practice

In Australia, the Divisions Data Quality Improvement Program is based at the Centre for General Practice Integration Studies (CGPIS) at the University of New South Wales (UNSW). The program provides resources, training, and support for division diabetes and cardiovascular shared-care programs, especially those with diabetes and/or cardiovascular-disease registers based on the diabetes (National Diabetes Outcomes Quality Review Initiative [NDOQRIN], 2002) and cardiovascular-disease data sets (CVDATA, 2002). The program has collated data from division registers in 1999 (Carter, Bonney, Powell Davies, & Harris, 2000) and in 2002 (covering the period of 2000 to 2002). Coverage of the estimated number of people with diagnosed diabetes for division registers was estimated to be 20.2% in 2002. Collective results were fed back to divisions

and workshops to facilitate quality and service improvement (Burns, Zingarelli, & Harris, 2002).

CRITICAL ISSUES

Privacy and Consent

Privacy and consent are important issues, especially in sending any identified data from the practice to a district or health-service-organization register. Patients need to be informed that information will be sent to the register and consent to the transfer of any identified information (Burns et al., 2000). Consumers and other stakeholders need to be involved in decisions about the data to be collected, who has access to them, and their reporting (CGPIS, 2004).

Data Ownership

Data ownership is also an issue for data collated from practices or local services to a district or primary-care organizational level (Cromwell et al., 2001). In Australia, there has been extensive debate on this issue. This has led to the development of policies for data extraction to the various levels (Carter et al., 2000).

Data Compatibility

Data compatibility is a critical issue for registers so that practices can exchange and compare data. This is dependent on a standardized minimum data set and a common coding system for clinical software (CGPIS, UNSW, 2004).

Data Capture

While the technology to capture clinical data is available, there is a need for a national interoperable clinical messaging infrastructure, messaging software that is minimally intrusive to the clinicians' work flow, and a seamless exchange of data between messaging systems (GPCG, 2004).

Data Quality

Data quality is critically important in any information system. Medical records that are the source of data for registers have significant limitations because of their quality (Del Mar, Lowe, Adkins, & Arnold, 1996).

Coverage

Participation in chronic disease registers is usually voluntary both for patients and providers. Data on such registers are therefore rarely representative of all providers or the population of people with chronic diseases. In general, such registers tend to include those with better quality of care (Nilasena & Lincoln, 1995).

Sustainability

The sustainability of regional registers is a critical issue. In Australia, the growth of division-based register-recall systems peaked in 2002 and may now be declining. Ironically, this decline may partly be due to the development of practice computer systems because of the difficulty of getting data from the practice to the division in electronic form. Other factors contributing to problems of sustainability include the lack of capacity within divisions, competing demands, or the lack of incentives for audits, which allow comparison between practices or services.

FUTURE DIRECTIONS

In Australia, we are likely to see a continued move of some functions, such as recall, from the regional or primary-care organizational level to services or practices. This will make issues of standardization and compatibility even more important in allowing the comparison of accessibility and the performance of services. At the primary-care-organization or district levels, we will see the development of at least three register models:

- A centralized database at the health-organization level with Web or intranet input of data from local services
- A practice register-recall system with the periodic extraction of data in identified or unidentified form for audit and quality improvement to the local or regional organization
- A data warehouse with linked data held in services and organizations (e.g., pathology providers)

Choices between such systems will be made on the basis of the resources required to set and maintain them over time both within individual practices and primary-care organizations. Both practices and primary-care organizations will require strong direction from government to develop the capacity to allow their wider implementation.

REFERENCES

Australian Institute of Health and Welfare (AIHW). (2002). *Australia's health 2002.* Canberra, Australia: Author.

Burns, J., Carter, S., Bonney, M., Powell Davies, G., & Harris, M. F. (2000). *National divisions diabetes program data collation project: Vol. 7. Policy framework for collation of data involving divisions of general practice.* Sydney, Australia: University of New South Wales, School of Community Medicine, Centre for General Practice Integration Studies.

Burns, J., Zingarelli, G., & Harris, M. F. (2002). *Quality improvement in diabetes at practice and division level.* General Practice and Primary Health Care Research Conference. Research: Making a Difference to Health and Health Care, Melbourne, Australia.

Carter, S., Bonney, M., Powell Davies, G., & Harris, M. F. (2000). *NDDP data collation project: Summary volume (Diabetes profiles).* Sydney, Australia: The Centre for General Practice Integration Studies.

Centre for General Practice Integration Studies (CGPIS), University of New South Wales (UNSW); Chronic Illness Alliance; & Australian Divisions of General Practice. (2004). *General practitioners' information data exchange divisions' capacity project final report* (GPCG Project 4 RFT 72/0203). Retrieved from http://www.gpcg.org/projects/CurrentProjects.html

Centre for General Practice Integration Studies (CGPIS), University of New South Wales (UNSW); Department of General Practice, University of Adelaide; Chronic Illness Alliance; Australian Divisions of General Practice; Collaborative Centre for e-Health, University of Ballarat; & Centre for Health Informatics, UNSW. (2004). *Chronic disease functionality project final report.* Retrieved from http://www.gpcg.org/projects/CurrentProjects.html

Cromwell, D., Arora, M., Dalley, A., Kreis, I. (2001). *The Epi-Beacon: A feasibility study on providing local epidemiological information to general practices within the Illawarra derived from routinely collected, computerised data. A second report on data analysis and GP reaction.* Report for the Commonwealth Department of Health and Family Services (p. 45). Wollongong: Centre for Health Services Development.

CVDATA. (2002). *A minimum clinical data set for the management of cardiovascular disease in primary care.* Melbourne, Australia: National Heart Foundation.

Del Mar, C., Lowe, J. B., Adkins, P., & Arnold, E. (1996). What is the quality of general practitioner records in Australia? *Australian Family Physician, 13,* S21-S25.

Dunn, N., & Pickering, R. (1998). Does good practice organization improve the outcome of care for diabetic patients? *British Journal of General Practice, 48*(430), 1237-1240.

Georgiou, A., Burns, J., Penn, D., Infante, F., & Harris, M. F. (2004). Register-recall systems: Tools for chronic disease management in general practice. *Health Information Management Journal, 33,* 31-35.

GPCG. (2004). *HL7 systems and services: GPs information and data exchange evaluating messaging project final report* (GPCG Project E RFT 72/0203). Retrieved from http://www.gpcg.org/projects/CurrentProjects.html

Harris, M. F., Priddin, D., Ruscoe, W., Infante, F. A., & O'Tool, B. I. (2002). Quality of care provided by general practitioners using or not using division based registers. *Medical Journal of Australia, 177,* 250-252.

Hunt, J. M., Gless, G. L., et al. (1998). Pap smear screening at an urban aboriginal health service: Report of a practice audit and an evaluation of recruitment strategies. *Australia and New Zealand Journal of Public Health, 22,* 720-725.

Mathers, C., Vos, T., & Stevenson, C. (1999). *The burden of disease and injury in Australia* (AIHW Cat. No. PHE 17). Canberra, Australia: Australian Institute of Health and Welfare.

Moher, M., Yudkin, P., Wright, L., Turner, R., Fuller, A., Schofield, T., et al. (2001). Cluster randomised controlled trial to compare three methods of promoting secondary prevention of coronary heart disease in primary care. *British Medical Journal, 322*, 1338.

Morris, A. D., Boyle, D. I. R., MacAlpine, R., Emslie-Smith, A., Jung, R. T., Newton, R. W., et al. (1997). The diabetes audit and research in Tayside Scotland (DARTS) study: Electronic record linkage to create a diabetes register. *British Medical Journal, 315*(7107), 524-528.

National Diabetes Outcomes Quality Review Initiative (NDOQRIN). (2002). *NDOQRIN national minimum data set for the management of diabetes.* Australia: Australian Diabetes Society.

National Health Data Committee. (2003a). Other data set specification: Cardiovascular disease (clinical) (AIHW Cat. No. HWI-46). In *National health data dictionary* (pp. 62-63). Canberra, Australia: Australian Institute of Health and Welfare.

National Health Data Committee. (2003b). Other data set specification: Diabetes (clinical) (AIHW Cat. No. HWI-47). In *National health data dictionary* (pp. 64-66). Canberra, Australia: Australian Institute of Health and Welfare.

Nilasena, D. S., & Lincoln, M. J. (1995). A computer-generated reminder system improves physician compliance with diabetes preventive care guidelines. *Proceedings of the Annual Symposium of Computer Applications in Medical Care 1995* (pp. 640-645).

Orstein, S. M., Garr, D. R., et al. (1991). Computer-generated physician and patient reminders: Tools to improve population adherence to selected preventive services. *Journal of Family Practice, 32*, 82-90.

Penn, D. L, Burns, J. R, Georgiou, A., Powell Davies, G., & Harris, M. F. (2004). Evolution of a register recall system to enable the delivery of better quality of care in general practice. *Health Informatics Journal, 10*, 163-174.

Pirkis, J., Jolley, D., et al. (1998). Recruitment of women by GPS for paper tests: A meta-analysis. *British Journal of General Practice, 48*, 1603-1607.

Wagner, E. H. (1998). Chronic disease management: What will it take to improve care for chronic disease? *Effective Clinical Practice, 1*, 2-4.

Weingarten, S. R., Henning, J. M., Badamagarau, E., Knight, K., Hasselblad, V., Gano, A., et al. (2002). Interventions used in disease management programmes for patients with chronic illness: Which ones work? Meta-analysis of published reports. *BMJ, 325*(7370), 925-932.

World Health Organization (WHO). (2001). *Innovative care for chronic conditions: Building blocks for action.* Retrieved from http://www.who.int/chronic_conditions/framework/en/

KEY TERMS

Audit: An analysis of data on patient care or the outcomes used to compare performance against standards or other services.

Chronic Disease: A disease present for 3 months or more.

Data Linkage: Linkage of individual health data from different databases using a common identifier.

Health Data Dictionary: Standard data definitions used in healthcare.

Physiological or Behavioral Risk Factors: They increase the risk of a chronic disease developing.

Recall: A database generates reminders for patients to receive planned care.

Register: A database of patients with chronic diseases used to identify patients for follow-up, reminders, or audit.

Section II
Standardization and Classification Systems in Medicine

For over 130 years, the systematic collecting and recording of medical information has been based on the use of traditional classifications, nomenclatures, and coding schemes of various kinds. Until relatively recently, such schemes were used mainly for recording causes of death and gathering minimal diagnostic information for statistical and epidemiological purposes. Despite their many limitations, schemes such as the International Classification of Diseases (ICD) have been successful in supporting the collation and comparison of national and international statistics on morbidity and mortality, and advancing our understanding of the distribution and causes of diseases.

Chapter VI
Standardization in Health and Medical Informatics

Josipa Kern
Andrija Stampar School of Public Health, Zagreb University Medical School, Croatia

ABSTRACT

Standard is a thing or quality or specification by which something may be tested or measured. The development of standards is organized on a global, international level, existing also on a national level, well harmonized with an international one. International developers are organizations working on this matter, like the International Organization for Standardization (ISO) or the European Committee for Standardisation (Comité Européen de Normalisation— CEN). Standards in health and medical informatics enable access to patient health records to read or to add some new data relevant to other healthcare providers taking care of a patient. Bad medical informatics can lead to patient deaths, and standardization in the field can prevent this from happening.

INTRODUCTION

When things go well, often it is because they conform to standards (International Organization for Standardization [ISO], 2005). In the Oxford Dictionary of Modern English, there is a lot of explanation of what the word standard means, but, in the context of the first sentence, the best meaning is the following: "standard is a thing or quality or specification by which something may be tested or measured." A personal computer is a standardized computer. This means that all of its components are made according to strictly defined specification. Consequently, it does not matter who produces the components or where they are produced.

Industry put in the first demand for standards. Standardization is especially important for electronics, and for ICT and its application in different areas. Nowadays, the developing of standards is organized on a global, international level, but it exists also on the national level, which is well harmonized with the international one.

Developers of standards are organizations and groups working on this matter. The leading standard developer in the world is the International Organization for Standardization. ISO is a nongovernmental organization that was established February 23, 1947. Its mission is to promote the development of standardization and related activities in the world with a view to facilitating the international exchange of goods and services, and to developing cooperation in the spheres of intellectual, scientific, technological, and economic activity (International Organization for Standardizaton, 2005). ISO collaborates with its partner in international standardization, the International Electrotechnical Commission (IEC), a nongovernmental body whose scope of activities complements ISO's. The ISO and the IEC cooperate on a joint basis with the International Telecommunication Union (ITU), part of the United Nations organization whose members are governments. The ISO standard can be recognized by the ISO logo, ISO prefix, and the designation "International Standard."

The European developer of standards is the European Committee for Standardisation (Comité Européen de Normalisation, CEN). It was founded in 1961 by the national standards bodies in the European Economic Community and EFTA countries. CEN promotes voluntary technical harmonization in Europe in conjunction with worldwide bodies and its partners in Europe, and the conformity assessment of products and their certification (Comité Européen de Normalisation, 2005). CEN cooperates with the European Committee for Electrotechnical Standardization (CENELEC) and the European Telecommunications Standards Institute (ETSI). A product of this cooperation is the European standard, which can be recognized by the prefix EN. Any added prefix to the existing one, for both the ISO and CEN standards, means that this standard is the result of cooperation with another standardization group or organization. The prefix ENV in European standardization means that this standard is not yet a full standard (it is under development by CEN).

ISO and CEN have technical committees working in specific areas. ISO/TC215, established in 1998, and CEN/TC251, established in 1991, are corresponding technical committees working on standardization in health and medical informatics. Both standardization bodies cooperate and mutually exchange their standards.

There are also a variety of other organizations and groups developing standards, either cooperating with ISO and CEN or acting as administrators and coordinators in standardization. For example, there are Health Level 7 (HL7); Digital Imaging and Communications in Medicine (DICOM); the American National Standards Institute (ANSI), a nonprofit organization that administers and coordinates the U.S. voluntary standardization and conformity assessment system, and so forth.

BACKGROUND

Definition

A standard is a set of rules and definitions that specify how to carry out a process or produce a product, or more precisely, a standard is a document established by consensus and approved by a recognized body that provides, for common and repeated use, guidelines or characteristics for activities or their results, aimed at the achievement of the optimum degree of order in a given context.

The main role of a standard is raising the levels of quality, safety, reliability, efficiency, and interchangeability, and consequently lowering costs (International Organization for Standardization, 2005).

Standard Creation Process

There are several phases in the process of standardization. The first phase of this process is characterized by demand for a standard.

There must be someone who needs a standard. Most standards are prepared at the request of industry. The European Commission can also request the standards bodies to prepare standards in order to implement European legislation. This standardization is mandated by the Commission through the Standing Committee of the Directive in support of the legislation. Groups of users can also ask for a standard in the field of their interest. The second phase of standardization is the developing of standards by following specifications based on the needs defined in the first phase. Experts of a specific field work on related standards. After the standard has been approved by the standardization body, it becomes a prototype and goes through testing and evaluation. Positive test results imply the dissemination of standards, and they start to take effect. It should be highlighted that a standard is dynamic, and it changes time after time. Most standards require periodic revision. Several factors combine to render a standard out of date: technological evolution, new methods and materials, and new quality and safety requirements. To take account of these factors, the general rule has been established that all standards should be reviewed at intervals of not more than a predefined time period. On occasion, it is necessary to revise a standard earlier (Hammond & Cimino, 2001).

Standardization in Health and Medical Informatics: Why and What

Standardization has been a major factor in companies' financial and clinical success, enabling faster implementation, greater quality control, and significant cost savings (Ball, Cortes-Comerer, Costin, Hudson, & Augustine, 2004). The contribution of the standardization process in healthcare terminology initiated by CEN/TC251 and supported now by the work of CEN/TC215/WG3 to this new approach can be summarized as the practical realization of ontology (Rodrigues, Trombert Paviot, Martin, Vercherin, & Samuel, 2002). The standard CEN ENV 12924 contains a security categorization model for information systems in healthcare, distinguishing six categories plus some refinements. For each category, it specifies the required protection measures (Louwerse, 2002). Standards support interoperability and electronic-health-record (EHR) communication. They support cooperative work among health agents when it is necessary to share health-care information about patients in a meaningful way. Examples of requirements for EHR are provided in four themes: EHR functional requirements; ethical, legal, and security requirements; clinical requirements; and technical requirements. The main logical building blocks of an EHR use the terminology of CEN/TC251 ENV 13606 (Lloyd & Kalra, 2003; Maldonado, Crespo, Sanchis, & Robles, 2004; Marley, 2002). Many specific medical records, like medical records of patients suffering from beta-thalassaemia, which are inevitably complex and grow in size very fast, are based also on ENV 13606 (Deftereos, Lambrinoudakis, Andriopoulos, Farmakis, & Aessopos, 2001). The wider electronic exchange of clinical information between heterogeneous information systems in the delivery of diabetes care demands a common structure in the form of a message standard and close cooperation with CEN/TC251 (Vaughan et al., 2000).

CURRENT STATUS OF STANDARDIZATION IN HEALTH AND MEDICAL INFORMATICS

All the standards developers work through their working technical committees in health and medical informatics and a number of working groups specialized in a specific area.

What are Specific Areas of Work and Results of the ISO/TC215?

Table 1 shows working groups acting in the ISO/TC215. Table 2 shows a list of standards given by this technical committee.

Table 1. Working groups of ISO/TC215

ISO/TC215 WG 1 Health records and modeling coordination
ISO/TC215 WG 2 Messaging and communication
ISO/TC215 WG 3 Health concept representation
ISO/TC215 WG 4 Security
ISO/TC215 WG 5 Health cards
ISO/TC215 WG 6 Pharmacy and medicines business

Table 2. Standards in health and medical informatics given by ISO/TC215

ISO/IEEE 11073-10101:2004	Health informatics—Point-of-care medical device communication—Part 10101: Nomenclature
ISO/IEEE 11073-10201:2004	Health informatics—Point-of-care medical device communication—Part 10201: Domain information model
ISO/IEEE 11073-20101:2004	Health informatics—Point-of-care medical device communication—Part 20101: Application profiles—Base standard
ISO/IEEE 11073-30201:2004	Health informatics—Point-of-care medical device communication—Part 30200: Transport profile -- Cable connected
ISO/IEEE 11073-30300:2004	Health informatics—Point-of-care medical device communication—Part 30300: Transport profile -- Infrared wireless
ISO/TR 16056-1:2004	Health informatics—Interoperability of telehealth systems and networks—Part 1: Introduction and definitions
ISO/TR 16056-2:2004	Health informatics—Interoperability of telehealth systems and networks—Part 2: Real-time systems
ISO/TS 16058:2004	Health informatics—Interoperability of telelearning systems
ISO/TS 17090-1:2002	Health informatics—Public key infrastructure—Part 1: Framework and overview
ISO/TS 17090-2:2002	Health informatics—Public key infrastructure—Part 2: Certificate profile
ISO/TS 17090-3:2002	Health informatics—Public key infrastructure—Part 3: Policy management of certification authority
ISO/TS 17117:2002	Health informatics—Controlled health terminology—Structure and high-level indicators
ISO/TR 17119:2005	Health informatics—Health informatics profiling framework
ISO/TS 17120:2004	Health informatics—Country identifier standards
ISO 17432:2004	Health informatics—Messages and communication—Web access to DICOM persistent objects
ISO 18104:2003	Health informatics—Integration of a reference terminology model for nursing
ISO/TR 18307:2001	Health informatics—Interoperability and compatibility in messaging and communication standards -- Key characteristics
ISO/TS 18308:2004	Health informatics—Requirements for an electronic health record architecture
ISO 18812:2003	Health informatics—Clinical analyser interfaces to laboratory information systems -- Use profiles
ISO/TR 21089:2004	Health informatics—Trusted end-to-end information flows
ISO 21549-1:2004	Health informatics—Patient healthcard data—Part 1: General structure
ISO 21549-2:2004	Health informatics—Patient healthcard data—Part 2: Common objects
ISO 21549-3:2004	Health informatics—Patient healthcard data—Part 3: Limited clinical data
ISO/TS 21667:2004	Health informatics—Health indicators conceptual framework
ISO/TR 21730:2005	Health informatics—Use of mobile wireless communication and computing technology in healthcare facilities—Recommendations for the management of unintentional electromagnetic interference with medical devices
ISO 22857:2004	Health informatics—Guidelines on data protection to facilitate trans-border flows of personal health information

ISO/TS is a normative document representing technical consensus within an ISO committee.
ISO/TR is an informative document containing information of a different kind from that normally published in a normative document (Beolchi, 2003).
IEEE is the Institute of Electrical and Electronic Engineers, USA.

Table 3. CEN/TC251 working groups

CEN/TC251 WG 1 Communications: Information models, messaging, and smart cards
CEN/TC251 WG 2 Terminology
CEN/TC251 WG 3 Security, safety, and quality
CEN/TC251 WG 4 Technology for interoperability (devices)

Table 4. Standards in health and medical informatics given by CEN/TC251

EN 14484:2003	International transfer of personal health data covered by the EU data protection directive—High level security policy
EN 14485:2003	Guidance for handling personal health data in international applications in the context of the EU data protection directive
EN 1828:2002	Categorial structure for classifications and coding systems of surgical procedures
EN ISO 18104:2003	Integration of a reference terminology model for nursing (ISO 18104:2003)
EN ISO 18812:2003	Clinical analyser interfaces to laboratry information systems—Use profiles (ISO 18812:2003)
EN ISO 21549-1:2004	Patient healthcard data—Part 1: General structure (ISO 21549-1:2004)
EN ISO 21549-2:2004	Patient healthcard data—Part 2: Common objects (ISO 21549-2:2004)
EN ISO 21549-3:2004	Patient healthcard data—Part 3: Limited clinical data (ISO 21549-3:2004)
EN 12251:2004	Secure user identification for healthcare - Identification and authentication by passwords—Management and security
EN 12252:2004	Digital imaging—Communication, workflow and data management (which endorses all of DICOM as a European Standard)

What are Specific Areas of Work and Results of the CEN/TC251?

The work carried out by CEN/TC251 is mentioned in Table 3.

CEN/TC251 has been operating for 10 years. By October 2004, it had created 10 full standards or EN (Table 4).

FUTURE TRENDS IN STANDARDIZATION IN HEALTH AND MEDICAL INFORMATICS

There is no doubt that candidates for standardization in medical informatics will be core data sets for healthcare speciality groups, decision-support algorithms and clinical guidelines, and vocabulary. The identification of patients, content, and structure of electronic patient records, and messages being communicating in the healthcare system are also candidates for international standards. Standard formats need to be defined for special kinds of data like images, signals and waveforms, sound and voice, and video, including motion video. Data security, the security of objects and communication channels, and data archiving, especially in case of a catastrophe of any kind, should be standardized. Some of these standards exist or have been under way, but standardization is a continuous process, depending on the development of information and communication technology, and therefore all standards need to be improved and adapted to new technology coming day after day.

CONCLUSION

Standards in health and medical informatics are means to enabling better healthcare. Healthcare is supposed to be better if healthcare providers can access data in a patient's health record, and can read it or add some new data relevant for other healthcare providers taking care of the patient. Information technology used in diagnostics produces data about a patient as images, signals, or waves, as well as classic alphanumeric data. The format of such data should be standardized, usable, and readable on any instrument of the same kind wherever it is in the world. Medical language should be standardized, and coding systems should be universal. The transfer of medical data should be secure, as well as data storage and communication. Some patient data should be portable by health cards, especially for patients suffering from chronic diseases. Bad medical informatics can kill a patient, and standardization in the field can help make this not happen.

REFERENCES

Ball, M. J., Cortes-Comerer, N., Costin, M., Hudson, K., & Augustine, B. (2004). HCA Inc.: Standardization in action. *Journal of Healthcare Information Management, 18*(2), 59-63.

Beolchi, L. (Ed.). (2003). *European telemedicine glossary of concepts, technologies, standards and users* (5th ed.). Brussels, Belgium: European Commission.

Comité Européen de Normalisation (CEN, European Committee for Standardisation). (n.d.). Retrieved February 11, 2005, from http://www.cenorm.be/cenorm/index.htm

Deftereos, S., Lambrinoudakis, C., Andriopoulos, P., Farmakis, D., & Aessopos, A. (2001). A Java-based electronic healthcare record software for beta-thalassaemia. *Journal of Medical Internet Research, 3*(4), E33.

Hammond, W. E., & Cimino, J. J. (2001). Standards in medical informatics. In E. H. Shortliffe & L. E. Perreault (Eds.), *Medical informatics: Computer applications in health care and biomedicine* (pp. 212-255). New York: Springer.

International Organization for Standardization. (ISO). (n.d.). *Why standards matter?* Retrieved February 11, 2005, from http://www.iso.org/iso/en/aboutiso/introduction/index.html#one

Lloyd, D., & Kalra, D. (2003). EHR requirements. *Studies in Health Technology and Informatics, 96*, 231-237.

Louwerse, K. (2002). Demonstration results for the standard ENV 12924. *Studies in Health Technology and Informatics, 69*, 111-139 (pp. 229-237).

Maldonado, J. A., Crespo, P., Sanchis, A., & Robles, M. (2004). Pangaea: A mediator for the integration of distributed electronic healthcare records. In M. Fieschi, E. Coiera, & Y. C. J. Li (Eds.), *Medinfo 2004* (p. 1738). Amsterdam: IOS Press.

Marley, T. (2002). Standards supporting interoperability and EHCR communication: A CEN TC251 perspective. *Studies in Health Technology and Informatics, 87*, 72-77.

Rodrigues, J. M., Trombert Paviot, B., Martin, C., Vercherin, P., & Samuel, O. (2002). Coordination between clinical coding systems and pragmatic clinical terminologies based on a core open system: The role of ISO/TC215/WG3 and CEN/TC2511/WG2 standardisation? *Studies in Health Technology and Informatics, 90*, 401-405.

Vaughan, N. J., Cashman, S. J., Cavan, D. A., Gallego, M. R., Kohner, E., Benedetti, M. M., et al. (2000). A detailed examination of the clinical terms and concepts required for communication by electronic messages in diabetes care. *Diabetes, Nutrition and Metabolism, 13*(4), 201-209.

KEY TERMS

ANSI (American National Standards Institute): The private, nonprofit membership organization responsible for approving official American national standards.

CEN (Comité Européen de Normalisation, European Committee for Standardisation): The European authority for standards.

CEN/TC251: CEN technical committee for standardization in health and medical informatics.

EN: European standard made by CEN.

European Standardization: Activity of the European authority for standards.

International Standardization: Activity of the world authority for standards.

ISO (International Organization for Standardization): World authority for standards. It is also the international standard made by the organization.

ISO/TC215: ISO technical committee for standardization in health and medical informatics.

Standard: A set of rules and definitions that specify how to carry out a process or produce a product.

Standardization: Process of producing of standards.

Chapter VII
Basic Principles and Benefits of Various Classification Systems in Health

Dimitra Petroudi
National and Kapodistrian University of Athens, Greece

Athanasios Zekios
National and Kapodistrian University of Athens, Greece

ABSTRACT

The introduction of information systems in health progressively led tï coding systems. The purposes of these systems are: recording causes of death, coding diseases and procedures, etc. The most important medical coding system in our days is ICD (International Classification of Diseases). Other coding systems that health professionals use are: SNOMED, LOINC, MeSH, UMLS, DSM, DRG and HCPCS. There are also many Nursing Classification Systems, such as: NANDA, NIC, NOC, ICNP, Omaha and HHCC. This chapter describes these coding systems and their advantages.

INTRODUCTION

Since the introduction of information systems in health, the demand for coding systems has been major. Medical coding systems are fundamental to medical record keeping as well as to gathering and communicating public health statistics. They are used for a variety of purposes: recording causes of death, coding diseases and procedures, and physician billing and reimbursement. The elements that make a coding system good are completeness, nonredundancy, clarity, stability, granularity, and the fact that it can be developed. Coding systems usually aim to be accurate, have unambiguous expressions, and are complete.

In classification systems, groups of words or terms are collected together and organised. Each of these terms will be associated with a particular concept. Systems of classification have typically been hierarchical, meaning that more detail is obtained the further down the hierarchy one proceeds, although ideas are still linked and organised around common attributes.

Each concept within a classification system can also be given a numeric or alphanumeric code. The more extensive the coding system, the more detail it can represent.

INTERNATIONAL CLASSIFICATION OF DISEASES

The most important medical coding system in our days is the ICD (International Classification of Diseases). The purpose of the ICD is to promote international comparability in the collection, classification, processing, and presentation of health statistics. Since the beginning of the 20th century, the ICD has been modified about once every 10 years, except for the 20-year interval between ICD-9 and ICD-10 (see Table 1). The purpose of the revisions is to stay abreast with advances in medical science.

The ICD is copyrighted by the World Health Organization (WHO), which owns and publishes the classification. Annual updates are published by the Health Care Financing Administration, now called the Centers for Medicare and Medicaid Services (CMS).

ICD-9 is the ninth version of ICD. ICD-9 is a classification system of diseases, health conditions, and procedures that represents the international standard for the labeling and numeric coding of diseases. These codes provide a worldwide standard for comparison of birth, death, and disease data.

ICD-9 includes diagnosis codes consisting of three to five numeric characters representing illnesses and conditions; alphanumeric E codes describing external causes of injuries, poisonings, and adverse effects; and V codes describing factors influencing health status and contact with health services.

Today, there is also the 10th version of ICD. The ICD-10 consists of:

- Tabular lists containing cause-of-death titles and codes (Volume 1),
- Inclusion and exclusion terms for cause-of-death titles (Volume 1),
- An alphabetical index to diseases, the nature of injuries, and external causes of injury, and a table of drugs and chemicals (Volume 3), and
- Descriptions, guidelines, and coding rules (Volume 2).

One benefit of ICD-10 is a more comprehensive scope. Table 2 gives examples of some of the subcategories provided in ICD-10 for the capture of risk factors to health, such as lifestyle, life management, psychosocial circumstances, and the occupational or physical environment. Another benefit is improved specificity and currency. The results of a mapping from ICD-

Table 1. Revisions of the ICD according to the year of the conference in which they were adopted and the years they were in use in the USA

Revision of the ICD	Year of Conference in which Adopted	Years in Use in USA
First	1900	1900-1909
Second	1909	1910-1920
Third	1920	1921-1929
Fourth	1929	1930-1938
Fifth	1938	1939-1948
Sixth	1948	1949-1957
Seventh	1955	1958-1967
Eighth	1965	1968-1978
Ninth	1975	1979-1998
Tenth	1992	1999-present

Table 2. Examples of some of the subcategories provided in ICD-10

ICD-10 Code	Code Title
Z56.3	Stressful work schedule
Z58.1	Exposure to air pollution
Z63.0	Problems in relationship with spouse or partner
Z72.4	Inappropriate diet and eating habits

9-CM (Clinical Modification) to ICD-10 carried out in Australia showed that of a total of 13,600 ICD-10 codes, 50.8% were more specific than the ICD-9-CM codes, 31.5% were as specific, and only 11.5% either were less specific or could not be compared. Other benefits of ICD-10 include ongoing maintenance and updating, a single set of national standards, international compatibility, a more effective structure, and better presentations and guidelines. Significant enhancements to the system's structure and presentation include an enlarged coding frame, hierarchic and logical presentation of codes, increased use of combination codes, and an improved format of the classification.

The estimated costs for adopting the new ICD-10 coding systems are given as follows.

Providers will incur costs for computer reprogramming; the training of coders, physicians, and code users; and for the initial and long-term loss of productivity among coders and physicians. The cost of sequential conversion (10-CM then 10-PCS [Procedure Coding System]) is estimated to run from $425 million to $1.15 billion in one-time costs plus somewhere between $5 million and $40 million a year in lost productivity.

A related classification, the International Classification of Diseases, Clinical Modification (ICD-9-CM), is used in assigning codes to diagnoses associated with inpatients, outpatients, and physician-office utilization in the United States. The ICD-9-CM is based on the ICD but provides for additional morbidity detail and is annually updated.

The ICD-9-CM consists of three volumes:

- A tabular list containing a numerical list of the disease code numbers (Volume 1),
- An alphabetical index to the disease entries (Volume 2), and
- A classification system for surgical, diagnostic, and therapeutic procedures (alphabetic index and tabular list; Volume 3).

Volumes 1 and 2 are used by physicians only to assign diagnosis codes. Physicians also use Current Procedural Terminology (CPT) to report medical and surgical procedures, and physician service codes rather than Volume 3 of the ICD-9-CM codes. The third volume of ICD-9-CM is used by hospitals for reporting inpatient procedures. The National Center for Health Statistics (NCHS) and the Centers for Medicare and Medicaid Services are the U.S. governmental agencies responsible for overseeing all changes and modifications to the ICD-9-CM. The aim of the diagnosis codes was epidemiological and not for billing functions, but now, in the United States, the codes are mostly used for billing and reimbursement purposes.

A clinical modification of ICD-10 (ICD-10-CM) has been developed by the NCHS. Revisions have been made to the draft of ICD-10-CM based on the comments received. An updated draft version of ICD-10-CM from June 2003 is now available for public viewing. However, the codes in ICD-10-CM are not currently valid for any purpose or use.

DIFFERENCES BETWEEN ICD-9 AND ICD-10

The tenth revision (ICD-10) differs from the ninth revision (ICD-9) in several ways despite the fact that the content is similar. First, ICD-10 is printed in a three-volume set compared to ICD-9's two-volume set. Second, ICD-10 has alphanumeric categories (A00-Z99) rather than numeric categories (001-999). Third, some chapters have been rearranged, some titles have changed, and conditions have been regrouped. Fourth, ICD-10 has almost twice as many categories as ICD-9. Fifth, some fairly minor changes have been made in the coding rules for mortality.

DIFFERENCES BETWEEN ICD-9-CM AND ICD-10-CM

The current draft of ICD-10-CM contains a significant increase in codes over ICD-10 and ICD-9-CM. Notable improvements in the content and format of ICD-10-CM include the addition of information relevant to ambulatory and managed-care encounters, expanded injury codes, the creation of combination diagnosis-symptom codes to reduce the number of codes needed to fully describe a condition, the addition of a sixth character, the incorporation of common fourth- and fifth-digit subclassifications, laterality, and greater specificity in code assignment.

ICD-10 is used to code and classify mortality data from death certificates, having replaced ICD-9 for this purpose as of January 1, 1999. ICD-10-CM is planned as the replacement for ICD-9-CM, Volumes 1 and 2.

ICD-10-PCS is currently designated to replace Volume 3 of ICD-9-CM for hospital inpatient use only. There is no intention for ICD-10-PCS to shape, form, or replace CPT

Table 3. Examples of differences between ICD-9-CM and ICD-10-CM

	ICD-9-CM	ICD-10-CM
Precordial Chest Pain	786.51	R07.2
Asthma, Acute Exacerbation	493.92	J45.21
Thumb Laceration	883.0	S61.011a

for the identification of physician work. Its only intention is to identify inpatient facility services in a way not directly related to physician work, but directed toward the allocation of hospital services.

OTHER CODING SYSTEMS

SNOMED (Systematized Nomenclature of Medicine) is a classification that is maintained by SNOMED International. SNOMED's design is based on detailed and specific nomenclature and has been successfully implemented internationally. The National Health Service in the United Kingdom has adopted a clinical version (SNOMED CT) as its preferred clinical terminology.

The LOINC (Logical Observation Identities, Names and Codes) database provides a set of universal names and ID codes for identifying laboratory and clinical observations. The aim of LOINC is to facilitate the exchange and pooling of clinical laboratory results, such as blood hemoglobin or serum potassium, for clinical care, outcomes management, and research.

MeSH was originally developed by the United States' National Library of Medicine (NLM) to index the world medical literature in MEDLINE (MeSH provides bibliographic headings for indexing). It also forms an essential part of the NLM's Unified Medical Language System (UMLS). MeSH is not an efficient indexing language for tasks such as classifying episodes of patient care.

The UMLS project is a long-term research and development project at the NLM whose goal is to help health professionals and researchers to intelligently retrieve and integrate information from a wide range of disparate electronic biomedical-information sources. This makes it easier for users to link information from patient record systems, bibliographic databases, factual databases, expert systems, and so forth. The UMLS Knowledge Services can also assist in data creation and indexing applications. UMLS is not itself a standard; it is a cross-referenced collection of standards and other data and knowledge sources. It gives the chance to exchange health-care information despite the multiplicity of coding systems in use today.

The UMLS metathesaurus contains mappings to MeSH, ICD-9-CM, SNOMED, CPT, and a number of other coding systems. The metathesaurus is organised by concepts, which means that alternate names (synonyms, lexical variants, and translations) for the same meaning are all linked together as one concept. The metathesaurus adds information to the concepts, including semantic types, definitions, and interconcept relationships.

DSM (Diagnostic and Statistical Manual of Mental Disorders) provides numeric codes, diagnostic criteria, and comprehensive definitions of mental disorders. The codes and terms in DSM-IV are fully compatible with ICD-9-CM and ICD-10.

CPT is a listing of descriptive terms and five-digit identifying codes for reporting medical, surgical, and diagnostic services performed by physicians and other health-care professionals. It first appeared in 1966 and is published annually by the American Medical Association.

DRGs (Diagnosis-Related Groups) are categories of clinically similar illnesses that require the same types of hospital resources to treat. Every patient can be classified into one of

511 categories. The purpose of DRGs is to reduce hospital costs and reimbursements.

HCPCS (Healthcare Common Procedure Coding System) was originally created for use under the Medicare program. Today, HCPCS is used by virtually every payer in the United States. HCPCS is comprised of three levels:

- **Level I:** CPT codes
- **Level II:** National codes (i.e., J codes, A codes, Q codes, C codes for OPPS only)
- **Level III:** Local codes

There are many nursing classification systems, such as, NANDA (North American Nursing Diagnosis Association), NIC, NOC, ICNP (International Classification of Nursing Practice), Omaha, and HHCC. The one that is most used is NANDA. It is a set of nursing diagnoses introduced by the North American Nursing Diagnosis Association in 1973. According to NANDA, the classification is based on "a selection of nursing interventions to achieve outcomes for which the nurse is accountable." ICNP first appeared in 1989 and was created by the International Council of Nursing (ICN). The purpose of this system was to place the common language of all nursing classification systems into an international frame.

BENEFITS OF CODING SYSTEMS

A coding system is important because, first of all, it groups, separates, abbreviates, and facilitates automated data processing and transmittal. Codes are used to help participants in the health-care system digitize information so that billing, record-keeping, and practice-management processes become more cost effective and reliable. Another important benefit is the fact that health professionals gain precious time during data recording and decision making. Classification systems improve the communication among health professionals and among health organisations. Coding makes it easier to handle medical insurance claims and to identify the provider on a predetermined basis. It also makes it easier for professionals to compare medical data internationally and do research. Plus, coding and classifications help to standardize a clinical language. Classification can therefore be used as another way of organising information and can act as a common language between health professionals, enhancing the quality and usefulness of the communication.

CONCLUSION

Automated coding systems hold the potential for increased coding speed and accuracy compared to unaided human coders. Coding and classification systems are developed rapidly today. Specialists tend to use more and more codes and classifications in order to create common international languages in all kinds of sciences so that research will become easier.

REFERENCES

Bakken, S., Campbell, K. E., Cimino, J. J., Huff, S. M., & Hammond, W. E. (2000). Toward vocabulary domain specifications for health level 7-coded data elements. *JAMIA, 7,* 333-342.

Bechhofer, S. K., Goble, C. A., Rector, A. L., Solomon, W. D, & Nowlan, W. A. (1997). Terminologies and terminology servers for information environments. *Proceedings of STEP '97 Software Technology and Engineering Practice.*

Campbell, J. R., Carpenter, P., Sneiderman, C., Cohn, S., Chute, C. G., & Warren, J. (1997).

CPRI Work Group on Codes and Structures, Phase II: Evaluation of clinical coding schemes: Completeness, taxonomy, mapping, definitions, and clarity. *J Am Med Inform Assoc., 4*(3), 238-250.

Chute, C. G., Cohn, S. P., & Campbell, J. R. (1998). A framework for comprehensive health terminology systems in the United States. *JAMIA, 5*(6), 503-510.

Chute, C. G., Elkin, P. L., Sheretz, D. D., & Tuttle, M. S. (1999). Desiderata for a clinical terminology server. *Proceedings of AMIA'99 Annual Symposium.*

Cimino, J. (1998). Desiderata for controlled medical vocabularies in the twenty-first century. *Methods Inf Med., 37*(4-5), 394-403.

ISO 1087-1:2000: Terminology work-vocabulary, Part 1: Theory and application.

Rector, A. L. (1999). Clinical terminology: Why is it so hard? *Methods Inf Med., 38*(4-5), 239-252.

URL REFERENCES

http://apt.rcpsych.org/cgi/content/full/8/3/165

http://citeseer.nj.nec.com/354766.html

http://faculty.washington.edu/momus/

http://rrc.gsk.com/ccp_issues/coding_systems.htm

http://secure.cihi.ca/cihiweb/dispPage.jsp?cw_page=codingclass_icd10bene_e

http://umls.nlm.nih.gov

http://www.acep.org/1,33890,0.html

http://www.amia.org/pubs/symposia/D005782.PDF

http://www.bacts.org.uk

http://www.biohealthmatics.com/health informatics/mlcls.aspx

http://www.cams.co.uk

http://www.cdc.gov/nchs/about/major/dvs/icd10des.htm

http://www.cdc.gov/nchs/about/otheract/icd9/abticd9.htm

http://www.cdc.gov/nchs/about/otheract/icd9/abticd10.htm

http://www.cdc.gov/nchs/about/major/dvs/icd10des.htm

http://www.cdc.gov/nchs/about/datawh/nchsdefs/icd.htm

http://www.cdc.gov/phin/data_models

http://www.cms.hhs.gov/medicare/hcpcs/.

http://www.defoam.net/hubris/hubris01.htm

http://www.hip.on.ca/search/160.html

http://www.hl7.org/standards/icd10.htm

http://www.hsl.unc.edu/services/guides/focusonmedcoding.cfm

http://www.medicalcodingandbilling.com/med_coding.htm

http://www.mwsearch.com/

http://www.opengalen.org

http://www.reimbursementcodes.com/medical_coding_d.html

http://www.snomed.org/products/content/mappings.html

https://wwws.soi.city.ac.uk/intranet/students/courses/mim/mi/lect2_2.htm

http://www.visualread.com

http://www.who.int/classifications/en

KEY TERMS

Classification: Systematic representation of terms and concepts and the relationship between them.

Clinical Classification: A method of grouping clinical concepts in order to represent classes that support the generation of indicators of health status and health statistics.

Codes: Numeric or alphanumeric abbreviations that can expand into some meaning.

Coding System: A terminology and context-free symbolic codes for each term.

Concept: An idea encompassing a class of objects ("A concept is a unit of knowledge created by a unique combination of characteristics"; ISO).

Health Information: Information about an identifiable individual that relates to his or her previous, current, and future health. It is also knowledge derived from statistics or data describing and enumerating attributes, events, behaviours, services, resources, outcomes, or costs related to health, disease, and health services.

Modification: A slight change or alteration made to improve something or make it more suitable.

Nomenclature: An agreed system of assigned names.

Terminology: A set of words or expressions together with a definition used within a certain field.

Section III
Virtual Reality Applications
in Medicine

*Medicine will see an enormous benefit from virtual reality. As shown in the
military, virtual reality can provide an excellent training mechanism when there
is no room for mistakes. Doctors will be able to practice alone or in teams to
fine-tune their skills for highly sensitive operations without having to risk a
human life. Virtual reality can improve the doctor's performance during
operations by superimposing vital information on the patient during an
operation. Superimposed images can increase the effectiveness of radiation
treatment and reduce the scarring of a surgery.*

Chapter VIII
Virtual Reality in Medicine

Theodoros N. Arvanitis
University of Birmingham, UK

ABSTRACT

This chapter explores the technological quest of virtual reality within the field of medicine. Although the author does not intend to provide an exhaustive review of the various health informatics applications of VR over the past 15 years of its development, he presents some of the major technological breakthroughs and their impact in the provision of healthcare services to the point-of-need (i.e., the patient).

INTRODUCTION

The continuing technological achievements of the modern era are changing dramatically the ways in which we conduct our daily activities and life. The medical field, through the provision of high-quality healthcare to the patient, is not an exception. The technological advances that we have witnessed during the past few decades have had an enormous impact on the manner in which we diagnose and treat dis-ease. Today's innovations in science and engineering raise the potential for medical technology to expand the frontier of healthcare delivery to unimaginable accomplishments. In this context, virtual-reality (VR) technologies have played an important role in revolutionising the practical provision of patient care. In recent years, VR technology and its application to medicine are not a research curiosity anymore; in several areas of clinical disciplines, the technology and innovation are developing in such a way that they can be adopted in routine practice, providing powerful tools in diagnostics, therapeutic planning, and interventions.

The enhancement of human health and, as a consequence, the improvement of the quality of human life, is one of the main objectives of scientific endeavour in the field of medicine. The provision of high-quality patient care is the ultimate outcome of any medical research and its related clinical implementation. The scientific advancements in medicine have always benefited from simultaneous developments in engineering and technology. Virtual reality is one of the important and recent technological innovations that have made a significant impact in medicine, more specifically in its quest for the high-quality provision of healthcare.

The medical applications of virtual reality originated in the early 1990s from the need of healthcare practitioners to visualise large amounts of complex medical data, particularly in surgical planning, preoperative training, and image-guided navigation during surgical procedures (Chinnock, 1994). Since the first surgical abdominal VR simulator in 1991 by Satava (1993), the scope of virtual reality in medicine has broadened, with applications ranging from 3-D (three-dimensional) immersive visualisation and manipulation of the cellular environment (Guan et al., 2004) to clinically applied diagnostic tools (e.g., virtual endoscopy technologies; Lorensen, Jolesz, & Kikinis, 1995), advanced medical education and training (Zajtchuck & Satava, 1997), augmented or enhanced surgery (Shuhaiber, 2004), medical therapy (Vincelli, Molinari, & Riva, 2001), and the virtual design of healthcare processes and environments (Kaplan, Hunter, Durlach, Schodek, & Rattner, 1995). Biomedical VR "has changed from [being] a research curiosity to a commercially and clinically important area of medical informatics technology" (Székely & Satava, 1999).

This chapter will explore the technological quest of virtual reality within the field of medicine. Although we do not intend to provide an exhaustive review of the various health-informatics applications of VR over the past 15 years of its development, we aspire to present and discuss some of the major technological breakthroughs and their impact in the provision of healthcare services to the point of need, that is, the patient. Our analysis will focus mainly on the research motivations and challenges in the routine use of the technology, while our argument will be about the socioeconomic effects and medicoethical concerns that relate to its implementation within the clinical practice.

THE CONCEPT OF VR IN THE CONTEXT OF MEDICINE

Traditionally, virtual reality is defined as a form of human-machine interaction technology, in which human users are fully immersed within a synthetic 3-D virtual environment (Ellis, 1994). Users can interact, through all their senses, with any virtual objects and scenes of such an environment as they are immersed in it with the assistance of appropriate graphical displays (usually, in the form of head-mounted display technologies, HMD) and other nonvisual technological modalities (e.g., auditory, haptic, etc.; Pratt, Zyda, & Kelleher, 1995). Such an interaction gives a full sense of virtual presence to the user.

This technology-oriented definition of VR, although valid for many scientific, industrial, and entertainment applications, is restrictive when considered within the context of the observed technological evolution of medical VR. Since the early years, many researchers and clinical practitioners have embraced the concept and technology of medical VR by adopting a broader definition and scope for its application in the field. Depending on the requirements of the healthcare application at hand, the implementation of immersion, in terms of technological devices used and sensory modalities involved, may vary. For instance, "in some applications, real and virtual objects need to be integrated making it necessary to present and manipulate them simultaneously in a single scene, leading to the development of hybrid systems referred to as augmented reality systems" (Székely & Satava, 1999). McCloy and Stone (2001) argue that "although this so called immersive technology is still evident today, only 10% of virtual reality applications warrant its use," while Riva (2003) states that only 20% of healthcare-related applications use immersive equipment. On the other hand, particular rehabilitation (Rizzo & Buckwalter, 1997) and clinical neuropsychology applications (Rizzo, Wiederhold, Riva, & Van Der Zaag, 1998) might benefit from an advanced immersive interactive environment, where users are active participants in the virtual world, interacting in real-time with the functionality of virtual objects and/or scenes (Schultheis & Rizzo, 2001). In such a scenario, the therapist can change, in a controlled manner, the conditions of the immersive interaction of a patient with the environment in order to study and manipulate any parameters of the patient's condition. Nevertheless, most biomedical VR practitioners advocate that the "key strength of virtual reality…is that it supports and enhances real time interaction on the part of the users" (McCloy & Stone).

This user-centric stance makes it futile to classify and study the bulk of medical VR applications in terms of their technological characteristics. Most authors in the current literature investigate such applications on the basis of their subject-matter categorisation within a specific subdiscipline of medical and clinical science (e.g., surgery, rehabilitation, metal

health, etc.) and their corresponding impact to such a knowledge domain. In this chapter, we aim to ascertain the revolutionary character of medical VR technologies in improving the appropriate provision of patient care. Thus, in the discussion that follows, we explore the relevant applications in terms of their innovation impact and clinical significance within the broad themes of medical diagnostics and visualisation, therapy interventions and planning, and medical education and training.

VR IN MEDICAL DIAGNOSTICS AND VISUALISATION

Medicine is an information-intensive field, where a large volume of real data is collected experimentally for the purposes of interpretation in order to understand the effects of disease in humans. To achieve such an interpretation of disparate and complex data, we commonly summarise all available and clinically related information through some form of meaningful visualisation. Traditional biomedical imaging techniques achieve the noninvasive visual representation of human anatomy and the functional mapping of human physiology from the cellular to the organism level. The advanced interactive 3-D-graphics technology of virtual reality (Haubner, Krapichler, Lösch, Englmeir, van Eimeren, & Kelleher, 1997) has further enhanced these visualisation possibilities by offering novel data-fusion approaches of human structural imaging with its corresponding functional mapping of human physiology and function (Soferman, Blythe, & John, 1998; Zajtchuck & Satava, 1997).

On the level of microcellular visualisation, we are currently experiencing a revolution in the 3-D representation of structural relationships within cells and human tissues, both in vivo and in vitro. Guan et al. (2004) recently developed novel VR visualisation that provides an intuitive, interactive way of viewing and manipulating 3-D cellular structures within an immersive synthetic environment. This breakthrough marks the beginning of further innovative visualisation for many other micromolecular imaging techniques, including electron microscopy (Frank, 2002) and NMR-based cellular imaging (Blackband, Buckley, Bui, & Phillips, 1999).

Novel VR visualisation of human anatomical structure has been rapidly realised since the completion of the Human Visible Project (Ackerman, 1991). The rich anatomical data sets have been acquired to serve as "a common reference point for the study of human anatomy, as a set of common public-domain data for testing medical imaging algorithms, and as a testbed and model for the construction of image libraries that can be accessed through networks" (Ackerman, 1998). A plethora of virtual-reality applications have been based on these data, many of which have been regularly reported in the conference series *Medicine Meets Virtual Reality* (e.g., Westwood, Haluck, Hoffman, Mogel, Phillips, & Robb, 2004; Westwood, Hoffmann, Robb, & Stredney, 1999).

The above-mentioned successes in human-anatomy visualisation have been more notable in a particular medical application of VR that has pushed the technology into the frontier of medical diagnostics. Virtual endoscopy (Lorensen et al., 1995; Rubino, Soler, Marescaux, & Maisonneuve, 2002; Wood & Razavi, 2002), one of the earlier endeavours in biomedical VR research, is now becoming a clinically acceptable new form of noninvasive screening for the diagnosis of structural abnormalities in internal organs. The concept of virtual endoscopy is based on the 3-D reconstruction of CT (computed tomography) or MRI (magnetic resonance imaging) data sets

of an internal organ of interest, followed by the execution of a visualisation "fly through" (Satava & Jones, 2002). The literature contains a vast amount of articles that successfully report the clinical implementation and use of virtual endocscopy in the organs of the colon (Vining, 1997), small bowel (Rogalla, Werner-Rustner, Huitema, van Est, Meiri, & Hamm, 1998), stomach (Springer et al., 1997), tracheo-bronchial tree (Jones & Athtanasiou, 2005), and so on.

The clinical significance of virtual endoscopy is currently being studied (e.g., Bhandari et al., 2004; Rapp-Bernhardt, Welte, Budinger, & Bernhardt, 1998) as it is becoming more and more urgent to use it in clinical diagnostic practice. Virtual endoscopy lacks any known complications (in contrast to known issues of perforation, bleeding, etc. found in traditional endoscopy), it is a totally noninvasive technique, and its implementation is far more cost effective in terms of materials and personnel when compared with traditional invasive screening methods (Dunkin, 2003).

VR IN CLINICAL THERAPY INTERVENTIONS AND PLANNING

The majority of current near-term therapeutic applications are identified in the areas of VR-technology-assisted surgical interventions (remote surgery and augmented- or enhanced-reality surgery; Marescaux & Rubino, 2003; Marmulla, Hoppe, Mühling, & Eggers, 2005), surgical planning, and surgical simulation (Satava & Jones, 1998). Remote surgery applications link research in robotics and virtual reality. Surgeons can manipulate equipment from a remote site while having full haptic-sensory feedback through the use of telerobotic equipment. VR-enhanced remote surgery applications have been beneficial for defence medicine and for solving the problem of providing emergency treatment at a distance, where there is no availability of specialists locally. Satava's (1995) original vision and concept of surgeons in the future being equipped with virtual-reality headsets and rehearsing real or robotic procedures, using advanced computer-generated images, has recently become a reality with the successful completion of a transatlantic robot-assisted surgical intervention. On September 7, 2001, surgeons in New York performed a laparoscopic cholecystectomy on a patient in France (Marescaux et al., 2001). Furthermore, many front-running concepts in image-guided surgery (augmented-reality concepts) are currently "undergoing consolidation through clinical validation" (McCloy & Stone, 2001). Most of these applications are used both as image-guided and planning surgical tools.

For the above-mentioned applications, there are still a few challenges to overcome. In order to achieve reliable real-time implementations of both remote and augmented-reality surgical procedures, further work is needed in ensuring that the technology will cope with the demands of the requirements for the procedures: The improvement of high-performance 3-D graphical visualisation and real-time image data-fusion algorithms, together with the robust and resilient distributed transmission of large and complex data sets, are still important requirements to be met (Satava & Jones, 1998).

In the area of surgical simulation, we can observe 15 years of continuous effort and development of surgical simulation technologies for planning and training (Chinnock, 1994; McCloy & Stone, 2001). Such systems can provide different levels of photo-realism in anatomical representations, different levels of fidelity in physical properties of tissue, and physiologic parameters (Satava & Jones, 1998).

Of the notable successes in VR surgical simulation applications, we should mention the progress of minimally invasive surgical trainers, such as the MIST system, "a product for training and assessment of surgical laparoscopic psychomotor skills" of trainee surgeons (McCloy & Stone, 2001) that is now commercially available (Mentice Corporation, n.d.). Currently, systems like MIST are undergoing clinical trials and validation and are slowly becoming useful tools for surgical skills certification. Nonetheless, McCloy and Stone are arguing that despite the technological achievement in the area of surgical training VR simulators, there is still a great need for objectively validating the acquisition of skills of individual surgeons during training: "The crucial factor that will determine the uptake of virtual reality technology by surgeons will be the demonstration that virtual reality is capable of delivering reliable and valid training and assessment systems." Various researchers are currently working toward the identification of objective metrics for the evaluation of surgical skills in real and virtual environments (Moody, Baber, & Arvanitis, 2002; Moody, Baber, Arvanitis, & Elliott, 2003).

VR technologies are now starting to play a crucial role as a clinical tool in the field of neuropsychological assessment and rehabilitation (Riva, 2003; Vincelli et al., 2001). A new era of clinical therapy interventions for clinical psychologists is at its beginning, in which the properties of immersive interactive environments are used by therapists to stimulate the real world of patients in a variety of flexible interventions on psychological-distress cases. Riva and Davide (1995) argue that the therapeutic effectiveness of VR clinical psychology interventions is most likely to be increased compared to traditional methods, while supporting their arguments by reporting current studies of the verification of the clinical effectiveness for six psychological disorders, including acrophobia, arachnophobia, panic disorders with agoraphobia, body-image disturbances, binge-eating disorders, and fear of flight (Riva, 2003). Even though the clinical potential is evident in this field, there are still some medicoethical issues to be resolved. Whalley (1995) argues that as this effort is still at a research stage, there is still

the possibility that some researchers place their own advancement above the interests of a particular patient. Some other researchers may be unduly paternalistic especially when making decisions about patients who because of mental impairment or illness are unable to give their informed consent. Potentially, VR machines may be prone to errors such that they introduce into the mental life of susceptible individuals specific distortions that serve to exacerbate the symptoms of mental illness or induce such symptoms when none were previously present.

Therefore, there is a need for an open ethical debate within the research community, while clearly medicoethical governance bodies have to regulate experimentation and application of the technologies.

VR IN MEDICAL EDUCATION AND TRAINING

It is evident from the above discussion that the visualisation, planning, and simulation aspects of VR technology have important implications for medical education and training (Riva, 2003; Székely & Satava, 1999). We could present a plethora of examples of successful applications of VR in medical education and training, relating to the study of anatomy, surgical training, and so forth. Many medical schools have successfully combined the use of VR technologies in established courses, such as the effort at the University of California at San Diego, where an established multimedia, computer-based education program on anatomy, pathology, and

radiology has been combined with virtual reality (Hoffman, 1992; Hoffman, Irwin, Ligon, Murray, & Tohsaku, 1995). There is a great potential of using VR with other established technologies, such as the Internet, in order to maximise the outputs of high-quality delivery of medical education (Samothrakis, Arvanitis, Plataniotis, McNeill, & Lister, 1997).

CONCLUDING REMARKS

Our brief exploration of medical VR technologies and their application in both basic medical research and clinical practice has shown that the impact of the technology can be simply characterised as revolutionary in the context of enhancing the quality of patient care. The informatics tools that VR has offered to the medical field are now widely accepted and validated for everyday use in clinical practice. The field of medical VR is not anymore a technological curiosity, but provides an appropriate and exemplar way of applying information and communication technologies in healthcare. However, despite the intensive research and development over the past 15 years, there is still great potential for the expansion of the capabilities that VR technology offers to medicine. The current successful clinical implementations show that VR has still the potential to offer a real value to further improving the appliance of informatics in healthcare and, as a consequence, the quality of human life.

REFERENCES

Ackerman, M. J. (1991). The visible human project. *The Journal of Biocommunication, 18*(2), 14.

Ackerman, M. J. (1998). The visible human project. *Proceedings of the IEEE, 86*(3), 504-511.

Bhandari, S., Shim, C. S., Kim, J. H., Jung, I. S., Cho, J. Y., Lee, J. S., et al. (2004). Usefulness of three-dimensional multidetector row CT (virtual gastroscopy and multiplanar reconstruction) in the evaluation of gastric cancer: A comparison with conventional endoscopy, EUS, and histopathology. *Gastrointestinal Endoscopy, 59*(6), 619-626.

Blackband, S. J., Buckley, D. L., Bui, J. D., & Phillips, M. I. (1999). NMR microscopy: Beginnings and new directions. *Magnetic Resonance Materials in Biology, Physics and Medicine, 9*(3), 112-116.

Chinnock, C. (1994). Virtual reality in surgery and medicine. *Hospital Technology Series, 13*(18), 1-48.

Dunkin, B. J. (2003). Flexible endoscopy simulators. *Seminars in Laparoscopic Surgery, 10*(1), 29-35.

Ellis, S. R. (1994). What are virtual environments? *IEEE Computer Graphics and Applications, 14*(1), 17-22.

Frank, J. (2002). Single-particle imaging of macromolecules by cryo-electron microscopy. *Annual Review of Biophysics and Biomolecular Structure, 31,* 303-319.

Guan, Y. Q., Opas, M., Cai, Y. Y., Zhang, X., Xiong, Z. W., Wong, S., et al. (2004). Application of virtual reality in volumetric cellular visualization. *Proceedings of the 2004 ACM SIGGRAPH International Conference on Virtual Reality Continuum and its Applications in Industry* (pp. 65-71).

Haubner, M., Krapichler, C., Lösch, A., Englmeir, K.-H., van Eimeren, W., & Kelleher, K. (1997). Virtual reality in medicine: Computer graphics and interaction techniques. *IEEE Transactions on Information Technology in Biomedicine, 1*(1), 61-72.

Hoffman, H. (1992). Developing network-compatible instructional resources for UCSD's core curriculum. In J. D. Westwood, H. M. Hoffman, R. A. Robb, & D. Stredney (Eds.), *Medicine meets virtual reality* (pp. 90-92). Washington, DC: IOS Press.

Hoffman, H., Irwin, A., Ligon R., Murray, M., & Tohsaku, C. (1995). Virtual reality-multimedia synthesis: Next-generation learning environments for medical education. *The Journal of Biocommunication, 22*(3), 2-7.

Jones, C. M., & Athanasiou, T. (2005). Is virtual bronchoscopy an efficient diagnostic tool for the thoracic surgeon? *The Annals of Thoracic Surgery, 79*(1), 365-374.

Kaplan, K., Hunter, I., Durlach, N. I., Schodek, D. L., & Rattner, D. (1995). A virtual environment for a surgical room of the future. In R. M. Satava, K. S. Morgan, H. B. Sieburg, R. Mattheus, & J. P. Christensen (Eds.), *Interactive technology and the new paradigm for healthcare* (pp. 161-167). Washington, DC: IOS Press.

Lorensen, W. E., Jolesz, F. A., & Kikinis, R. (1995). The exploration of cross-sectional data with a virtual endoscope. In R. M. Satava, K. S. Morgan, H. B. Sieburg, R. Mattheus, & J. P. Christensen (Eds.), *Interactive technology and the new paradigm for healthcare* (pp. 221-230). Washington, DC: IOS Press.

Marescaux, J., Leroy, J., Gagner, M., Rubino, F., Mutter, D., Vix, M., et al. (2001). Transantlantic robot-assisted telesurgery. *Nature, 413*(6854), 379-380.

Marescaux, J., & Rubino, F. (2003). Telesurgery, telemonitoring, virtual surgery and telerobotics. *Current Urology Reports, 4,* 109-113.

Marmulla, R., Hoppe, H., Mühling, J., & Eggers, G. (2005). An augmented reality system for image-guided surgery. *International Journal of Oral and Maxillofacial Surgery, 34*(6), 594-596.

McCloy, R., & Stone, R. (2001). Science, medicine and the future: Virtual reality in surgery. *British Medical Journal, 323*(7318), 912-915.

Mentice Corporation. (n.d.). *Procedicus MIST™*. Retrieved August 15, 2005, from http://www.mentice.com/

Moody, C. L., Baber, C., & Arvanitis, T. N. (2002). Objective surgical performance evaluation based on haptic feedback. In J. D. Westwood, H. M. Hoffman, R. A. Robb, & D. Stredney (Eds.), *Medicine meets virtual reality 10* (pp. 304-310). Amsterdam: IOS Press.

Moody, C. L., Baber, C., Arvanitis, T. N., & Elliott, M. (2003). Objective metrics for the evaluation of simple surgical skills in real and virtual domains. *Presence, 12*(2), 207-221.

Pratt, D. R., Zyda, M., & Kelleher, K. (1995). Virtual reality: In the mind of the beholder. *IEEE Computer, 28*(7), 17-19.

Rapp-Bernhardt, U., Welte, T., Budinger, M., & Bernhardt, T. M. (1998). Comparison of three-dimensional virtual endoscopy with bronchoscopy in patients with oesophageal carcinoma infiltrating the trancheobronchial tree. *British Journal of Radiology, 71*(852), 1271-1278.

Riva, G. (2003). Applications of virtual environments in medicine. *Methods of information in medicine, 42*(5), 524-534.

Riva, G., & Davide, F. (2001). *Communications through virtual technologies: Identity, community and technology in the communication age*. Amsterdam: IOS Press.

Rizzo, A. A., & Buckwalter, J. G. (1997). Virtual reality and cognitive assessment and

rehabilitation: The state of the art. In G. Riva (Ed.), *Virtual reality in neuro-psycho-physiology* (pp. 123-146). Amsterdam: IOS Press.

Rizzo, A. A., Wiederhold, B., Riva, G., & Van Der Zaag, C. (1998). A bibliography of articles relevant to the application of virtual reality in the mental field. *Cyberpsychology and Behaviour, 1*(4), 411-425.

Rogalla, P., Werner-Rustner, M., Huitema, A., van Est, A., Meiri, N., & Hamm, B. (1998). Virtual endoscopy of the small bowel: Phantom study and preliminary clinical results. *European Radiology, 8*(4), 563-567.

Rubino, F., Soler, L., Marescaux, J., & Maisonneuve, H. (2002). Advances in virtual reality are wide ranging. *British Medical Journal, 324*(7337), 612.

Samothrakis, S., Arvanitis, T. N., Plataniotis, A., McNeill, M. D. J., & Lister, P. F. (1997). WWW creates new interactive 3D graphics and collaborative environments for medical research and education. *International Journal of Medical Informatics, 47*, 69-73.

Satava, R. M. (1993). Virtual reality surgical simulator: The first steps. *Surgical Endoscopy, 7*, 203-205.

Satava, R. M. (1995). Medicine 2001: The king is dead. In R. Morgan, R. M. Satava, H. B. Sieburg, R. Matthews, & J. P. Christensen (Eds.), *Interactive technology and the new paradigm for healthcare* (pp. 334-339). Amsterdam: IOS Press.

Satava, R. M., & Jones, S. B. (1998). Current and future applications of virtual reality for medicine. *Proceedings of the IEEE, 86*(3), 484-489.

Satava, R. M., & Jones, S. B. (2002). Medical applications of virtual reality. In K. M. Stanney (Ed.), *Handbook of virtual environments:*

Design, implementation and applications (pp. 368-391). Mahwah, NJ: Lawrence Erlbaum Associates, Inc.

Schultheis, M. T., & Rizzo, A. A. (2001). The application of virtual reality technology in rehabilitation. *Rehabilitation Psychology, 46*(3), 296-311.

Shuhaiber, J. H. (2004). Augmented reality in surgery. *Archives of Surgery, 139*(2), 170-174.

Soferman, Z., Blythe, D., & John, N. W. (1998). Advanced graphics behind medical virtual reality: Evolution of algorithms, hardware, and software interfaces. *Proceedings of the IEEE, 86*(3), 531-554.

Springer, P., Dessl, A., Giacomuzzi, S. M., Buchberger, W., Stoger, A., Oberwalder, M., et al. (1997). Virtual computed tomography gastroscopy: A new technique. *Endoscopy, 29*(7), 632-634.

Székely, G., & Satava, R. M. (1999). Virtual reality in medicine. *British Medical Journal, 319*(7220), 1305-1309.

Vincelli, F., Molinari, E., & Riva, G. (2001). Virtual reality as clinical tool: Immersion and three dimensionality in the relationship between patient and therapist. *Studies in Health Technology and Informatics, 81*, 551-553.

Vining, D. J. (1997). Virtual colonoscopy. *Gastrointestinal Endoscopy Clinics of North America, 7*(2), 285-291.

Westwood, J. D., Haluck, R. S., Hoffman, H. M., Mogel, G. T., Phillips, R., & Robb, R. A. (Eds.). (2004). *Medicine meets virtual reality 12: Building a better you. The next tools for medical education, diagnosis, and care.* Amsterdam: IOS Press.

Westwood, J. D., Hoffman, H. M., Robb, R. A., & Stredney, D. (Eds.). (1999). *Medicine meets virtual reality 7.* Amsterdam: IOS Press.

Whalley, L. H. (1995). Ethical issues in the application of virtual reality in medicine. *Computational Biology in Medicine, 2*, 107-114.

Wood, B. J., & Razavi, P. (2002). Virtual endoscopy: A promising new technology. *American Family Physician, 66*(1), 107-112.

Zajtchuck, R., & Satava, R. M. (1997). Medical applications of virtual reality. *Communications of the ACM, 40*(9), 63-64.

Chapter IX
Modelling and Simulation of Biological Systems

George I. Mihalas
"Victor Babes" University of Medicine and Pharmacy, Romania

ABSTRACT

It is unanimously accepted that a theoretical approach of a system or phenomenon reveals new features and offers a deeper insight into the intimate mechanisms. In life science, this approach is mainly based on mathematical modeling, followed naturally by computer simulation. The chapter presented here tries to give the reader a comprehensive view over the main issues arising when attempting to build models of biological systems. A series of applications is shortly presented. The second half of the chapter is dedicated to one of the most interesting models: protein synthesis regulation. The example follows the classical steps: the scheme of the processes to be described, the set of differential equations and the results, including their possible interpretation.

INTRODUCTION

Mathematical modelling proved to be a useful research tool, offering an elegant and simple description of a system (Ingram & Bloch, 1984). The computer's advent stimulated its use also in complex systems, like biomedical systems (Garfinkel, 1965). There are several ways to approach a formal description of biological systems, yielding several types of models (Brown & Rothery, 1993, Fishwick & Luker, 1991). We can classify the models from various viewpoints (Mihalas, Lungeanu, Kigyosi, & Vemic, 1995):

a. A system's structure
   - Continuous models
   - Discrete models
b. An input-output relationship
   - Deterministic models (subdivided into analytical models and models based on differential equations)
   - Stochastic models

c. A modeled feature
- Models for structure
- Models for function

BUILDING MATHEMATICAL MODELS OF BIOLOGICAL SYSTEMS

There are several typical steps followed for building mathematical models (Keen & Spain, 1992).

- Defining and delimiting the system and the process to be modelled
- Selecting the variables, both independent and dependent variables
- Establishing the relations between the variables
- Defining the input and output
- Setting initial conditions and the values of parameters and constants
- Choosing the results representation
- Establishing the validation mode

APPLICATIONS IN BIOMEDICAL RESEARCH

The results of a simulation are usually presented as a graphical plot representing the system evolution over time; the experimental conditions are represented by a set of input parameters.

There are several possible applications of mathematical models and their corresponding simulation programs in biomedical research (Mihalas, 1998).

- **Experimental Design:** The system behaviour for various values of input parameters is analyzed, letting us choose the best set of parameters corresponding to the experimental conditions that yield measurable results.
- **Testing Hypotheses:** Sometimes there are no direct experimental procedures to test two different hypotheses concerning a certain phenomenon or process; in this case, we can simulate a system's behaviour under the two conditions and compare the simulation output with the real behaviour.
- **Determining Parameters:** For the parameters that are not (easily) accessible by direct measurements, we can simulate the process for a wide range of values of the studied parameter. By comparing the results with the real experimental behaviour, we can estimate the parameter.
- **Prognosis:** It is one of the largest applications and lets us analyze possible system evolution.
- **Feeling the Phenomenon:** A better understanding of the process is achieved when a system's behaviour is analyzed over several conditions.
- **Didactic Applications:** These are used for educational purposes.

AN EXAMPLE: COMPUTER SIMULATION OF PROTEIN-SYNTHESIS REGULATION

Delimiting the System and the Process

The system is represented by a reduced (simplified) cell (Mihalas, Niculescu-Duvaz, & Simon, 1985). We take into account only three components (Figure 1).

- A DNA sequence on which we can distinguish two genes: the synthesis gene (SG) and the control gene (C)

Figure 1. Scheme of a protein synthesis control system. The variables and parameters are also denoted here.

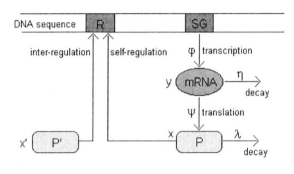

- the messenger ribonucleic acid (mRNA)
- the synthesized protein (P)

The process is the protein synthesis, which comprises the following major steps:

- mRNA is produced in the nucleus when the SG is activated with a rate dependent on the activation degree.
- mRNA migrates into the cytoplasm and bounds to a ribosome; we should also consider the mRNA degradation, with a decay rate proportional to its concentration.
- The protein P is synthesized on the ribosome with a rate proportional to the mRNA concentration; again, we will also consider the protein decay.
- The activation degree of the SG is regulated by the control gene C, whose state is controlled either by the synthesized protein P (self-regulation), or by another protein P' (interregulation).

Selecting the Variables and Defining the Parameters

- Concentrations are dependent variables; let [mRNA] = x and [P] = y.

- The activation degree, A, is also a dependent variable.
- Parameters include proportionality constants for synthesis rates (φ for mRNA and ψ for protein) and for decay rates (λ for mRNA and η for protein), and the coupling process between the protein P and the control gene C for the autoregulated process.

To establish the relations between variables, the processes described can be formally written as:

$$\begin{cases} \dfrac{dx}{dt} = \varphi A - \lambda x \\[2mm] \dfrac{dy}{dt} = \psi x - \eta y \\[2mm] A = \dfrac{1}{1 + y/k} \end{cases}$$

Defining the Input and the Output

- The input represents the starting conditions, that is, all parameters (φ, ψ, λ, η, k) and initial values for the variables (x_0, y_0).
- The output is represented by the time evolution of the two major components (variables), that is, x(t) and y(t).

Setting Initial Conditions, (i.e., Associating values to φ, ψ, λ, η, k, x_0, and y_0)

We also set now in the iteration step a value for dt, which is usually very small. It is important to note that for qualitative simulations, we do not need exact values for the parameters and initial concentrations; it would suffice to work with relative values (to consider one parameter as a unit). However, when absolute values are available, we will use them.

Figure 2. Time evolution of a protein (y) on an arbitrary time scale

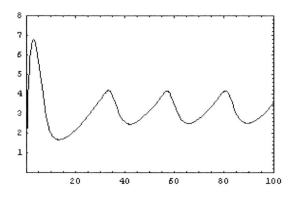

Figure 3. Phase diagram (Oscillatory behaviour is visible)

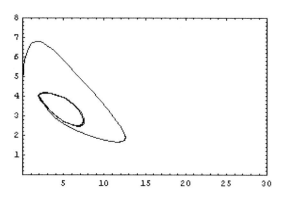

Choosing the Results Representation

Usually, the time evolution is preferred: x(t) and y(t) (Figure 2).

However, we can also draw a phase diagram y = f(x) (Figure 3), which is convenient for oscillatory systems or systems with multiple steady states.

Stating the Validation Mode

When experimental data are available, a comparison of simulated data with real data is recommended. However, we often consider also the type of behaviour as a validation mode: evolution toward steady state(s), damped or sustained oscillations, and so forth (Mihalas, Simon, Balea, & Popa, 2000).

TRENDS FOR FUTURE DEVELOPMENTS

The specific requirements for a convenient simulation program have encouraged software development, from simple forms (Mendes, 1993;

Tomita et al., 1999) to more advanced software (Loew & Schaff, 2001; Tomita et al.); some developers also pay special attention to the user interface (Ichikawa, 2001).

An important step was taken when dedicated programming languages were proposed (Cuellar, Lloyd, Nielsen, Bullivant, Nickerson, & Hunter, 2003; Hucka et al., 2003), which bring the formal descriptions of biological processes to a higher level.

Our example was taken from molecular biology, but the use of modeling and simulation in life sciences covers a much wider range, from physiology (Randall, 1987) to integrated approaches (Moolgavkar, 1986) and even healthcare systems.

CONCLUSION

Computer simulations of biological processes are convenient tools for biomedical research, and are easy to handle with various applications. The complexity of biological systems imposes limits in their use; most often the results are limited to a small number of variables and cover just certain relations, always neglecting others. However, the programs will become more and more complex, covering more and more variables, trying to get closer to the great challenge in this field in the (near) future: to simulate an entire cell.

REFERENCES

Brown, D. B., & Rothery, P. (1993). *Models in biology: Mathematics, statistics and computing.* Chichester, UK: John Wiley & Sons.

Cuellar, A. A., Lloyd, C. M., Nielsen, P. F., Bullivant, D. P., Nickerson, D. P., & Hunter, P. J. (2003). An overview of CellML 1.1: A biological model description language. *SIMULATION: Transactions of the Society for Modeling and Simulation International, 79*(12), 740-747.

Fishwick, P. A., & Luker, P. A. (Eds.). (1991). *Qualitative simulation, modeling and analysis.* New York: Springer Verlag.

Garfinkel, D. (1965). Simulation of biochemical systems. In R. W. Stacy & B. D. Waxman (Eds.), *Computers in biomedical research* (Vol. 1, pp. 111-134). New York: Academic Press.

Hucka, M., et al. (2003). The systems biology markup language (SBML): A medium for representation and exchange of biochemical network models. *Bioinformatics, 19*(4), 524-531.

Ichikawa, K. (2001). A-Cell: Graphical user interface for the construction of biochemical reaction models. *Bioinformatics, 17*(5), 483-484.

Ingram, D., & Bloch, R. (1984). *Mathematical methods in medicine.* Chichester, UK: John Wiley & Sons.

Keen, R. E., & Spain, J. D. (1992). *Computer simulation in biology.* New York: Wiley-Liss.

Loew, L. M., & Schaff, J. C. (2001). The virtual cell: A software environment for computational cell biology. *Trends in Biotechnology, 19*(10), 401-406.

Mendes, P. (1993). Gepasi: A software package for modeling the dynamics, steady states, and control of biochemical and other systems. *Computer Applications in Biosciences (CABIOS), 9*(5), 563-571.

Mihalas, G. I. (1998). Modelling and simulation in medicine and life sciences. *Medical Informatics, 23*(2), 93-96.

Mihalas, G. I., Kigyosi, A., Lungeanu, D., & Vernic, C. (1998). Modeling and simulation in molecular pharmacology. *MEDINFO'98*, 372-375.

Mihalas, G. I., Lungeanu, D., Kigyosi, A., & Vernic, C. (1995). Classification criteria for simulation programs used in medical education. *MEDINFO'95, 2*, 1209-1213.

Mihalas, G. I., Macovievici, G., Simon, Z., & Lungeanu, D. (1999). MOBISIM: Package for simulation in molecular biology. *Medical Informatics Europe '99*, 617-620.

Mihalas, G. I., Niculescu-Duvaz, I., & Simon, Z. (1985). Trigger with positive control for gene activity regulation: Computer simulation. *Studia Biophysica, 107*(3), 223-229.

Mihalas, G. I., Simon, Z., Balea, G., & Popa, E. (2000). Possible oscillatory behaviour in P53-MDM2 interaction: Computer simulation. *Journal of Biological Systems, 8*(1), 21-29.

Mihalas, G. I., Zaharie, D., & Kigyosi, A. (2004). Step-wise or continous activation in cell regulation? A comparative study of p53-mdm2 interaction by computer simulation. *MEDINFO2004*, 1758.

Moolgavkar, S. H. (1986). Carcinogenesis modeling: From molecular biology to epidemiology. *Annuual Review of Public Health, 7,* 151-169.

Randall, J. E. (1987). *Microcomputers and physiological simulation.* New York: Raven Press.

Tomita, M., Hashimoto, K., Takahashi, K., Shimizu T. S., Matsuzaki, Y., Miyoshi, F. et al. (1999). E-CELL: Software environment for whole cell simulation. *Bioinformatics, 15*(1), 72-84.

KEY TERMS

Computer Simulation: A computer program that mimics the behaviour of the model variables for a set of values of the model parameters, and initial values of the independent variables.

Deterministic Model: A mathematical model based on a relation between the dependent and independent variables; for each set of values of the independent variables, there is only one well-defined possible value of the dependent variable.

Mathematical Modelling: A method to describe system behaviour by a set of relations between the system's characteristic variables and parameters.

Model: A simplified representation of a system (a conventionally defined part of the universe), keeping only a set of features (variables, parameters, and relations) considered relevant and neglecting irrelevant features.

Stochastic Model: A mathematical model based on probabilities for which there are several possible values for a set of values of the independent variables; the model computes the probabilities of various output values.

Chapter X
Virtual Reality Simulation in Human Applied Kinetics and Ergo Physiology

Bill Ag. Drougas
ATEI Education Institute of Epirus, Greece

ABSTRACT

Virtual reality is today an excellent tool for a full simulated experience in a modern environment where any researcher or any individual scientist may work with vital experimental environments or use parameters that sometimes does not really exist. It is already a vital step for the future of science and for the modern experiment. Ergo physiology today has many applications for research. We can find new unknown parameters for the human body searching biokinetics and ergo physiology, and it is time to use modern technologies and applications. The vital issues discussed in this chapter may offer many applications for human kinetics and movement and may also discuss biokinetics research using the physical laws and parameters in various biokinetics and physiology fields.

INTRODUCTION

Virtual reality is today an important part of modern scientific methodology and research, using modern high-speed computers of lately designed technologies for research and simulation in various scientific fields such as ergo physiology and biokinetics. This is a new field in contemporary science, methodology, and experimentation, and we can recognize that during the past years, it has continued with great success. An important field using this new way of research is the simulation of human movement in ergo physiology and applied biokinetics science. Virtual reality is very useful for researchers in these fields because they can have simulations of the physical human body at any time they want for study or experimentation.

BACKGROUND

One of the first authors who wrote about virtual reality was Howard Rheingold (1991), who wrote about data visualization and 3-D CAD (computer-aided design) in which someone may use his or her hands and fingers. Many applications can be found from the middle war period by the U.S. Air Force to create flying simulations.

Myron Krueger, during the '60s, worked on the affiliation of human and computer with special research in computer-controlled responsive environments, which were named by him artificial reality (Krueger, 1993). He also designed the video place, a system that contains a projection screen and a video camera that is controlled by a computer. By this method, human movements in each activity are transferred to computer graphics in software (Boudouridis, 1994).

So, there can be a connection between human and technical things in space with computer graphics. This was one of the first methodologies in human-kinetics research and applications.

Tom Furness was another scientist who designed the Super Cockpit for the U.S. Air Force after many years of research. In a small place, a human could use computers and a HMD (head-mounted display) to understand vital secrets of the flight without any danger (Furness, 1991).

But the man who is the father of the terms virtual reality and reality engine is Jaron Lanier, an informatics scientist who, with another young man named Tom Zimmerman, established the Visual Programming Language Research Inc in 1980 (Boudouridis, 1994). This company was the first to make important tools for virtual reality programs and applications, such as data gloves and HMDs.

ISSUES

In the beginning, many other scientists worked with computer data for virtual reality applications in various fields with very big success.

Today, there are many different fields and applications of virtual reality technology. Table 1 summarizes some of the virtual reality applications similar to those of ergo physiology.

Especially in the fields of ergo physiology and biokinetics, virtual reality is used in many applications. Some of the characteristics of human movement, the human body, and parameters such as space, geometry, color, and sound may help virtual reality programs become more effective in various methodologies of research and virtual applications.

The importance of this is to find a methodology for using virtual reality and a way to recognize the results, such as some of the official physiology results that can give to researchers many new discoveries in existing science and theory, or future science research in finding new signals from the human body during simulations.

Today we have all the modern technology to make better simulations for the human body

Table 1. Summary of the virtual reality applications similar to those in ergo physiology fields

- Human behavior in flying simulations
- Human behavior in space simulations
- Learning and human-movement programs in kinetics
- Neurodisease science
- Rehabilitation
- Physical behavior in space
- Step-correction learning and research
- Adapted methodologies in kinetics
- Special gymnastics programs
- Study of the human senses and their characteristics
- Pain confrontment
- Continuing education

Table 2. Important parameters in virtual reality simulations for ergo physiology and human movement

- Length
- Height
- Time
- Sound frequency
- Color frequency
- Wave length
- Velocity
- Pressure
- Area
- Energy
- Power

and to see new fields that had not previously existed. This is, of course, the future of research.

For example, it is not possible for anyone to fly at high speeds without any danger so that scientists can see the behavior of the human body or parameters such as blood pressure, the behavior of the heart, muscle energy, signals or other problems in the eyes, and so forth. But with virtual reality simulations, we can today register many of these parameters and standards, see how they change after the experimentation, and see it is used in our theories.

The very best aspect of this method is that we can stop the experiment when we must or when we want to begin the experiment again from the last step, or, if we want, we can design another model with new parameters. So, we can always put something new into our experimentation and theory, and this is important because every person is different from every other. By this methodology, we can register statistical effects or make a very good mathematical analysis of the problem to continue with advanced research and measurements or to make other project experiments.

So many past methodologies or past technologies will be changed after these experiments. Ergo physiology and applied human

kinetics today use many important laws of physics, physiology, mathematics, statistics, and, of course, medical data, and it is important to continue to grow using new technologies like virtual reality. Table 2 summarizes some of the parameters that are important in virtual reality simulation for the human body and movement.

In some experiments, all of the parameters in Table 2 can be used, and in some others, only a few of them can be used. However, the parameters in the simulations are very near to those of physics, and the philosophy is about the same in similar experiments.

Table 3 summarizes some of the fields in which virtual reality can help to recognize and study the physical parameters of Table 2.

In every subject of the study of human abilities, there are various techniques and methodologies. However, the philosophies of all methodologies are about the same and have similar directions.

So it is important to understand that with virtual reality simulations in ergo physiology, we may simulate human models in an environment that does not really exist physically. In this way we can find new and unknown parameters of the basics of human biokinetics and ergo physiology. In the same way, a researcher can establish new models of experiments and fields for research using many parameters of the modern population and all the modern kinetic problems that appear in people. Researchers

Table 3. Summary of the fields of the physical parameters in virtual reality

- Kinetics conception
- Space-creation parameters
- Relative-movement creation
- Color-conception studies
- Sound-conception studies
- Kinetics-parameters registration
- Study of velocity
- Study of frequency
- Study of space parameters
- Study and registration of time

can include these problems in the data of the simulation and study the methodology or the effects within the simulation. For example, the influence of a brain problem on human kinetics ability can be registered from various kinetics parameters and/or kinetics behavior and movement in various daily skills. Many years before, this was not so clear, and many of these problems seemed like they didn't exist. In simulations, we have two bodies: the virtual and the real.

It is important to understand that two human bodies in the same experiment are the same but also different.

We have two human bodies during the experiment that we can use, or many more if it is possible with the program. Virtual reality biokinetics research programs must have both human bodies: the real and the virtual one. The parameters and simulations must be very close between these two categories. These two bodies are different persons, but closely exhibit the same movements. It is very important to recognize the abilities of the bodies. The information about kinetics behavior or any other information from any data structure that defines the behaviors of the movement and kinetic parameters of one virtual human can be passed directly to all the other virtual humans if there is more than one human in the program of the experiment. In this way, we can have parameters and measurements from various kinetic models at the same time and study many different behaviors. This is the philosophy of a multiple experiment.

Two or more students or researchers can work with two or more models at the same time and give different conclusions and different theories. Virtual humans are real models that can be used many times for the same work and for the same or a different research. This is very good for the physiology studies and medicine experiments for human biokinetics and

Table 4. Summary of some of the simulated and virtual applications

- Simulation of ergonomic environments
- Simulation-based training
- Rehabilitation and modern orthopedics
- Virtual patients and human organs for surgery
- Psychotherapy and applied physiology
- Sports simulations
- Physiological behavior with various phobias
- Biomechanical walking
- Virtual training for balance

behavior, and, of course, for education programs for researchers or students at the graduate or postgraduate levels.

Table 4 summarizes some of the simulated and virtual applications to human abilities.

Many of the methodologies that exist today began first in front of a computer screen and, with the help of modern programs of simulation in physiology, biology, and mathematics, they continue to establish some of the new theories.

Today, electronic methods give us the opportunity to continue our research in a safer work environment; in the past, various experimental problems in the physical environment were impossible to avoid. Virtual reality and its development are currently underway in a number of organizations such as NASA, IBM, Boeing, and so forth, and also in many official research programs of famous university laboratories and technological educational institutes. In many of these institutes, there exist many new international programs of human study and ergo physiology research.

CONCLUSION

Virtual reality is today an excellent tool for a fully simulated experience in a modern environment where the researcher or simple scientist may work with vital experimental environments or use any parameter that sometimes does not really exist. This is important for people who are researching the abilities of the human body. The vital issues discussed in this article may offer many applications for human kinetics and movement, and biokinetics research using physical laws and parameters. In the same philosophy, any researcher may propose or design new models for informatics scientists. Ergo physiology today has many applications for research, and the modern computer systems for simulations and virtual reality give us many applications and the opportunity to work in easier experimental environments to make and design experiments using real and unreal parameters without any danger for us or any other human. This is already a step toward the future of science and the experiments.

REFERENCES

Boudouridis, M. (1994). *The technology of virtual reality.* Presentation to the International Summer School of Communications, Athens, Greece.

Computers: Artificial intelligence. (n.d.). *Time Life,* 73-77.

Deisinger, J., Breining, R., & Robler, A. (n.d.). ERGONAUT: A tool for ergonomic analysis in virtual environments. In J. D. Mulder & R. van Liere (Eds.), *Virtual Environments 2000, Proceedings of the 6th Eurographics Workshop on Virtual Environments,* Amsterdam, The Netherlands. New York: Springer Wien.

Drougas, B. Ag. (n.d.). Rehabilitation by new technologies. *Research and Theory Journal,* 12-15.

Drougas, B. Ag. (2003). *Theory and laboratory applications for the lesson of teleinformatics and applications in medicine.* ATEI of Epirus, Department of Teleinformatics.

Drougas, B. Ag. (2004a). *Home care and the modern technologies* (1st ed.). D-publications Arta Greece.

Drougas, B. Ag. (2004b). *Telemedicine applications in a contemporary environment.* D-publications Arta Greece.

Drougas, B. Ag. (2004c). *Virtual reality and health: Manual of the Laboratory of the Teleinformatics and Applications in Medicine.* ATEI of Epirus, Department of Teleinformatics.

Furness. (1991). Harnessing virtual space. *Society for Information Display Digest of Technical Papers* (1st ed.).

Hoffman, H. G. (2004). Therapy applications of virtual reality. *Scientific American* (Greek ed.), 28-36.

Koutsuris, D., Nikita, K., & Pavlopoulos, S., (2004). *Medical represented systems.* Thesaloniki, Greece: Tziolas Publications.

Koutsuris, D., Pavlopoulos, S., & Prentza, A. (2003). *Introduction into biomedical technology and analysis of medical signals.* Thesaloniki, Greece: Tziolas Publications.

Krueger, M. (1993). *Artificial reality.* New York: Addison-Wesley.

Rheingold, H. (1991). *Virtual reality.* New York: Simon & Schuster.

Thalmann, D. (n.d.). *Animating autonomous virtual humans in virtual reality.* Swiss Federal Institute of Technology, Computer Graphics Lab.

Zeimbekakis, G., (2003). Telematics applications. Athens: Modern Season Publications.

KEY TERMS

Biokinetics: A scientific division of ergo physiology for the research and recognition of physical laws, standards, and existing parameters of human movement and kinetics, or the changes from any external or internal effect that can change any physiological movement. The creation of a physical model helps researchers to understand the problems of movement and kinetics and their relation with various pathological problems.

Ergo Physiology: A division of physiology that searches physiological and physical parameters, constants, and standards for the creation of energy, power, balance, velocity, and other physical changes in the human body. This division includes a vital search for the physical and physiological laws related to various kinetics problems for humans.

Kinetics Behavior: A number of characteristics of human movement including the physical behavior of the human body in movement and kinetics. These characteristics draw a behavior model for the physical body and offer the opportunity to researchers in the area of physiology and biokinetics to search the behavior of humans and to create scientific programs for rehabilitation.

Physical Biokinetics Parameters: A number of different parameters, laws, and measurements that are recognized from a physical model from physiology and human movement. We can use this model in various applications recognizing human behavior and movement.

Rehabilitation: A scientific methodology using physical methods, especially applied movements, kinetics, and modern psychology applications, to change the human body and mind behavior, helping people to recreate their energy levels and their physical ability, or to use the near environment in the best way to live with their problems for a better life.

Simulation: A number of presentations of different parameters for things, models, or environments designed from physical standards and laws. In this virtual presentation, one can use his or her experience to have an interactive participation and use this virtual environment for personal training, education, rehabilitation, and so forth.

Virtual Human: A virtual human body in a 3-D immersive, interactive simulation, created by computer software, for the parallel presentation of reality in the virtual using any influence from the real environment.

Virtual Reality: An immersive, interactive simulation for real and unreal environments. We can also use this term for simple interactive models that cannot offer to a user any immersive presentation in a virtual environment. Virtual reality is the most useful tool in medicine today, with many applications in various fields, especially in rehabilitation, education, and so forth.

Visualization: A medicine application using a 3-D human body model that has been made from a number of different 3-D scans from a medical computed tomography.

Section IV
Virtual Learning Environments in Healthcare and Biomedicine

The application of computer technology to education is often referred to as computer-assisted learning (CAL), computer-based education (CBE), or computer-aided instruction (CAI). Computer-based learning has been developed for the beginning medical student and the experienced practitioner, for the lay person and the medical expert. This section presents examples of actual programs that are being used to support medical education for each of these categories of learners.

Chapter XI
Care2x in Medical Informatics Education

Andreas Holzinger
Medical University Graz (MUG), Austria

Harald Burgsteiner
Graz University of Applied Sciences, Austria

Helfrid Maresch
Graz University of Applied Sciences, Austria

ABSTRACT

In this chapter the authors report about their experiences in education of both students of healthcare engineering at Graz University of Applied Sciences, and students of medicine at the Medical University Graz, gained during the winter term 2004. Care2x is an open source Web-based integrated healthcare environment (IHE). It allows the integration of data, information, functions, and workflows in one environment. The system is currently consisting of four major components, which can also function independently: hospital information system (HIS), practice management (PM), a central data server (CDS) and a health exchange protocol (HXP). Although the components are under heavy development, the HIS has reached a degree of stability, where one can use it at least for educational purposes. Various groups also report the usage of enhanced versions of Care2x in real life settings. Our experiences in both—very different—student groups have been very promising. In both groups the acceptance was high and Care2x provided good insights into the principles of a hospital information system. The medical students learned the principal handling of a HIS, whereas the engineering students had the possibility to go deeper into technical details.

INTRODUCTION

In this chapter, the authors report about their experiences in the education of students of healthcare engineering (HCE) at Graz University of Applied Sciences, and students of medicine at the Medical University Graz, gained during the winter term of 2004. Care2x is an open-source Web-based integrated healthcare environment (IHE). It allows the integration of data, information, functions, and work flows in one environment. The system currently consists of four major components, which can also function independently: the hospital information system (HIS), practice management (PM), a central data server (CDS), and a health exchange protocol (HXP). Although the components are under heavy development, the HIS has reached a degree of stability so that one can use it at least for educational purposes. Various groups also report the usage of enhanced versions of Care2x in real-life settings. Our experiences with both—very different—student groups have been very promising. In both groups, the acceptance was high and Care2x provided good insights into the principles of a hospital information system. The medical students learned the principal handling of an HIS, whereas the engineering students had the possibility to go deeper into technical details.

How to prepare both medical and engineering students in the best possible way for their later work with modern HISs is a common question. Whereas students of engineering are rather enthusiastic about IT, students of medicine are skeptical in general about using it. However, HISs are not widely accepted by healthcare professionals; that is, barriers to the use of HIS are primarily sociological, cultural, and organizational rather than technological (Moore, 1996).

It seems plausible to not only give students theoretical background about the structure, func-tions, and common tasks of an HIS, but to also let them work with a fully functional HIS during lectures. This is essential, particularly if students are required to be able to work with possibly any HIS in practice after only a short period of vocational adjustment. However, it depends on many different factors regarding which HIS to choose. One of the most important is whether it is necessary to teach (with) a particular HIS of a certain vendor, for example, if this system is deployed in a network of local hospitals. Another key factor, especially for noncommercial educational institutions, is the economic impact of the introduction of a commercial HIS at the university. Third, for the education of students of medical informatics, it might also be reasonable to teach the process of developing (parts of) a bigger software engineering project. Hence, the need for an open-source system arises if one does not want to start the development of his or her own HIS. Although there are many more factors to consider in general, we chose Care2x as our primary educational HIS for the following reasons.

CARE2X

Care2x is a generic multilanguage, open-source project that implements a modern hospital information system (the Web page of Care2x is located at http://www.care2x.org/). The project was started in May 2002 with the release of the first beta version of Care2x by a nurse who was dissatisfied with the HIS in the hospital where he was working. As of today, the development team has grown to over 100 members from over 20 countries. Care2x is a Web-based HIS that is built upon other open-source projects: the Apache Web server from the Apache Foundation (http://www.apache.org/), the script language PHP (http://www.php.org/), and the re-

Figure 1. Help page describing the clinical path for starting a new surgery-operation document

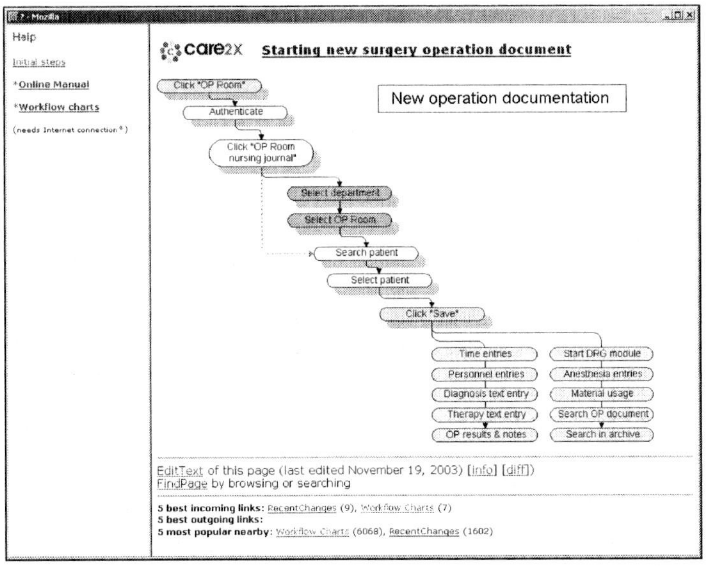

lational database-management system (RDMS) mySQL (http://www.mysql.com/). There exist several source-code branches that try to integrate the option to choose from other RDBMSs like Oracle and postgreSQL. The latter one is already supported in the current version at the time of this writing (Deployment 2.1). For our investigations, we chose the most feature-rich version that was available from the Care2x Web page in early fall of 2004. This release had the version number 2.0.2. Some minor deficiencies that we report later may already be fixed in the current version, Deployment 2.1.

Care2x is a very feature-rich HIS that is fully configurable for any clinical structure. It is built upon different modules, which include, for example, in and outpatient administration, admission, pharmacy, radiology (including DICOM [Digital Imaging and Communications in Medicine] image uploads), laboratories, ambulatories, nursing, medics, DRGs (diagnosis-related groups), and so forth. Online help is available for some clinical paths. See Figure 1 for an example.

REVERSE ENGINEERING

The reverse engineering of existing complex software packages starting at the source-code level has a higher value for practical education than a new development. Bothe (2001) argues that groups of students will rarely be able to develop a project further than to a prototype stage during a single lecture. Access to the source code is not available for most commercial HISs, which is another advantage of using Care2x as an educational system. In our first lecture, the students of HCE were asked to test all functions and paths of Care2x. They had to set up a small virtual clinic and employ doctors, nurses, and technical stuff. Finally, patients had to be admitted, attended to, and dismissed at all stations. In a second lecture in the upcoming semester, our students have the assignment to analyze a fully functional HIS at the source-code level. Since Care2x is built upon a modular structure, small teams of programmers have tasks like finding and fixing bugs in the current version, adding simple modules for special functions not included in the official version, or implementing interfaces to other existing information systems or medical equipment. In the spirit of open-source projects, reasonable additions and modifications can and should be published to the Care2x community Web page.

LESSONS LEARNED

Approximately 100 students from medicine and 25 from HCE participated (Figure 2). The whole lecture was built in the following way:

1. Theoretical foundations of HIS in traditional lectures
2. Principles of Care2x explained (HCE group's lecture was more technology orientated)
3. Familiarization with Care2x in practical sessions
4. Practical work, specific work flows
5. Applying reverse engineering (HCE group only in the second part of the lecture)
6. Examination (both theoretical and practical)

During the education, the students were faced with the following strengths and weaknesses of Care2x.

Strengths:

- Everyone can make his or her own tools
- Work does not have to be done in a strict order
- Very flexible
- Easy to handle
- Continuing design and development
- Open source
- Lots of different languages
- Bg community that takes care of Care2x
- Easy to select the different departments and stations

Figure 2. Students at work with Crae2x (We assigned groups of 2-3 students with different tasks related to the administration of a virtual hospital)

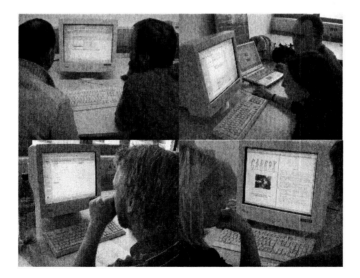

Weaknesses:

- No real standard between the modules
- Documentation is only rudimentary
- A few tools are not really easy to interpret
- Lack of security measures
- Not a state-of-the-art user interface
- There is no global list of patients from which to select one

OBSTACLES IDENTIFIED

During our lectures and trainings, there emerged several problems while using Care2x. There are a lot of small bugs that caused troubles. The biggest problem was that sometimes the browser responded with an "inactivity error" and the session would time out. Most of the time this error message was shown, the last click had not been made but one single minute ago. The next problem with the handling was that sometimes the back button on the Web browser would lead to nowhere because Care2x does not manage this. Much later, we found out that the back button of the browser is unnecessary because the program has included this function. That did not solve the problem completely: Every now and then the integrated back button of Care2x led to nowhere, too. In addition, some pages did not include the Care2x back button (inconsistency), resulting in a blank page. This required the user to restart at the very beginning and click through all the menus once again, which was boring for the students.

The general software problems that did not concern the running process were not severe. However, there is a serious problem when it is possible to admit a patient to more than one station, or when it is possible to alter a patient's record after his or her death.

A severe problem that has to be solved is that patients have to be discharged and then hospitalized again when we just want them to be transferred from the ambulatory to a station.

There are some translation errors and missing notes. For example, if a new patient record is being applied, there are red stars above some properties. Although this is an obvious sign for experienced users, it is not noted anywhere why these stars appear. The students found out that these stars show the minimum amount of

Figure 3. Example of a graphically embedded complex form, the diagnostic test order

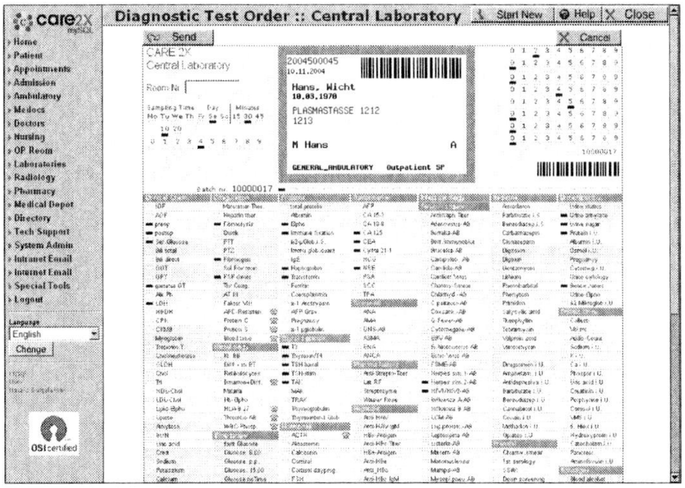

Figure 4. Nursing information about stationary occupancy for one of our virtual wards

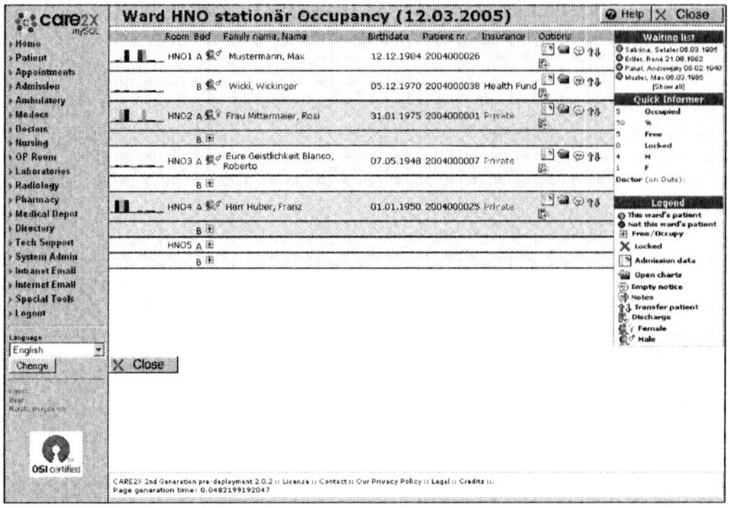

data that is required to create a patient record, but how would the students of medicine with little experience in IT know this fact?

It is also sometimes annoying that bits of information are hidden behind a link. For example, if you want to hospitalize a patient, you have to remember the social insurance number because it is not shown in the place it is needed. This is due to the fact that Care2x works with only one window. Sometimes there might just be too little space to provide all the information needed, and then the user has to write this information down or remember it; this cannot be the aim of an HIS.

CONCLUSION

Care2x is flexible open-source software. Although there are some bugs, it has the potential to become functional software to support work flows within a (real) hospital. We think the biggest problems are the documentation and the deduction of treatments. Working with Care2x as a beginner is not very comfortable,

and the software is not very intuitive. However, if one trains with Care2x, the work flows become clearer and more logical. The online help of Care2x should be better and more comprehensive. Working with the software was very fun because you really can play with a virtual hospital. Care2x is a very good possibility for training with work flows in a hospital. Further improvement of Care2x will open new areas to work with this software.

REFERENCES

Alpay, L., & Murray, P. (1998). Challenges for delivering healthcare education through telematics. *International Journal of Medical Informatics, 50*(1-3), 267-271.

Bemmel, J. H. v., & Musen, M. A. (2000). *Handbook of medical informatics*. Berlin, Germany: Springer.

Bothe, K. (2001). Reverse engineering: The challenge of large-scale real-world educational projects. *14ᵗʰ Conference on Software Engineering Education and Training* (p. 115).

Fieschi, M. (2002). Information technology is changing the way society sees health care delivery. *International Journal of Medical Informatics, 66*(1-3), 85-93.

Haux, R. (1998). Health and medical informatics education: Perspectives for the next decade. *International Journal of Medical Informatics, 50*(1-3), 7-19.

Haux, R. (2002). Health care in the information society: What should be the role of medical informatics? *Methods of Information in Medicine, 41*(1), 31-35.

Haux, R., Hasman, A., Leven, F. J., Protti, D. J., & Musen, M. A. (1997). Education and training in medical informatics. In J. Bemmel, J. V. Bemmel, & M. A. Musen (Eds.), *Handbook of medical informatics* (p. 537ff). Heidelberg, Germany: Springer.

Haux, R., & Knaup, P. (2000). Recommendations of the International Medical Informatics Association (IMIA) on education in health and medical informatics. *Methods of Information in Medicine, 39*(3), 267-277.

Hovenga, E. J. S. (2004). Globalisation of health and medical informatics education: What are the issues? *International Journal of Medical Informatics, 73*(2), 101-109.

Moore, M. B. (1996). Acceptance of information technology by health care professionals. *Symposium on Computers and the Quality of Life* (pp. 57-60).

KEY TERMS

Care2x: An open-source HIS available from http://www.care2x.org/. Care2x is a quite mature and stable product that can be used at least for educational purposes for both students of medicine and students of medical informatics. Some groups report the deployment of enhanced and adopted versions in real hospitals.

Diagnosis-Related Group (DRG): The DRG system is an inpatient classification system based on several factors: the principal diagnosis, secondary diagnosis, surgical factors, age, sex, and discharge status. Under the Medicare prospective payment system, hospitals are paid a set fee for treating patients in a single DRG category, regardless of the actual cost of care for the individual.

Digital Imaging and Communications in Medicine (DICOM): The DICOM image format is commonly used for the transfer and storage of medical images. Visit Chris Rorden's DICOM page for information about the format and free software to view and manipulate it.

Hospital Information System (HIS): It is the central medical information system in most hospitals in which most healthcare-related data (e.g., personnel, stations, patients and their medical history, etc.) are stored.

Medical Informatics: The rapidly developing scientific field that deals with biomedical information, data, and knowledge: their storage, retrieval, and optimal use for problem solving and decision making. The emergence of this new discipline has been attributed to advances in computing and communications technology, to an increasing awareness that the knowledge base of medicine is essentially unmanageable by traditional paper-based methods, and to a growing conviction that the process of informed decision making is as important to modern biomedicine as is the collection of facts on which clinical decisions or research plans are made (Shortliffe, 1995).

Open Source: The idea of sharing the source code of applications or tools for free. Other people are invited to elaborate on future extensions and improvements. Most open-source projects are committed to one of the Gnu public licenses (see http://www.gnu.org/licenses/licenses.html).

RDBMS (Relational Database Management System): A software package that manages a relational database, optimized for the rapid and flexible retrieval of data. It is also called a database engine.

Reverse Engineering: Taking apart an existing system to analyze smaller or single parts. The reduced complexity simplifies the process of enhancing or understanding its functions.

Chapter XII
An Object–Oriented Approach to Manage E–Learning Content Using Learning Objects

Andreas Holzinger
Medical University Graz (MUG), Austria

Josef Smolle
Medical University Graz (MUG), Austria

Gilbert Reibnegger
Medical University Graz (MUG), Austria

ABSTRACT

Learning objects (LO) are theoretically based on granular, reusable chunks of information. In this chapter the authors argue that LOs should consist of more than just content, that is, they should include pre-knowledge questions on the basis of the concept of the advanced organizer, of self-evaluation questions (assessment), and finally of appropriate metadata. The used metadata concept must be based on accepted standards, such as learning object metadata (LOM) and the shareable object reference model (SCORM). A best practice example of the realization of these concepts is the Virtual Medical Campus Graz (VMC-Graz), which actually is the realization of an information system to make a new curriculum digitally accessible.

INTRODUCTION

Learning objects (LOs) are theoretically based on granular, reusable chunks of information. In this article the authors argue that LOs should consist of more than just content; that is, they should include preknowledge questions on the basis of the concept of the advanced organizer, self-evaluation questions (assessment), and finally appropriate metadata. The used metadata concept must be based on accepted standards, such as learning object metadata (LOM) and the shareable object reference model (SCORM). A best-practice example of the realization of these concepts is the Virtual Medical Campus Graz (VMC-Graz), which actually is the realization of an information system to make a new curriculum digitally accessible.

We regard LOs as having a historical foundation in the object-oriented paradigm of computer science. Object orientation basically values the creation of components (called objects) that can be reused (Booch, 1994; Dahl & Nygaard, 1966).

Cisco (n.d.) defines such a learning object as "a granular, reusable chunk of information that is media independent." The term *information chunk* reaches back to Miller (1956); in his sense, a chunk is an information unit that can be perceived at one time by the individual and stored in the short-term memory (STM). Chunks are generally information units that can be individually complex and intra-individually very different (Simon, 1974).

Generally, the term *media object* is also often used, and for the purpose of e-learning, this type of object is further defined as "digital media designed and/or used for instructional purposes" (South & Monson, n.d.). Such objects range from simple text to video demonstrations and interactive simulations (Holzinger & Ebner, 2003).

According to Wiley (2001), however, the main idea of LOs is to break educational content down into small chunks so that they can be (re)used in various learning environments, in the spirit of object-oriented programming. The Learning Object Metadata Working Group of the IEEE Learning Technology Standards Committee (LTSC) refers to an LO as "any entity, digital or non-digital, which can be used, reused or referenced during technology enhanced learning" (Robson, n.d.). Some authors use other terms; for example, they speak of e-

learning objects (ELOs; e.g., Muzio, Heins, & Mundell, 2002) or reusable learning objects (RLOs; e.g., Polsani, 2003).

Within the VMC-Graz, we use LOs as a new way of considering and handling learning content. They include at least the following four characteristics (compare also with the Center for International Education of the University of Milwaukee; Beck, n.d.):

- They must be much shorter than traditional learning units, typically ranging from 2 minutes to 15 minutes (absolute maximum within the VMC-Graz is 45 minutes).
- They must be self-contained: Each learning object can be used independently.
- They must be tagged with metadata, which contain descriptive information allowing them to be easily found.
- They can be aggregated: Learning objects can be grouped into larger collections of content, including traditional course structures.

INSTRUCTIONAL DESIGN THEORY AND LEARNING OBJECTS

Instructional design theories (IDTs) describe methods of instruction and the situations in which these methods should be used. The methods can be broken into simpler component methods and are probabilistic (Reigeluth, 1999). IDT, or instructional strategies and criteria for their application, play an important role in the application of learning objects. Combination and granularity are two factors that we consider vital:

- **Combination:** Whilst the LTSC promotes international discussion around the tech-

Figure 1. A learning object within the VMC-Graz typically consists of four parts

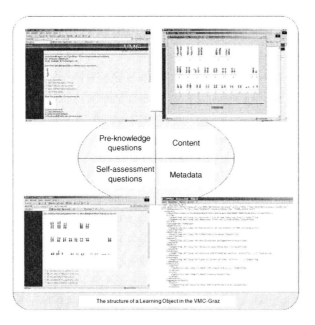

The structure of a Learning Object in the VMC-Graz

nology standards necessary to support learning-object-based instruction, and many people are talking about the financial opportunities about to come into existence, there is astonishingly little conversation concerning the instructional design implications of learning objects (Wiley, 2001).

• **Granularity:** The discussion of the problem of combining learning objects in terms of sequencing leads to another connection between learning objects and IDT. The most difficult problem facing the designers of learning objects is that of granularity (Wiley, 2001). How big should a learning object be?

The IEEE LTSC leaves room for an entire curriculum to be viewed as a single learning object, but such a large object view diminishes the possibility of learning-object reusability. Due to the fact that reusability should always

be considered as the core learning-object notion, this question must be answered cautiously. Luckily, within the VMC-Graz, this problem was relatively easy to solve due to the modular and strict logic of the curriculum.

Within the VMC-Graz, a LO can have any granularity with the maximum didactical duration of a lecture unit of 45 minutes. In any case, the produced LO must fit into this lecture unit. For example, this is in close accordance with Reigeluth's (1999) elaboration theory. Wiley (2001) synthesized this and other IDTs into a learning-object-specific instructional design theory called the learning object design and sequencing theory.

PRACTICAL APPLICATION OF LOs IN THE VMC-GRAZ

The general objective of the Virtual Medical Campus Graz (http://vmc.meduni-graz.at) is

Figure 2. The logical structure of the VMC-Graz. The atomic unit is an LO that is then assembled in lecture hours. An LO can have a maximum didactical size of one lecture hour.

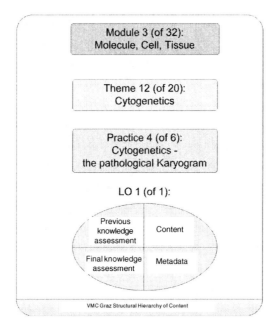

not a new learning platform, but the realization of a tailor-made information system to make the curriculum digitally accessible and to support the end users in the creation of individual work flows. Consequently, it is not aiming at providing traditional distance learning courses, but it contains accompanying material that supports the students before (e.g., prereadings), during (e.g., hands-on experiments or simulations), and after the real lectures with corresponding material. Thus, the system does not replace any lecture but supports every lecture, and the system can be used in any learning scenario.

Technically, the departmental knowledge covering the different disciplines is stored in LOs and can be accessed via teaching and learning module catalogs. The target audience of the Virtual Medical Campus Graz is about 4,500 students and 600 teachers of the medical university. This high number of users justified a custom-made system, which was specially designed and developed by using a user-centered development process (Holzinger, 2003, 2004).

The content is developed by medical domain experts in close cooperation with media specialists. The project, as such, should not be regarded in isolation, but rather as a part of the development of an e-learning strategy for the whole medical faculty. The solution of didactic problems is central to this type of software project, and multimedia is one of the many possible elements of the solution (Holzinger, 2002).

An LO within the VMC-Graz consists usually of four parts:

1. Preknowledge questions,
2. Learning material (content),
3. Self-evaluation questions, and
4. Metadata.

LOs form atomic units. These are grouped within the VMC-Graz in lecture units (45-minute lecture blocks, called lecture hours or lessons), thematic groups (topics, themes), and modules (see Figure 3 and Figure 4). An LO is technically unrestricted in the amount of data. The only limitation is didactical; that is, an LO must not exceed a maximum of 45 minutes in didactical size. The longest LO fills one lecture hour with material. However, this didactical length is determined by the lecturers themselves. They must know which material they wish to supply to the students as support for a 45-minute lecture block.

Preknowledge Questions

The preknowledge questions serve in our LOs as advance organizers that are used as frameworks for helping students to understand what is to be learned. The term advance organizer was originally used by Ausubel (1960) to describe a process of linking the upcoming unfamiliar learning material to the learners' previously acquired knowledge. Generally, advance organizers are defined as a kind of appropriately relevant and inclusive introductory material, introduced in advance of the learning material itself and used to facilitate the establishment of a meaningful set of learning (cf also with Ausubel, 1968; Corkill, Buring, & Glover, 1988; Kralm & Blanchaer, 1986).

Advance organizers are closely related to the schema model of cognitive processing. The schema theory suggests that students learn better when information is presented in an associative organization. Students build new information on information that is already mastered, thus scaffolding new knowledge on top of old. In other words, learning progresses from what is already known to what is unfamiliar, and then finally to the relationship between the two. When the prior knowledge is linked to the

new material, a connection is made cognitively and the information is processed into long-term memory (Bruning, Ronning, & Schraw, 1999).

Schema theory is a cognitive learning theory that was introduced by Bartlett (1932). Piaget (1961) described schemas as the basic building blocks of knowledge and intellectual development. Schemas are extremely interesting in the field of human-computer interaction, for example, to include knowledge structures that store concepts in human memory, including procedural knowledge of how to use concepts (Chalmers, 2003; Satzinger, 1998; Shapiro, 1999).

The Content of an LO

Taxonomy of Content

Similar to Bloom's (1956) famous taxonomy of educational objectives, Wiley (2001) also developed a taxonomy of LOs and differentiated between five learning-object types, which we also used within the VMC-Graz.

- A fundamental LO can include as content either an image (JPEG, GIF, or others; in medical education, images play an important role), a document (DOC, PDF, PPT, etc.), a movie (MPEG, AVI, etc.), or any other file, for example, a simple text entry (containing only a literature reference to a hard-copy library book).
- A combined-closed LO can contain, for example, a video with accompanying audio.
- A combined-open LO contains, for example, an (external) link to a Web page dynamically combining JPEG and QuickTime files together with extraneously supplied textual material.
- A generative-presentation LO can contain, for example, a JAVA applet.

- A generative-instructional LO may include, for example, an execute instructional transaction shell (Merrill, 1999), which both instructs and provides practice for any type of procedure.

The purpose of the taxonomy of Wiley (2001) was to differentiate between possible types of learning objects available for use in instructional design. This taxonomy is not all encompassing in that it includes only those LO types that facilitate high degrees of reusability. Types of learning objects that hamper or even prevent reusability (e.g., an entire digital textbook created in a format that prevents any of the individual media from being reused outside of the textbook context) have been purposefully excluded.

The Content

The main content contribution comes from each of the 600 teachers. Mostly, they use their available material, which encompasses written scripts (PDF, DOC), transparencies (PPT), images (GIF, JPEG, etc.), videos (AVI, MOV, etc.), and any combination of these. For the support of good content development, we provide special training courses and written tutorials, as well as a hotline and a FAQ (frequently asked question) section that is based on previous experience. We also make sure that the teachers include their preknowledge questions, self-evaluation questions, and the proper metadata.

Of course, multimedia content must be designed effectively in order to maximize the true capabilities that multimedia has for enhancing human learning (Holziner, 2002). Within the VMC-Graz, the cooperation of the domain specialists together with media experts ensures appropriate content development. This functional separation secures qualitatively high-qual-

ity content on the one hand and a professional, media-didactic, and technical realization on the other hand.

Self-Evaluation Questions

Self-evaluation methods make it possible for learners to check their progress (Bloom, Hastings, & Madaus, 1971). Due to the fact that multiple choices have been used at our medical facility for a long time, we also support all questions in a multiple-choice test style (Gathy, Denef, & Haumont, 1991; McDonald, 2002). According to Burton, Sudweeks, Merril, and Wood (n.d.), the difficulty of multiple-choice items can be controlled by changing the alternatives since the more homogeneous the alternatives, the finer the distinction the students must make in order to identify the correct answer. Normally, it takes much longer to respond to an essay test question than it does to respond to a multiple-choice test item. Consequently, students are able to answer many multiple-choice items in the time it would take to answer a single essay question. Teachers can use this feature to assess a broader sample of the course content in a shorter time. An essential point is grading because multiple-choice accelerates the reporting of test results to the student; thus, any follow-up clarification of instruction may be done before the course has proceeded much further (Burton et al., n.d.).

Metadata

Experience from other projects has generally shown that these are mostly technology driven without enough commitment to content, content management, and above all metadata strategies (Holzinger, Kleinberger, & Müller, 2001). On the one hand, it is necessary to provide all users (in our case, students and teachers) with the possibility to find relevant material quickly; on the other hand, we aim for interoperability of the learning material within an international context. Consequently, such a project can only be successful when it is fully committed to the implementation of metadata activities. It is not just a project but a strategy, which raises awareness of the possibilities of these metadata.

Correspondingly, our LOs are developed according to accepted standards for international education as a basis for worldwide networking in the form of RLOs. These LOs are stored in the repository and are arranged in lectures, themes, and modules by the VMC logic.

We consistently used the SCORM, Version 1.2. SCORM is a reference model that defines a Web-based-learning content model, which consists of a set of interrelated technical specifications. In November 1997, the U.S. Department of Defense (DoD) and the White House Office of Science and Technology Policy (OSTP) launched the Advanced Distributed Learning (ADL) initiative (ADLNet, n.d.). The metadata model of the LOM standard integrated in the SCORM supports the retrieval of learning objects in varying constellations. SCORM denominates the smallest unit that can be administered by a learning-management system (LMS) as a sharable content object (SCO). An SCO represents so-called assets, which use the SCORM run-time environment to communicate with different systems.

This SCO represents the lowest level of content granularity that can be tracked by any system. An SCO should be principally independent of the learning context and therefore be reusable in different learning situations. Moreover, several SCOs can be assembled to form learning or exercise units on a superordinate level. To make a potential reuse practicable, SCOs should be small units. They can be the basis for sharable content repositories that

facilitate their exchange. Only an LMS may launch an SCO. An SCO itself is not allowed to launch other SCOs (Dodds, n.d.).

CONCLUSION AND LESSONS LEARNED

Generally, the auspicious theoretical concept of learning objects was not easy to carry out in practice. It needs a lot of awareness rising amongst the teachers and the provision of information to realize the advantages of these new concepts. As an incentive, we always pointed out the future advantages that the successful completion of learning material would bring.

The handling of the LO editor proved to be successful, although we weakened our strict concepts (originally, teachers were forced to fill in every part), providing prefilled sections (with default settings) and allowing the postponed production of the preknowledge and self-evaluation questions (although we personally recommend strictness).

We found that most of the teachers did not like the creation of the preknowledge questions. Some even refused to provide any questions. Thus, we also had to weaken our previous concept wherein the creation of preknowledge questions was obligatory. We advocate strongly the advantages of the advance-organizer concept and provide pay-off possibilities within special VMC courses. The dislike of the preknowledge-question section is easy to explain: The teachers, mainly medical doctors, lack the exorbitant time required to construct questions that reflect exactly the content and the necessity for assessing the students' understanding of the material. However, once they had created the questions, they gained a deeper understanding of their material and of the knowledge they expected from their students. Consequently, the students benefit from this effort. Also, if the teachers get feedback about possible troubles of the students, eventually they will also get a return on their investment. However, the self-evaluation questions were regarded as useful and important by every student. The students like to see their own progress and thus are able to reflect about the content.

There is still scientific research to be carried out, including extensive research in the exchange of LOs in an international context, in measuring and benchmarking the quality of the content, and in gaining understanding of the optimal granularity of such LOs with the aim to support maximum exchangeability and usability.

REFERENCES

ADLNet. (n.d.). *Advanced distributed learning*. Retrieved from http://www.adlnet.org

Ausubel, D. P. (1960). The use of advance organizers in the learning and retention of meaningful verbal material. *Journal of Educational Psychology, 51*, 267-272.

Ausubel, D. P. (1968). *Educational psychology: A cognitive view*. New York: Holt, Rinehart & Winston.

Bartlett, F. C. (1932). *Remembering*. London: Cambridge University Press.

Beck, R. J. (n.d.). *University of Milwaukee, Center for International Education: Learning objects*. Retrieved from http://www.uwm.edu/Dept/CIE/AOP/LO_what.html

Bloom, B. S. (1956). *Taxonomy of educational objectives, handbook 1: Cognitive domain*. New York: Longmans Green.

Bloom, B. S., Hastings, J. T., & Madaus, G. F. (1971). *Handbook on formative and summative evaluation of student learning*. San Francisco: McGraw Hill.

Booch, G. (1994). *Object-oriented analysis and design with applications*. Redwood City, CA: Benjamin/Cummings.

Bruning, R. H., Ronning, R. R., & Schraw, G. J. (1999). *Cognitive psychology and instruction* (3rd ed.). Upper Saddle River, NJ: Prentice-Hall.

Burton, S. J., Sudweeks, R. R., Merrill, P. F., & Wood, B. (n.d.). *How to prepare better multiple-choice test items: Guidelines for university faculty*. Retrieved from http://testing.byu.edu/faculty/handbooks.asp

Chalmers, P. A. (2003). The role of cognitive theory in human-computer interface. *Computers in Human Behavior, 19*(5), 593-607.

Cisco. (n.d.). *E-learning glossary*. Retrieved from http://www.cisco.com/warp/public/10/wwtraining/elearning/pdf/elearn_glossary.pdf

Corkill, A. J., Bruning, R. H., & Glover, J. A. (1988). Advance organizers: Concrete versus abstract. *Journal of Educational Research, 82*, 76-81.

Dahl, O.-J., & Nygaard, K. (1966). SIMULA: An ALGOL-based simulation language. *Communications of the ACM, 9*(9), 671-678.

Dodds, P. (n.d.). *Advanced distributed learning, sharable content object reference model (SCORM): ADL version 1.3 application profile working draft 1.0, March 26, 2003, version 1.2, release 2001*. Retrieved from http://www.adlnet.org

Gathy, P., Denef, J.-F., & Haumont, S. (1991). Computer-assisted self-assessment (CASA) in histology. *Computers & Education, 17*(2), 109-116.

Holzinger, A. (2002). *Multimedia basics: Vol. 2. Learning. Cognitive fundamentals of multimedial information systems*. New Delhi, India: Laxmi.

Holzinger, A. (2003). Experiences with user centered development (UCD) for the front end of the virtual medical campus Graz. In J. A. Jacko & C. Stephanidis (Eds.), *Human-computer interaction, theory and practice* (pp. 123-127). Mahwah, NJ: Lawrence Erlbaum.

Holzinger, A. (2004). Application of rapid prototyping to the user interface development for a virtual medical campus. *IEEE Software, 21*(1), 92-99.

Holzinger, A., & Ebner, M. (2003). Interaction and usability of simulations & animations: A case study of the Flash technology. *Interact 2003*, 777-780.

Holzinger, A., Kleinberger, T., & Müller, P. (2001). Multimedia learning systems based on IEEE learning object metadata (LOM). *ED-Media World Conference on Educational Multimedia, Hypermedia and Telecommunications* (pp. 772-777).

Kralm, C., & Blanchaer, M. (1986). Using an advance organizer to improve knowledge application by medical students in computer-based clinical simulations. *Journal of Computer Based Instruction, 13*, 71-74.

McDonald, M. E. (2002). *Systematic assessment of learning outcomes: Developing multiple-choice exams*. Sudbury, MA: Jones & Bartlett.

Merrill, M. D. (1999). Instructional transaction theory (ITT): Instructional design based on knowledge objects. In C. M. Reigeluth (Ed.), *Instructional design theories and models: A new paradigm of instructional theory* (pp. 397-424). Hillsdale, NJ: Erlbaum.

Miller, G. A. (1956). The magical number seven, plus or minus two: Some limits of our capacity for processing information. *Psychological Review, 63*, 81-97.

Muzio, J. A., Heins, T., & Mundell, R. (2002). Experiences with reusable e-learning objects: From theory to practice. *The Internet and Higher Education, 5*(1), 21-34.

Piaget, J. (1961). *On the development of memory and identity*. Worchester, MA: Clark University Press.

Polsani, P. R. (2003). Use and abuse of reusable learning objects. *Journal of Digital Information, 3*(4).

Reigeluth, C. M. (1999). *Instructional design theories and models: A new paradigm of instructional theory*. Hillsdale, NJ: Erlbaum.

Robson, R. (n.d.). *IEEE learning technology standards committee (LTSC)*. Retrieved from http://ltsc.ieee.org

Satzinger, J. W. (1998). The effects of conceptual consistency on the end user's mental models of multiple applications. *Journal of End User Computing, 10*(3), 3-14.

Shapiro, A. M. (1999). The relationship between prior knowledge and interactive overviews during hypermedia-aided learning. *Journal of Educational Computing Research, 20*(2), 143-167.

Simon, H. A. (1974). How big is a chunk? *Science, 183*, 482-488.

South, J. B., & Monson, D. W. (n.d.). A university-wide system for creating, capturing, and delivering learning objects. Retrieved from http://reusability.org/read/chapters/south.doc

Wiley, D. A. (n.d.). Connecting learning objects to instructional design theory: A definition, a metaphor, and a taxonomy. *The instructional use of learning objects.* Retrieved from http://reusability.org/read/chapters/wiley.doc

Wiley, D. A. (Ed.). (2001). *Agency for Instructional Technology and the Association for Educational Communications and Technology.* New York.

KEY TERMS

Aggregated Learning Object (ALO): A combination of learning objects that can be broken down into separate parts without losing the integrity of each part.

Assessment: Any process used to systematically evaluate the knowledge level of learners.

Content Aggregation: Any process of building a new learning object from one or more existing objects or assets. For example, if a pretest reveals that students are missing some key skills or core knowledge, an instructor might locate a series of objects and link them using a common interface as a strategy for remediation.

Curriculum: A set of courses, modules, or other organized learning experiences that constitute a complete, cohesive, and coherent program of study.

Digital Asset: Any audio, animation, graphic, photograph, text, or video that may convey information, does not have a learning objective attached, and is not multimedia.

Granularity: The breadth and depth of an object's content as it relates to reusability.

Learning Object: Any digital resource that can be reused to mediate learning.

Metadata: Descriptive information and designed to help users and managers locate, organize, access, and use objects effectively.

Module: A grouping of readings, activities, tasks, and assignments that are organized around a central topic or theme. Breaking content into components supports the organization of knowledge and reduces the cognitive load of the learner. For example, a beginning algebra course includes the following modules:

Multimedia: A combination of text, graphics, audio, animation, video, and/or simulation. Typically, combinations of media can provide deeper explanations or illustrations of content than data presented in one medium.

Reusable: To be placed in different situations, environments, or locations for different purposes or functions by different end users.

Shared Content Object Reference Model (SCORM): Defines a Web-based-learning content-aggregation model and run-time environment for learning objects. The SCORM is a collection of specifications adapted from multiple sources to provide a comprehensive suite of e-learning capabilities that enable the interoperability, accessibility, and reusability of Web-based learning content.

Chapter XIII

Motivating Healthcare Students in Using ICTs

Boštjan Žvanut

College of Healthcare Izola, University of Primorska, Slovenia

ABSTRACT

Motivating and teaching healthcare students to use information and communication technologies represent a challenge. For the successful integration of healthcare and technology, there must be an investment in the organization, but particularly in its people. Motivation and a lot of practical work are mandatory for teaching informatics in healthcare. A practical knowledge of informatics is an investment for healthcare students that can improve their quality of study, work efficiency, and everyday life. In this article, four examples of connecting healthcare jobs with informatics are presented. Connecting healthcare students' work and everyday lives is an efficient way of motivating them to use information and communication technologies.

INTRODUCTION

The usage of modern information and communication technologies in healthcare became mandatory. Services and technologies like telemedicine, e-learning, medical and pharmaceutical databases, robotized tele-operating systems, computer-assisted radiology, and so forth can provide healthcare professionals with access to the latest knowledge and help them in their everyday work.

Working as a lecturer of informatics in healthcare at the College of Healthcare Izola, University of Primorska, I realized that the majority of my students, particularly the older ones, are afraid of new technologies and try to avoid them. The causes can be the following:

- Inappropriate education in information technologies
- No opportunity to do practical work with computer applications and services like the World Wide Web and e-mail
- The opinion that healthcare specialists are not computer specialists
- The belief that they are too old to learn and use information technologies

- Not knowing that the usage of information technologies in healthcare can reduce costs, increase productivity, and help healthcare professionals stay focused on their patients

The research in computer applications applied to healthcare is intensified. The proper information system at the right time can be a competitive advantage. On the other hand, inadequate information systems can be disastrous to an institution. The development and implementation of information technology into an organization is no easy matter and, particularly in healthcare, where users of these systems may be patients, the successful introduction of systems may be difficult. Often this is not because of technological problems; typically, the technologies employed are relatively mature as they have been in service for some time and have been tested in commerce or industry (Fitch, 2004). For the successful integration of healthcare and technology, we have to invest in people and the organization. As a lecturer of informatics in healthcare, I have the opportunity to teach students to use information and communication technologies. Connecting their work and everyday lives is an efficient way of motivating healthcare students to use them.

In this chapter, some practical examples of the motivation of students in learning information and communication technologies, and using them in everyday life, are described. Motivation is an internal process that creates and maintains the desire to move toward goals (http://www.psychadvantage.com/glossary.html). Our aim is to transform students into advanced users, capable to use the computer and operating system, determine a simple bug, use the Internet and so forth, and apply their knowledge of information and communication technologies in healthcare.

PRACTICAL EXAMPLES OF MOTIVATING HEALTHCARE STUDENTS TO LEARN ABOUT ICT

Example 1: Von Neuman Model of the Computer with a Screwdriver and Medical Input-Output Devices

When we have a class full of healthcare students and we try to explain to them the Von Neuman model of the computer, we soon notice that 90% of them are not interested in the topic at all. First, we must motivate them by bringing in a personal computer and a screwdriver. Physical contact with the computer and its parts reduces the fear of the computer that some students have.

Then we try to link the model of the computer to the everyday life of a healthcare professional. After we explain what input and output devices are, we present them with the monitor, mouse, printer, keyboard, and other devices specific to healthcare and medicine, such as the following:

- Electrocardiograms (ECG or EKG)
- Radiography devices
- Ultrasound devices
- Laboratory devices

Figure 1. Input-output devices that are specific to healthcare and medicine

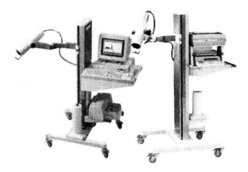

Students often have the wrong ideas about the computer. They see it as a box with a monitor, mouse, and keyboard. We must to explain them that the computer can also be a blood-pressure monitor, a pulse-meter watch, a complex laboratory device, and so forth. In this way, a student extends the term computer with more familiar terms: We make the computer more familiar to them.

Example 2: Software is a Tool that Prevents the Worst Scenarios

Teaching healthcare students to use Excel, Calc, SPSS, and similar tools can be very difficult. For instance, when they open Excel, they find several sheets, toolbars, and menus, and they usually do not know how to use these tools and cannot imagine how this application can possibly facilitate their work. My tactic is to prepare a scenario and make them realize the power of these tools. I usually prepare a table with the data of 5,000 people, including their names, surnames, personal identification numbers, sex, blood groups, birth dates, home addresses, telephone numbers, and so forth. I print the table and also save it somewhere on the server.

After that, the students must pretend there is a car accident and that in 30 minutes they need 100 blood donators with blood type AB+ who are older than 18 years. Those students who are not familiar with the computer will probably try to find the donators manually and run out of time. Then I explain to them that they are responsible for their patients and must find the right way to accomplish the task in time. In this way, we can explain to them that using tools like filters can help them find a solution and solve the problem in someone's life.

With examples like this, students realize that computer applications can solve problems faster and in an efficient way. The aim is to make

Figure 2. Searching the data by hand or with the help of a computer

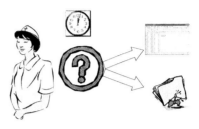

these scenarios as real as possible and motivate students to use the computer efficiently.

Example 3: The Internet and Its Services

When you explain to healthcare students the definition of the Internet, you must not start out with using terms like protocols, packets, routers, servers, gateways, DNS servers, DDNS, DHCP servers, modems, optical fibers, satellite communication, TERENA, certificates, IPSec, sources of information, and so forth. We have to keep in mind that our aim is to make healthcare students advanced users and not information and communication technology experts. Too much technical details can de-motivate them.

My aim is to explain what the Internet is, what services it offers to users, and how these services can help healthcare professionals in their jobs and private lives.

The World Wide Web, e-mail, file transfer protocol, Telnet, and so forth—all these terms must be connected with students' everyday lives. When explaining the World Wide Web, we must show to the students the possibilities that this service offers. We can start with searching pages like http://www.altavista.com, http://www.google.com, http://www.yahoo.com, and then search healthcare, nursing, pharmaceutical, and medical home pages.

Real-life scenarios must be included in the study. For instance, a patient from the USA spends the holidays in Europe and accidentally needs a doctor. After the visit, the patient asks a nurse to prepare the bill in U.S. dollars because of the formality of his or her insurance company. The nurse can immediately find the recent exchange rate and edit the bill. Another example is when a patient from South Africa uses a special medicine and you are not able to find a substitution for it in your documentation.

If we want to give our students the idea of how big the Internet is, we can explain it by telling them that Internet services are used by millions of people all over the world. We can explain that there are hundred of thousands of servers, routers, switches, and so forth. But the most effective way is to give them simple tasks. For example, with the help of the World Wide Web, we can have them do the following:

- Find the telephone numbers of three colleges of healthcare in Venezuela
- Find the picture of the lighthouse Kereon in France

- Find the address and telephone number of a friend in New Zealand
- Find what the price is of a train ticket from Budapest to Moscow
- Find the three main pharmaceutical companies in China
- Find some important Web pages and Internet portals about healthcare
- Find databases of libraries
- Find the most important healthcare conferences in Central and Eastern Europe

Students can be up to date with recent research in healthcare and medicine with the help of newsgroups in nursing (e.g., sci.med.nursing), pharmacy (e.g., sci.med.pharmacy), nutrition (e.g., sci.med.nutirtion), and informatics in medicine (e.g., sci.med.informatics). It is very important to show the students Web portals like Mediline, Web of Science, and so forth, where students can find recent publications. We can also present students with the possibilities of e-learning and include it in their study.

Figure 3. Data encryption (Žvanut, 2003)

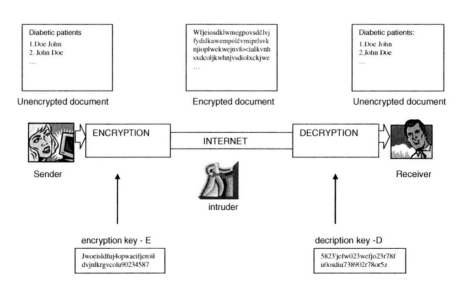

Example 4: Data Encryption

When you start to explain to students the problem of encrypting data, they often ask, "Why do I have to encrypt and decrypt the data?" Fortunately, there exists a good example for this: a list of diabetic patients that must be sent to the clinic immediately. Pharmaceutical companies would pay millions for such lists and they will do anything to find them. Sending these lists by e-mail unencrypted can be very dangerous because the companies can get them.

In this way, the principles of encryption and decryption, and public and private keys can be explained to the students. We need three personal computers—a sender, a receiver, and an intruder—a hub, a program like Network Analyzer, which runs on an intruder computer, and a list of diabetic patients. First, we send the data from the sender to the receiver unencrypted. With the help of a program like Network Analyzer, we can receive all the packets sent from the sender computer and show to the students the unencrypted data captured from the intruder computer.

Then we repeat the scenario with encrypted data and explain to the students the following:

- The sender can encrypt the data without knowing the receiver's private key.
- The intruder will spend many years decrypting the data, and the data will be certainly be unusable because the patients may all be deceased by that time.
- The receiver can easily decrypt the data with the private key.

This way, students can realize that sending unencrypted information over the Internet can be a danger for data confidentiality, and that if we want to protect the data, we must take into account the fact that intruders will do anything to access them.

CONCLUSION

An information system is made of hardware, software, data, the organization, and people. People are a very important part of every information system. As a lecturer of informatics in healthcare, I have the goal to motivate my students to use information and communication technologies by connecting healthcare with informatics and computer science. The examples in this chapter are efficient ways to motivate students and are also good chances for lecturers to learn about healthcare and medicine.

REFERENCES

Fitch, C. J. (2004). Information systems in healthcare: Mind the gap. *Proceedings of the 37th Hawaii International Conference on System Sciences,* Waikoloa, HI.

Sriæa, V., Teven, S., & Pavliæ, M. (1995). *Informacijski sistemi: Gospodarski vestnik.* Ljubljana, Slovenia: Gospodarski vjestnik.

Žvanut, B. (2003). *Informatics in healthcare.* Koper, Slovenia: Author.

KEY TERMS

Data Encryption: Scrambling data by the use of a key and a transformation technique, which protects the confidentiality of the information being transferred.

Information and Communication Technologies: The study of developing and using technology to process information and aid communication.

Motivation: Internal process that creates and maintains the desire to move toward goals.

Organization: A formal group of people with one or more shared goals.

World Wide Web: A system of Internet servers that support specially formatted documents in a language called HTML (HyperText Markup Language), which supports links to other documents as well as graphics, audio, and video files.

Von Neuman Model: The most common conceptual model of a computer, in which a computer is considered to consist of linear memory and a central processor.

Chapter XIV

The User Agent Architecture and E–Learning in Healthcare and Social Care

Konstantinos M. Siassiakos
University of Piraeus, Greece

Stefanos E. Papastefanatos
University of Piraeus, Greece

Athina A. Lazakidou
University of Piraeus, Greece

ABSTRACT

E-learning is developing rapidly worldwide. The volume of the information that e-learning systems render grows, too. Nowadays, the critical issue is to acquire more knowledge using less time and effort. Contemporary e-learning systems, although they embody up-to-date technology, artificial-intelligence techniques, and pedagogical methods, address too flat a spectrum of users. The user agents deal with this weakness. E-learning has the potential to transform learning for healthcare and social care, supporting the aims of the National Health System Plan and raising standards of care for patients and service users across healthcare and social care. The solution proposed is based upon the user-agent architecture and confronts the individual issues of the health and social sector.

INTRODUCTION

Society is entering into an era where the future essentially will be determined by people's ability to use knowledge wisely. Knowledge is a precious global resource that is the embodiment of human intellectual capital and technology. As people begin to expand their understanding of knowledge as an essential asset, they are realizing that in many ways the future is limited only by imagination and the ability to leverage the human mind. As knowledge increasingly becomes a key strategic resource, the need to develop comprehensive understanding of knowledge processes for the creation, transfer, and deployment of this unique asset is becoming critical.

The issue about the difference between knowledge and information is today the subject of much literature, discussion, planning, and some action. Moreover, the involvement of knowledge management in e-learning systems is a crucial matter: Contemporary e-learning systems increasingly take advantage of knowledge-management techniques to utilize the great volume of information that they render.

On the other hand, nowadays the academic community is addressing more and more the rise of the online community that will be instrumental in the realization of advanced learning societies. Internet online environments enable new and interesting designs for the support of traditional learning and for the development of new forms of learning. Ideally, users will be able to access all forms of knowledge in any combination, from any location at any time. This, of course, implies considerable complexity in the software design and a substantial level of intelligence across the systems: from the servers to the networks, to the user interfaces. Although e-learning environments can be used widely either for educational or for training purposes, the problem that still exists is the efficient management of content and effectiveness for users.

E-learning has the potential to transform learning for health and social care, supporting the aims of the NHS Plan and raising standards of care for patients and service users across health and social care. The solution proposed is based upon the user-agent architecture and confronts the individual issues of the health and social sector.

HEALTH AND SOCIAL SECTOR PARTIES

As the health and social sector holds great significance in society, the spectrum of the parties involved is wide and manifold. A system willing to provide knowledge to this spectrum must be flexible, accurate, effective, and direct, and at the same time it must be able to accept and elaborate information from this spectrum. Only by recording the involved parties and their specifications can an e-learning system have success.

The spectrum discussed above can be broken down into the following parties (user groups):

- Individuals
- Employers
- Managers
- Healthcare professionals
- Providers
- Organizations
- Patients and service users
- All staff

These groups have different properties that induce the specifications of an integrated e-learning environment. By developing a unified set of internal mechanisms and an interface, an e-learning environment cannot have equal success throughout the whole spectrum of users.

The answer to the problem is the appropriate formation of the learning-content structure, but also the creation of respective procedures regarding the interaction between the content and the user.

Before proceeding to the presentation of the solution proposed, it is useful to introduce the Gagne model of learning and recall (Figure 1). The model is based on the theory of information elaboration. It represents the procedure of knowledge generation within the human brain. The interaction between the environment and

Figure 1. Gagne model of learning and recall

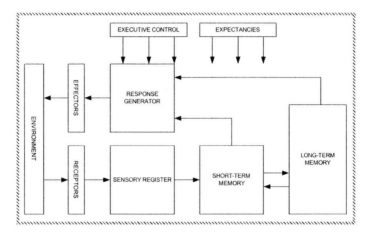

the human is performed through receptors and effectors (input and output); the data are saved in the temporary (short-term) memory, while repeating and performing save them in the long-term memory. Then, the response generator performs actions, using data from memory and controlling them by executive control and expectancies. The mechanisms of knowledge acquisition (or the learning procedure) can be managed by using the appropriate methods and tools.

The architectural model proposed (Figure 2) is a coordinated cooperation of user agents, content management, learning-objects metadata, and e-learning models. The goal of this model can be divided into the following axes.

• Categorization of the information according to the user's needs. The information will have a different hierarchy and will be sorted according to the user's personal needs. This will be achieved with metadata tags, which will categorize the content with the support of the user agents.

• Users' progress monitoring and support. The user agents will be the entrance point of the users in the e-learning environment.

The user agents will monitor the input and output data of the environment. So, they will be able to record the users' steps, interests, and needs, and also the feedback of the environment. After a period of training, the user agents will be able to propose, filter, search, and present the appropriate information to the user.

• Rapid, reliable, and accurate content restore and presentation.

• Compatibility with pedagogical and e-learning models.

Before the information is saved in the content database, the metadata assignment procedure takes place. This procedure does not identify the data directly, but assigns several property metadata tags. These tags are used by the user agents to categorize the data. Then, the data are saved in the content database along with their metadata tags.

The user agents are the users' representatives: They forward their selections, record their steps, filter information, and collect the environment's feedback. This is achieved through the elaboration of the metadata tags. The users' agents are trained, for an initial

Figure 2. Architecture of the proposed model

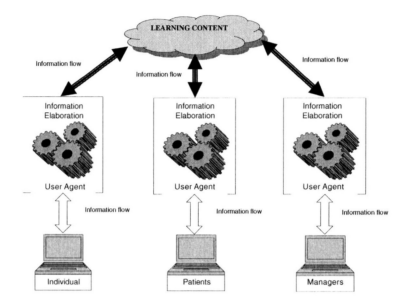

period of time, to identify the correct data by searching through their metadata tags.

After the training period, the users' agents have a complete view of their users' needs, selections, interests, and so forth. Then, they are able to work online even if the user is off line. They can perform searches, filter the results, and present them to the user when he or she connects back to the system.

According to the above, the users' agents are a part of Gagne's learning and recall model. They simulate the learning and facilitate the recall process. The technology used for the implementation of the users' agents is based on artificial neural networks and associative memories.

USER AGENTS' CUSTOMIZATION AND ADVANTAGES

The user-agent architecture has great benefits regarding the customization of the learning

mechanisms. Since the user is authorized to use the e-learning environment, a profile is created that matches his or her status. There will be a pool of profiles (templates) that will be determined and created by experts. This pool will cover the whole spectrum of health and social sector parties. Each profile will describe the party (user-group) properties (interests, needs, job descriptions and specifications, skills, etc.). The profile templates will be the basic entities of the e-learning environment. When a user creates a profile (by selecting a template and filling in the information required), a new instance of the template begins to live in the environment. The representative of the profile is the user agent. The user agent is always online, whether the user is connected to the environment or not. When the user is online, the agent monitors the user's steps and paths, filters the information flow, suggests useful information, brings similar users together, and so forth. When the user is off line, it searches for useful information, updates the user profile according to the progress made, streamlines the information flow in order to form the next e-learning course, and so forth.

There are several advantages to the sector parties. First of all, the information stored in the environment (especially by the passing of time) is categorized and starts to form knowledge. As the user proceeds to acquiring knowledge, he or she helps the other users with similar profiles to improve their learning procedure because the user agents communicate with each other, exchanging experience. Since there is feedback to the user-agent mechanisms, by the passing of time the results improve and the searches for information become more and more accurate and successful.

Another great advantage is the automation of the formation of learning courses. By streamlining and elaborating the information, the user agents are able to form a learning course that will cover a thematic unity. Moreover, the course can be reviewed and adjusted by the experts (e.g., system administrators, authors, etc.), and even be exported as a single course to a CD-ROM. Another benefit of the user agents is the transformation of information to knowledge. Knowledge is not a set of information. Although the definition of knowledge is beyond the framework of this chapter, it is widely acknowledged that the information needs to be elaborated to conduct knowledge. Such an elaboration is being performed by the user agents, producing knowledge.

DISCUSSION

As computer and communications technologies are incorporated as teaching tools, traditional materials and technologies are being adapted. Histology and pathology slides that previously required a microscope are now digitized for study on a computer. Course-management soft-

ware has become integral for both on-campus and distance learning classes due to its ability to organize syllabi, lecture materials, handouts, and assignments.

Physicians and medical students on a clinical rotation may soon be able to attend on-campus seminars or lectures from a laptop across town, across the state, or across the country. Telehealth programs designed to improve medical education for students in rural healthcare areas are developing rotations that link several community hospitals with a sponsoring medical school.

Distance learning is still in its infancy with little standardization, but most academic medical centers have or are planning some type of distance learning programs. The availability of technical support for both instructors and students is a critical issue for all technology-mediated learning.

Distance learning and telehealth are still new concepts. However, communications technologies available today (though dependent on individual systems' capacities) are able to connect healthcare professionals (with patients and other healthcare professionals) and information systems (for data and information exchange) located at distant sites. Emerging medical applications that can occur between geographically dispersed locations include initial and continuing medical education, clinical services delivery and consultation, patient education, and healthcare management and administration.

With increasing demands on physicians with regards to their knowledge base and productivity, distance learning and telehealth may provide an opportunity for busy clinicians to meet clinical responsibilities to a more dispersed and diverse population while still participating in educational activities. These teleprograms may take more time and be more expensive in the short term; however, as the technology becomes more prevalent and the number of users increases, these programs may offer an efficient alternative to meet the escalating demands of a rapidly changing healthcare environment.

CONCLUSION

E-learning is developing rapidly worldwide. The volume of the information that e-learning systems render grows, too. Nowadays, the critical issue is to acquire more knowledge in less time and effort. The chaotic volumes of information provided must be elaborated and transformed into knowledge. Contemporary e-learning systems, although they embody up-to-date technology, artificial-intelligence techniques, and pedagogical methods, address too flat a spectrum of users. The user agents deal with this weakness. Also, the wide and manifold spectrum of the health and social sector parties will definitely benefit from the architecture proposed as most e-learning systems lack this feature.

REFERENCES

Berridge, E., et al. (2000). Computer-aided learning for the education of patients and family practice professionals in the personal care of diabetes. *Comput Methods Programs Biomed., 62*(3), 191-204.

Devitt, P., Smith, J. R., & Palmer, E. (2001). Improved student learning in ophthalmology with computer-aided instruction. *Eye, 15*(5), 635-639.

Hubbs, P. R., Rindfleisch, T. C., & Godin, P. (1998). Medical information on the Internet. *JAMA, 280*, 1363.

Meyen, E. L. (2000). *Using technology to move research to practice: The online academy. Their world 2000.* New York: National Center for Learning Disabilities.

Pulido, P., & Requena, J. (2003). *PAFAMS: Panamerican Federation of Associations of Medical Schools. Alternatives in "e-learning" for health professionals in Latin America and the Caribbean.*

Rosenberg, H. (2003). The effectiveness of computer-aided, self-instructional programs in dental education: A systematic review of the literature. *J Dent Educ., 67*(5), 524-532.

Rosenberg, M. J. (2001). *E-learning: Strategies for delivering knowledge in the digital age.* McGraw-Hill.

Sakai, S., Mashita, N., Yoshimitsu, Y., Shingeno, H., Okada, K., & Matsushita, Y. (n.d.). *An efficient method of supporting interactions for an integrated distance learning system.*

Schreiber, D. A., & Berge, Z. L. (1998). *Distance training: How innovative organizations are using technology to maximize learning and meet business objectives.* San Francisco: Jossey-Bass.

Zahm, S. (2000). No question about it e-learning is here to stay: A quick history of the e-learning evolution. *E-Learning, 1*(1), 44-47.

URL REFERENCES

http://agelesslearner.com/intros/elearning.html

http://derekstockley.com.au/elearning-definition.html

http://www.brandonhall.com/public/glossary/glossary.html

http://www.emeraldinsight.com/Insight/html/
Output/Published/EmeraldFullTextArticle/Articles/0460100403003.png

http://www.iste.org/research/reports/tlcu/internet.html

http://www.ochsnerjournal.org/ochsonline/
?request=get-document&issn=1524-5012&volume=003&issue=01&page=0022

KEY TERMS

Asynchronous E-Learning: Asynchronous e-learning happens when communication between people does not occur simultaneously. Some examples of asynchronous e-learning include taking a self-paced course, exchanging e-mail messages with a mentor, and posting messages to a discussion group.

Distance Learning: Instruction provided by a human separated by place from the learner.

E-Learning: The delivery of a learning, training, or education program by electronic means. E-learning involves the use of a computer or electronic device (e.g., a mobile phone) in some way to provide training, educational, or learning material.

Learning-Content Management System (LCMS): A learning-content management system is an environment where developers can create, store, reuse, manage, and deliver learning content from a central object repository, usually a database. LCMS generally works with content that is based on a learning-object model. These systems usually have good search capabilities, allowing developers to find quickly the text or media needed to build training content.

Synchronous E-Learning: Synchronous or live e-learning means that communication occurs at the same time between individuals, and information is accessed instantly. Examples of synchronous e-learning include real-time chat, and video or audio conferencing.

User Agent: A program or device that can be used to access the Web. This includes browsers, Web robots, intelligent agents, advanced hardware, specialized software, and so on.

Chapter XV
E–Learning in Healthcare and Social Care

Maria Kalogeropoulou
National and Kapodistrian University of Athens, Greece

Maria Bastaki
National and Kapodistrian University of Athens, Greece

Polyxeni Magoulia
National and Kapodistrian University of Athens, Greece

ABSTRACT

E-learning has the potential to transform learning for healthcare and social care, supporting the aims of the NHS Plan and raising standards of care for patients and service users across health and social care. This chapter sets out a vision of healthcare and social care services in the 21ˢᵗ century, and a strategy for making it a reality. The authors present and discuss here the basic principles and benefits of e-learning for healthcare professionals, medical students, and patient education.

INTRODUCTION

E-learning is the use of interactive technologies to support and improve learning. It is not just about online courses. E-learning can include a range of technologies from CD-ROMs (compact disc read-only memory) to electronic whiteboards or online simulations. It should usually include some form of support, whether face to face or electronic, and can often be blended with classroom methods. It can offer learners and tutors many services, including access to resources, information, and advice. It can reduce the time spent on administration, and help with the planning, recording, and tracking of learning and development. An e-learning strategy is therefore really an aspect of a strategy for effective learning.

E-learning has the potential to transform learning for health and social care, supporting the aims of the NHS Plan and raising the standards of care for patients and service users across health and social care. This document sets out a vision of health- and social-care services in the 21st century and a strategy for making it a reality. The vision is of a health and social sector in which:

- Patients and service users have the information they need to be involved in their own care, and know that staff have the skills and expertise to give them the highest standards of care,
- All health- and social-care staff can access the learning opportunities and support they need to develop personally and professionally,
- Flexible learning is a central part of everyday work for everyone,
- The highest standards of professionalism are found throughout all occupations and communities,
- People share knowledge, resources, expertise, and good practice within and across their communities, and
- Resources are used effectively to provide lifelong learning and continuous development opportunities for all staff now and in the long term.

In the past, involvement in learning has been largely a matter of personal preference and opportunity, governed by the individual's own motivation, their seniority, the availability of suitable learning, and the support of colleagues and supervisors. Increasingly, factors such as the ones listed here mean that learning is becoming a central part of everyone's working life:

- The rapidly changing workplace
- A more competitive job market
- Increased emphasis on teamwork
- Informal learning
- Technology
- The need for professionalism

E-learning is increasingly widely used by learners in schools, colleges, and universities. It is also widely used in work-based learning and corporate education, and in industry and the public sector. E-learning is therefore a significant factor in the personal and professional development of the 1.2-million-plus people who work in the health sector, and the 1.4 million who work in social care. Clearly, e-learning is important when it comes to acquiring job-related knowledge and skills.

CAPABILITIES AND BENEFITS OF E-LEARNING

E-learning strategy sets out generic e-learning capabilities for the education sector. It is useful to look at how these could apply to health and social care.

- **Individualized Learning:** Meeting the needs of all staff, including those working in remote locations, in the home, or in small organizations, or whose work requires them to be mobile
- **Personalized Learning Support:** Exploring learning pathways and resources, finding the right courses and materials, and tracking work-based learning
- **Collaborative Learning:** Including collaboration between learners on work-based projects or action research (on, for example, national service frameworks), and supporting health informatics commu-

nities or health- and social-care interprofessional groups

- **Tools for Educators and Employees:** Support for innovation by customizing or creating learning resources or simulations
- **Virtual Learning Worlds:** Online master's classes and simulations, and access to virtual campuses or wider learning environments
- **Flexible Study:** On-demand learning, which people can access when and where they need it
- **Online Communities of Practice:** Bringing together specialist communities, practitioners, learners, community or voluntary workers, and service users and care givers
- **Quality at Scale:** Providing access to e-learning resources and services right across the sector, without variations in standards, that are linked to information, and HR (human-resource) and management systems

E-learning can offer huge practical benefits. The value of e-learning for all parties is clear:

- **For Individuals:** Freedom to develop, both personally and professionally, through accessible learning opportunities
- **For Employers:** Engaging staff and promoting a sense of ownership and involvement
- **For Managers:** Achieving business and performance targets
- **For Health Professionals:** Better collaboration and communication, and creating more development opportunities
- **For Providers:** Widening participation in learning, at work, in the community, and at home

- **For organizations:** Becoming partners in workforce-development functions and promoting knowledge management
- **For Patients and Service Users:** Getting individuals and communities involved in improving care outcomes
- **For all Staff:** Interlinking the technologies used for learning and for work

E-LEARNING FOR HEALTHCARE PROFESSIONALS

In recent years, as the demand for lectures without the limitations of time and place by those who have jobs and require lifelong education grows, there are more and more expectations on the implementation of distance learning systems (Sakai, Mashita, Yoshimitsu, Shingeno, Okada, & Matsushita, n.d.). There is a double source of demand for services: institutional and personal. Initially, the demand will basically arise from the public education system of health professionals and technicians. In this initial phase, recipients of information and courses will be of two kinds: technical staff of health divisions or institutions in every state, and managing, medical, and nursing staff of hospitals and ambulatories in individual states (Pulido & Requena, 2003).

Until now, professionals were required to take time away from their practices and personal lives to attend in-person training sessions. The introduction of an Internet-based training curriculum provides physicians with the flexibility and convenience of learning at their own pace and on their own time.

In-depth, efficient training for physicians enables them to deliver an even higher standard of care to patients. E-Learning provides physicians with the means to address their training needs immediately (Raz, 2002). The e-learning program will help participants assimilate the basic principles and practices of therapies, including patient selection, where the treatment should be positioned in the care continuum for diseases, and the significant symptoms of these diseases. The e-learning curriculum consists of modules, and some of them are free for physicians. The modules are interactive and include animation and streaming video, as well as exercises and review questions. In addition, participants receive a CD-ROM containing educational surgical or other kinds of videos, and audio programs on patient-physician communication. Finally, physicians have the option of communicating with e-learning faculty members.

E-LEARNING FOR MEDICAL STUDENTS

It is important to note that a lot of people believe that traditional training combined with a strong implementation process and coaching can create measurable results for students. E-learning can increase the retention of learned information by an additional 35% to 45% when blended with other training approaches and technologies.

Undergraduate medical students are a group of individuals who often have a list for knowledge along with the skills and opportunities to use information technology. Furthermore, as the doctors of the future, they will be increasingly involved with technology in their professional practice.

Past experience in developing e-learning packages for students learning tutorials has shown them to be powerful tools for learning as there are exciting opportunities for the use of images, video, and links to external sites or relevance. However, they are extremely labour intensive to set up and, unless created judi-

ciously, can lead to information overload. Furthermore, whilst they are valuable for developing learning in the cognitive domain, they are less useful for improving interpersonal skills and changing attitudes (Marshall & Kirwan, 2004).

The best balance seems to be reached by providing small-group sessions with a facilitator to consolidate the subject, and to place it within the current clinical context. Furthermore, the involvement of the students in the production of e-learning packages helps to impart a sense of ownership to the students and overcome any resistance to the use of alternative teaching methods. General Medical Council (GMC) guidance on reducing the amount of information imparted to students (GMC & Tomorrow's Doctors, 2003) must be squared with ever increasing amounts of information freely available on the Internet—human contact is vital for this.

The University of Hull's School of Nursing, Social Work, and Applied Health Studies has developed an interdisciplinary, part-time module called Facilitating E-Learning in Health and Social Care Education and Practice to provide health- and social-care professionals involved in education with the opportunity of considering how they can integrate e-learning into their practice and teaching. A major step in implementing the university's e-learning strategy within the school has been to implement a virtual learning environment: an integrated set of electronic teaching tools that are available to students and teachers online, allowing information transfer, learning-material delivery, and communication through e-mail, discussion, and chat to support student learning (Santy, 2003).

The module has the potential to attract students not only nationally, but also internationally because the module can be delivered at any time to any place with an Internet connection. E-learning can make these students more independent and lifelong learners. New technology has been transforming the way we think about education in health and social care, and the increasing use of technology in practice settings.

E-LEARNING FOR PATIENT EDUCATION

GeneEd develops new e-learning systems for patient education for major pharmaceutical clients. As the leading provider of advanced e-learning solutions for the life-science industry, it announced that it has extended its e-learning curriculum to span all subject areas, from drug discovery and molecular medicine to patient education.

The GeneEd patient-education curriculum that was announced (in addition to the over-100 therapeutic courses released over the last two quarters) represents a significant expansion of GeneEd's product line. GeneEd products are extensively used in the research, development, and sales divisions of major global pharmaceutical organizations. In combination with the soon-to-be-released regulatory and compliance curriculum, the patient-education program greatly enhances the GeneEd product portfolio to address all of the mission-critical training needs of modern life-science organizations. As the role of molecular medicine broadens its reach within pharmaceutical organizations, employees, physicians, and patients alike are required to absorb the complex scientific and medical issues this new science brings. GeneEd is the only organization providing validated e-learning across the spectrum. These techniques range from genomics and proteomics, through disease states, all the way to physician and patient education. GeneEd is utilizing its award-winning, proprietary Repurposing™ and View-

ing™ engine technology to offer compelling, intuitive, and effective e-learning to some of the most demanding users of information: everyday patients trying to better understand their diseases and the therapeutics that may help them (Patel, 2003).

Patient-education e-learning courses empower physicians, allied health professionals, and patients alike with the knowledge critical to the understanding of diseases and the therapeutic regimens used to treat them. E-learning courses are actively responding to the ever-changing training needs of the life-science industry, and the introduction of this new patient-education curriculum reiterates the strength of our science-focused curriculum design.

DISCUSSION

While there are clearly many benefits and advantages to e-learning, we also need to take into account the barriers, challenges, and disadvantages associated with it. These include high development costs, barriers to access for disadvantaged learners or those with disabilities, and the misconception that online learning is a solitary and unsupported activity. It is particularly important to address any barriers relating to potential users so that e-learning really does benefit all target groups. To gain full benefit, we will need to take steps to guard against a potential digital divide by addressing both access and skills. We also need to achieve the right balance between e-learning and traditional methods. While e-learning can make a powerful contribution to large-scale engagement in learning, as well as the tailoring of learning to individual needs, it should not and cannot replace all other approaches to learning. An e-learning strategy should be one aspect of a wider learning strategy.

CONCLUSION

E-learning is developing rapidly worldwide. Any strategy will therefore need to have an international dimension so that e-learning for the NHS can be genuinely world class. We may need to harness international knowledge and best practice, and use research to benchmark NHS e-learning against the very best globally. Furthermore, with the increasing pace of globalization, learning resources and opportunities that originate abroad will increasingly be available, and health and social care will require systems that are compatible and interoperable with those in use in other fields at home and abroad.

E-learning is not an end in itself, nor is it a marginal activity related only to online courses or distance learning. It will increasingly embrace all aspects of learning and will therefore form a fundamental part of how people will learn in 10 or 20 years. Although we cannot predict exactly which technologies or which models of learner support will be most widely used, existing examples of leading practice, whether in the United Kingdom or elsewhere in the world, provide some indications. These examples, as well as alternative scenarios, should inform the emerging e-learning strategy for health and social care.

REFERENCES

Department of Education and Skills (DfES). (2003). *Towards a unified learning strategy.*

Department of Health (DOH), Cheshire and Merseyside, Cumbria and Lancashire, and Greater Manchester WDCs. (2003). *Delivering e-learning in the NHS. Getting the blend right: A strategic approach for the north west.*

General Medical Council (GMC) & Tomorrow's Doctors. (2003). *Recommendations on undergraduate medical education.*

Marshall, R. W., & Kirwan, J. R. (2004). *Development of e-learning tutorials in rheumatology.*

Pulido, P., & Requena, J. (2003). *Alternatives in "e-learning" for health professionals in Latin American and the Caribbean.* Panamerican Federation of Associations of Medical Schools (PAFAMS).

Sakai, S., Mashita, N., Yoshimitsu, Y., Shingeno, H., Okada, K., & Matsushita, Y. (n.d.). *An efficient method of supporting interactions for an integrated distance learning system.*

URL

http://www.cmwdc.nhs.uk/elearning/elearningstrategy.pdf

http://www.dfes.gov.uk/consultations2/16/

http://www.dfes.gov.uk/elearningstrategy/

http://www.edu.gov.mb.ca/ks4/tech/wbc/wbcgloss.html

http://www.geneed.com

http://www.google.com

http://www.interstim.com

http://www.medtronic.com

http://www.nhsu.nhs.uk./webportal/learning/elearning/StrategyDocument.pdf

http://www.training.interstim.com

http://www.UniversityofHull.com

KEY TERMS

CD-ROM: High-capacity optical storage medium.

Distance Learning: Learning in which students and instructors are separated by distance or time.

E-Learning: A wide set of applications and processes including Web-based training, virtual classrooms, digital collaboration, and computer-based training.

Face to Face (F2F): Students and teachers are in the same location at the same time.

Internet-Based Learning or Training: Courses delivered via Internet technologies (these were text based before the Web).

Learning Networks: Communities of learners connected via computer networks.

Learning Objects: Course materials developed according to a standard (e.g., IMS) that allows the easy sharing of materials. Materials are modular and can be used for a variety of purposes and outputs.

Online: Connected to a computer network.

Online Community: Learners who, although separated by distance and time, share a common experience.

Online Conferencing: Communications happening over a network. They can be synchronous via chat or asynchronous via discussion groups.

Web-Based Course (WBC): Distance education course materials supported by computer-mediated communications and delivered asynchronously via the World Wide Web. Ancillary materials such as print, videos, and CD-ROMs may be required.

Chapter XVI
Potential Benefits and Challenges of Computer–Based Learning in Health

Athina A. Lazakidou
University of Piraeus, Greece

Christina Ilioudi
University of Piraeus, Greece

Andriani Daskalaki
Max Planck Institute of Molecular Genetics, Germany

ABSTRACT

Computer-based learning has been developed for the beginning medical student and the experienced practitioner, for the lay person and the medical expert. There are many advantages to online and computer-based learning when compared to traditional face-to-face courses and lectures. Information technologies are providing new opportunities for linking medical schools around the world for sharing computer-based learning materials. In this chapter, the authors present examples of actual programs that are being used to support medical education for each of these categories of learners.

INTRODUCTION

Information technology is an increasingly important tool for accessing and managing medical information: both patient-specific knowledge and more general scientific knowledge. Medical educators are aware of the need for all medical students to learn to use information technology effectively. Computers can play a direct role in the education process; students may interact with educational computer programs to acquire factual information and to learn and practice medical problem-solving techniques. In addition, practicing physicians may use computers to expand and reinforce their professional skills throughout their careers (Shortliffe & Perreault, 2001).

The application of computer technology to education is often referred to as computer-assisted learning (CAL), computer-based education (CBE), or computer-aided instruction (CAI).

Computer-based learning has been developed for the beginning medical student and the experienced practitioner, for the lay person and the medical expert. In this article, we present examples of actual programs that are being used to support medical education for each of these categories of learners.

TYPES OF COMPUTER-BASED TRAINING

There are four levels of computer-based training (CBT), each based on the application's complexity and its level of interactivity with the user (Dulworth & Carney, 1996):

- **Level I. Customized Linear Presentation:** Training similar to a standard PowerPoint overhead presentation with little interactivity
- **Level II. Instructor-Led, Nonlinear Presentation:** Training by a facilitator accompanied by navigation through the information on a computer without the use of multimedia
- **Level III. Facilitator-Led Training:** A multimedia presentation accompanied by classroom-based training
- **Level IV. Self-Paced Training:** A multimedia presentation that trainees use independently with minimal assistance (also known as stand-alone training). Individuals can train at their own pace, either at an outside lab or on their own desktop com-

puter, and complete the exam provided in the program.

Levels I, II, III, and IV are the types of computer-based training that would be most effective in addressing performance gaps among international health workers. To qualify for these levels, a computer-based training program must meet the following commonly accepted criteria (Dickelman, 1994).

- Be easy to enter and exit
- Provide a simple way to move forward and backward (i.e., from screen to screen)
- Be consistent in its key conventions
- Offer context-sensitive prompts and helps
- Provide tracking feedback (e.g., where have I been? Where am I now? How much more is there to go?)
- Offer bookmarks (i.e., quit now, resume later)
- Always offer a way out

COMPUTER-BASED TRAINING IN HEALTHCARE

In the health setting, CBT can be delivered in a preservice or in-service mode, as follows:

- **Preservice Training:** Computerized training delivered in health-education, nursing, and medical-school curricula through the use of software tutorials with or without professor facilitation, followed by examinations programmed in the computer program or given by an instructor
- **In-Service Training:** Health workers use CD-ROMs independently on their own computers for stand-alone training, meet at a computer lab where facilitator-led courses are coupled with the computer program, or attend the lab according to

their own schedules and review the materials at their own pace

Research has shown that computer training is particularly well suited to visually intensive, detail-oriented subjects, such as anatomy and kinesiology. This is because it allows text to be combined with still and moving graphics, with the display of this information controlled by the learner (Toth-Cohen, 1995). For example, computers can be particularly effective in presenting the following (Phillips, 1996):

- Subjects that are difficult to conceptualize, such as microscopic processes
- Material that is three dimensional and difficult to visualize on traditional two-dimensional media such as books or whiteboards
- Simulations of expensive or complex processes, where the mechanical details of performing the process or the impossibility of using the real equipment may hinder understanding

BENEFITS OF COMPUTER-BASED LEARNING

Students may be learning more from using their computers than from attending lectures, according to a study published in July 2004 at studentbmj.com (http://www.studentbmj.com/back_issues/0800/news/265a.html).

Research psychiatrists at the School of Medicine, University of Leeds, compared students' use of a computer-based multimedia package with lecture-based teaching on the subject of anxiety. They found that even though students felt they learned more in the lecture theatre, they gained more from using a computer package.

There are many advantages to online and computer-based learning when compared to traditional face-to-face courses and lectures. There are a few disadvantages as well.

Main Advantages of Online or Computer-Based Learning

- Class work can be scheduled around work and family.
- It reduces the travel time and travel costs for off-campus students.
- Students may have the option to select learning materials that meet their level of knowledge and interest.
- Students can study anywhere they have access to a computer and an Internet connection.
- Self-paced learning modules allow students to work at their own pace.
- There is the flexibility to join discussions on the bulletin-board threaded discussion areas at any hour, or visit with classmates and instructors remotely in chat rooms.
- Instructors and students both report that e-learning fosters more interaction among students and instructors than in large lecture courses.
- E-learning can accommodate different learning styles and facilitate learning through a variety of activities.
- It develops knowledge of the Internet and computers skills that will help learners throughout their lives and careers.
- Successfully completing online or computer-based courses builds self-knowledge and self-confidence, and encourages students to take responsibility for their learning.
- Learners can test out of or skim over materials already mastered and concentrate their efforts on mastering areas containing new information and/or skills.

Main Disadvantages of Online or Computer-Based Learning

- Learners with low motivation or bad study habits may fall behind.
- Without the routine structures of a traditional class, students may get lost or confused about course activities and deadlines.
- Students may feel isolated from the instructor and classmates.
- The instructor may not always be available when students are studying or need help.
- Slow Internet connections or older computers may make accessing course materials frustrating.
- Managing computer files and online learning software can sometimes seem complex for students with beginner-level computer skills.
- Hands-on or lab work is difficult to simulate in a virtual classroom.

THE INTERNATIONAL VIRTUAL MEDICAL SCHOOL

The International Virtual Medical School (IVIMEDS, http://www.ivimeds.org) is a major international collaboration created to meet the challenge facing medical education through innovative approaches that exploit developments in educational thinking and information and communication technologies. Currently, 37 leading medical schools located in 14 countries have committed financial and human resources, and have agreed to share learning resources to make a reality of the IVIMEDS vision.

The International Virtual Medical School provides the following:

- A comprehensive medical-education resource, the Medical Education Service, available to teachers and learners worldwide. It will provide users with educationally and technologically state-of-the-art medical-education resources and services at low cost.
- A cost-effective alternative-track curriculum for undergraduate medical students for the early years of the undergraduate program, and the right to complete the clinical stages of their training in a partner medical school.
- Customized postgraduate and continuing professional development (CPD) programs that can be taken at the time and place of choosing of the learner, thereby facilitating convenient and cost-effective lifelong learning.
- Customised medical and multiprofessional health education through the IVIMEDS Foundation appropriate to the needs and circumstances of developing countries in regard to curriculum, localization, language, and mode of delivery.

Benefits to Partner Institutions

IVIMEDS offers membership to an international network of partner institutions sharing resources to enrich individual member curriculums and to enhance the ability to deliver cost effectively high-quality medical-education programs. Benefits include the following:

- Improved finances and assets by providing the means to develop an enhanced curriculum with additional topics and approaches to learning, open access to medical training for students of different backgrounds, and a global market for home-grown educational resources and strategies.

- Rapid, effective execution of new approaches that may be beyond the budget and scope of any one institution, drawing upon a global body of expertise in subject matter, educational theory, and technology.
- Reduced risk associated with curriculum changes by sharing innovative thinking and benefiting from other schools' experiences in curriculum planning and their use of learning technologies and learning-management systems.
- Quality resources and innovative approaches to medical education, which can contribute to the creation of a curriculum that is coherent, integrated, student centered, and authentic.

Benefits to Students, Trainees, and Practicing Doctors

IVIMEDS will provide an innovative curriculum and/or curriculum elements tailored to the changing educational needs of students, trainees, and medical professionals. Benefits include the following:

- A learner-centered approach with students exposed to just-in-time learning with theory closely linked to practice.
- Adaptive learning or "just-for-you" learning catering to individual learning styles and interests.
- Curriculum frameworks provided by established learning outcomes, a broad curriculum map, and a bank of virtual patients.
- Blended learning including anytime, anywhere electronic study guides, face-to-face and online tutors, and peer-to-peer learning.
- Flexible learning based in a variety of settings (e.g., a university teaching hospital, a local health centre, or home-based

study), best suited to the financial, personal, and educational circumstances of individual students.

Benefits to Society

IVIMEDS offers an approach to medical education and training that is both adaptable and cost effective. Benefits to society include the following:

- Flexibility to expand and contract numbers of learners to meet changing circumstances.
- Wider access to medical education for students, including disadvantaged and mature students.
- Training doctors to focus on the needs of particular communities, with the potential that qualified doctors will return to work in these communities.
- Training doctors with an appropriate high level of competence in information handling and an aptitude for self-directed learning and continuing professional development.
- Cost-effective training with schools working together to blend e-learning with face-to-face learning in a variety of educational and clinical settings.

CONCLUSION

We recognize that technology impacts healthcare-education, research, and science educators in the areas of research, classroom teaching, and distance education. While the overall effect is not yet fully assessable, the presence of technology in so many different aspects of the profession makes it important to more clearly recognize and appreciate its current and potential role.

Information technologies can be educators' tools in finding creative ways that encourage students to self-test, self-question, and self-regulate learning and in helping them to create solutions to complex problems. Information technologies are providing new opportunities for linking medical schools around the world for sharing computer-based learning materials. They open a wide horizon for acquiring and expending medical knowledge originated in any part of the world without the limitations of time, space, or distance.

The use of computers and information technology in medical education should be regarded as an additional tool and must never be a goal in itself but part of flexible learning. On the contrary, clinical medical education should always be centered on direct patient contact and bedside education. While we urge for direct patient contact, we believe that using stimulations would also benefit the student in training.

REFERENCES

Dickelman, G. J. (1994). Designing and managing computer-based training for human resource development. In C. E. Schneier, C. J. Russell, R. W. Beatty, & L. S. Baird (Eds.), *The training and development sourcebook.* Amherst, MA: Human Resource Development Press.

Dulworth, M. R., & Carney, J. (1996). *Improve training with interactive multimedia: Infoline 9601.* Alexandria, VA: American Society for Training and Development.

Evans, L. A., Brown, J. F., & Heestand, D. E. (1994). Incorporating computer-based learning in a medical school environment. *Journal of Biocommunication, 21*(1), 10-17.

Henry, S. B., & Waltmire, D. (1992). Computerised clinical simulations: A strategy for staff development in critical care. *American Journal of Critical Care Nursing, 1*(2), 99-107.

Jaffe, C. C., & Lynch, P. J. (1993). Computers for clinical practice and education in radiology. *Radiographics, 13*(4), 931-937.

Johannson, S. L., & Wertenberger, D. H. (1996). Using simulation to test critical thinking skills of nursing students. *Nurse Education Today, 16,* 323-327.

Lauri, S. (1992). Using a computer simulation program to assess the decision making process in child health care. *Computers in Nursing, 10*(40), 171-177.

Lauriland, D. (1995). Multimedia and the changing experience of the learner. *The British Journal of Educational Technology, 26*(3), 179-189.

Phillips, R. (1996). *Developers guide to interactive multimedia: A methodology for educational applications.* Perth, WA: Curtin University.

Romiszowski, A. (1994). Individualization of teaching and learning: Where have we been? Where are we going? *Journal of Special Education Technology, 2,* 182-194.

Shortliffe, E. H., & Perreault, L. E. (2001). *Medical informatics: Computer applications in health care and biomedicine* (2nd ed.). New York: Springer.

Toth-Cohen, S. (1995). Computer-assisted instruction as a learning resource for applied anatomy and kinesiology in the occupational therapy curriculum. *American Journal of Occupational Therapy, 49*(8), 821-827.

FURTHER READING

http://www.asme.org.uk/

http://www.cdlhn.com

http://www.chime.ucl.ac.uk/

http://www.dso.iastate.edu/dept/asc/elearner/advantage.html

http://www.emedicine.com

http://www.health.state.mn.us/divs/hrm/dl/compbased.html

http://www.ifmsa.org/partners/wfme_he.htm

http://www.interactive-designs.com/cbl1.htm

http://www.ivimeds.org

http://www.lib.uiowa.edu/commons/cbl.html

http://www.med.cam.ac.uk/html/teaching/DepMed/Phase1/computer.html

http://www.personal.dundee.ac.uk/~cdvflore/

http://www.qaproject.org/pubs/PDFs/researchcbtx.pdf

http://www.sph.umn.edu/publichealthplanet

KEY TERMS

Computer-Aided Instruction (CAI): The application of computer technology to education (also called computer-assisted learning and computer-based education).

Computer-Assisted Learning (CAL): The application of computer technology to education (also called computer-aided instruction and computer-based education).

Computer-Based Education (CBE): The application of computer technology to education (also called computer-assisted learning and computer-aided instruction).

Multimedia Content: Information sources that encompass all common computer-based forms of information, including texts, graphics, images, video, and sound.

Simulation: A system that behaves according to a model of a process or another system; for example, a simulation of a patient's response to therapeutic interventions allows a medical or nursing student to learn which techniques are effective without risking human life.

Tutoring System: A computer program designed to provide self-directed education to a student or trainee.

Section V
Computer–Assisted Diagnosis

Digital imaging still remains one of the key technologies for progress in healthcare. With further advances in the processing, display, and communication of medical imaging, it becomes the key to solving many problems in diagnosis and therapy. As well as computer-assisted diagnosis, computer-assisted surgery relies increasingly on some type of image management. Typical examples can be found in craniofacial surgery, neurosurgery, orthopaedic surgery of the hip and spine, plastic and reconstructive surgery, otolaryngology, and so forth.

Chapter XVII
Brain Mapping in Functional Neurosurgery

George Zouridakis
University of Houston, USA

Javier Diaz
University of Houston, USA

Farhan Baluch
University of Houston, USA

ABSTRACT

Functional brain mapping is a procedure that can be used to identify cortical areas that mediate sensorimotor and higher cognitive brain functions, such as language, attention, memory, and cognition. Clinically, it is currently used for preoperative surgical planning in patients suffering from intractable epilepsy and brain tumors, and may soon have significant applications in brain injury, stroke, dementia, and developmental disorders. Functional brain mapping is also a very powerful research tool in the area of cognitive neuroscience and, lately, in psychiatry. Recent technological advances in neuroimaging techniques, the development of large sensor arrays, the use of sophisticated computer systems and superior graphics, gradually make more apparent the relevance of this technique in providing answers to complex questions about the structural and functional connectivity of the brain, and the way it represents and processes information.

INTRODUCTION

Functional neurosurgery refers to those surgical interventions that are intended to improve the function of the central or peripheral nervous system. It is usually reserved for chronic neu-rological diseases resistant to drug therapy, such as refractory epilepsy, Parkinson's disease, essential tremor, and intractable chronic pain. Ablative procedures entail the permanent disconnection of certain neural pathways, while augmentative ones make use of implantable devices that modulate the function of dysfunctional neuronal assemblies through the chronic electrical stimulation of specific neuronal pathways.

In all cases, accurate localization of the intended surgical target and of the cortical areas that are responsible for vital brain functions, such as sensation, movement, and speech, is of paramount importance because resection of such critical brain areas can have devastating results. The procedure employed is called functional brain mapping and aims at visualizing the relationship between neural structures and their function.

BACKGROUND

During the past several years, a number of noninvasive functional imaging modalities, including functional magnetic resonance imaging (fMRI; Binder, Frost, Hammeke, Cox, Rao, & Prieto, 1997), positron-emission tomography (PET; Peterson, Fox, Posner, Mintun, & Raichle, 1998), regional cerebral blood flow (rCBF; Friberg, 1993), and single-photon-emission computed tomography (SPECT; Gomez-Tortosa, Martin, Sychra, & Dujovny, 1994), have been used to map brain function with varying degrees of success. However, the most reliable approach to date still relies on direct electrical stimulation of the exposed cortex (Ojemann, Ojemann, Lettich, & Berger, 1989), a procedure that is highly invasive and unpleasant, and is performed mostly intraoperatively on an awake patient.

More recently, however, completely noninvasive procedures have been successfully used for brain mapping (Ebersole & Wade, 1990; Peterson et al., 1998; Zouridakis, Simos, Breier, & Papanicolaou, 1998). These procedures rely on the fact that the performance of certain brain functions involves only a small population of cortical neurons whose activation gives rise to electromagnetic signals that can be recorded outside the head. The electrical aspects of brain activation can be recorded in an electroencephalogram (EEG) by placing a set of electrodes on the scalp, while the corresponding magnetic aspects can be captured in a magnetoencephalogram (MEG) by placing an array of coils in close proximity to the head. Brain-mapping procedures based on the combination of high-resolution MRI and EEG or MEG recordings are known as electrical source imaging and magnetic source imaging, respectively.

In general, MEG systems are expensive as they require special cryogenic equipment, a magnetically shielded room, and daily monitoring and maintenance. They are also only available in a handful of places around the world, so the clinical usefulness of MEG is limited. On the other hand, EEG equipment is portable, does not require any special maintenance, is readily available in practically all clinical settings, and even the most sophisticated systems that incorporate dense-array sensors are at least one order of magnitude less expensive than MEG. Moreover, recent advances in hardware and the development of new mathematical tools for modeling the intracranial sources and the head make dense-array EEG (*d*EEG) a very attractive methodology because it can provide a temporal resolution of one millisecond or less and a very high spatial sampling. Therefore, brain mapping based on *d*EEG and MRI can have a significant impact on patient care. A state-of-the-art *d*EEG system (ActiveTwo, BioSemi, The Netherlands) that is available in our lab features 256 recording channels for whole head coverage at a sampling rate of 5 kHz per channel and uses active electrodes with built-in preamplifiers for noise cancellation.

Figure 1. Somatosensory (squares), language (circles), and epileptogenic (triangles) cortical areas in an epileptic patient

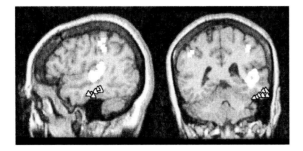

APPLICATION EXAMPLES

Medically intractable epilepsy and brain cancer are two of the most debilitating diseases that severely affect the quality of life of those suffering from the conditions, and they also have a heavy impact on the lives of those caring for, and supporting, the patients.

Refractory epilepsy is a neurological disorder characterized by recurrent seizures originating from abnormal electrical activity in the brain. Patients experience a variety of symptoms, which can recur many times in a day, including loss of consciousness and possibly a fall, rigidity, jerking motions, incontinence of urine, weakness or paralysis, and even visual and sensory hallucinations. Usually these symptoms are followed by a period of confusion and deep sleep. Recurrent seizures severely limit school achievement, employment prospects, and normal daily activities, such as driving a vehicle or operating machinery.

Brain cancer is a life-threatening disease that typically has a debilitating unremitting course until the patient eventually expires: The physical mass of the tumor is disruptive, the tumor cells cannot carry out normal cell functions, and the fast-growing cells place an extraordinary metabolic demand on the brain. Cancer-related fatigue is the most common and debilitating side effect of cancer and its treatment.

Typically, brain tumors and medically intractable epilepsy require surgical treatment, but there is a narrow therapeutic window between treatment and debilitating side effects due to surgery. Accurate preoperative brain mapping is of paramount importance because resection of functionally vital brain areas can have devastating results.

BRAIN-MAPPING PROCEDURES

Several brain functions can be studied using recordings of spontaneous neurophysiological activity and of evoked responses (Zouridakis & Iyer, 2003). The primary auditory, somatosensory, and visual cortices can be identified by analyzing responses to auditory, somatosensory, and visual stimuli, respectively. Epileptogenic brain areas can be identified by analyzing spontaneous activity containing interictal spikes, while brain areas that contribute to language function can be identified using evoked responses obtained, for example, with a task for the continuous recognition of single words presented either visually or aurally. The intracranial sources of the externally recorded responses can be modeled, for example, as a series of dipoles, whose locations can be visualized by projecting the estimated sources onto a participant's MRI.

An example of a brain map (Zouridakis & Iyer, 2003) obtained using MEG recordings is shown in Figure 1, in which the somatosensory, language, and epileptogenic cortical areas are shown as squares, circles, and triangles, respectively. Figure 2 shows an example of mapping the primary auditory cortex based on *d*EEG (Zouridakis & Iyer, 2003). Shown are the evoked responses obtained from 256 recording elec-

Figure 2. N1 component (left), surface potentials around the N1 peak (middle), and cortical areas activated (right) after auditory stimulation with tones of 1 kHz

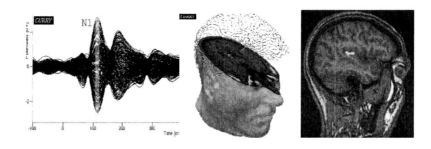

trodes and the N1 component used to fit the single-dipole model (left), the 3-D distribution of surface potentials at the N1 peak (middle), and the estimated intracranial sources (right).

After mapping, surgical treatment may consist of the implantation of a Vagus nerve stimulator or the surgical resection of the epileptogenic cortical areas. In the latter case, the functional maps estimated from the surface neurophysiological recordings can be verified intraoperatively through direct electrical stimulation of the exposed cortex to avoid postoperative deficits associated with inadvertent resection of eloquent cortex.

FUTURE TRENDS

The previous paragraphs give some examples of how functional source imaging can be used for clinical purposes. Both MEG and EEG large-array systems have received Food and Drug Administration (FDA) approval for clinical and research use, and they are gradually becoming available in many centers around the world. In particular, in the case of epilepsy surgery, the usefulness of source imaging as a noninvasive tool to preoperatively delineate the extent of a lesion (to be resected) and of the eloquent cortex (to be preserved) has already

been recognized (Papanicolaou et al., 1999; Zouridakis, Simos, Breier, et al., 1998; Zouridakis, Simos, & Papanicolaou, 1998).

A very important part of the mapping procedure is the processing of the signals that represent brain activation, namely, the ongoing EEG and the evoked potentials out of which the intracranial sources are estimated. Thus, the development of advanced mathematical tools is of paramount importance. We have recently developed procedures (Zouridakis & Iyer, 2004) that can reliably separate the scalp recordings into the neuronal activation that results from the experimental task and other activity that includes the ongoing background rhythm and artifacts. Our methodology is based on independent component analysis (ICA) and employs single-trial recordings in an iterative fashion to obtain improved estimates of the true evoked response embedded in each single trial. This procedure, termed iterative ICA (*i*ICA), was used with single-trial auditory responses obtained from normal participants to demonstrate the existence of aberrant (positive-going) N100 components that were intermixed with the expected normal (negative-going) ones (Zouridakis & Iyer, 2005b). When the same procedure was applied to recordings from schizophrenic participants, it was found that the percentage of aberrant responses was much

Figure 3. Series of expected (value 0) and aberrant (value 1) responses obtained from a normal (left) and a schizophrenic (right) participant after auditory stimulation with tones of 1 kHz

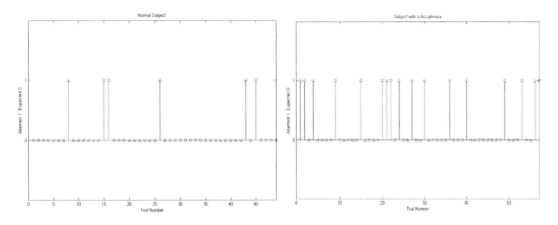

higher in the schizophrenia patients than in the normal controls (Iyer & Zouridakis, 2004; Zouridakis & Iyer, 2005a). Thus, we believe that this measure may be used as a noninvasive biological marker of schizophrenia. Figure 3 shows an example of the classification patterns obtained from typical normal controls and a schizophrenic participant.

In an effort to understand information processing and brain dynamics, and how the brain's connectivity influences its function, we are investigating the concept of functional connectivity, in which we employ descriptive measures of similarity to study the various spatiotemporal patterns of brain activation formed between spatially distinct regions of the cerebral cortex during specific tasks.

A simple example is shown in Figure 4. Single-trial responses obtained from 24 channels around the head were processed with the *i*ICA procedure mentioned earlier and averaged to produce clean evoked potentials, one from each channel, which are shown superimposed in the middle panel of Figure 4. Then, the coherence between all possible pairs of channels in a 20-millisecond sliding window was computed as a function of time, and the average

Figure 4. Spatiotemporal pattern of brain activation quantified by channel coherence. Average coherence across all channels (top), the N100-P200 complex of the auditory evoked responses recorded from 24 channels (middle), and the cortical areas that are synchronized before stimulation (bottom left) and at the N100 peak (bottom right)

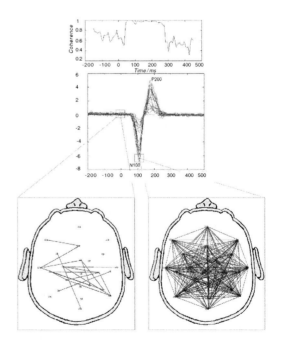

computed across all channels is shown in the top panel of Figure 4. As it can be seen, the coherence function shows very high values during the evolution of the N100-P200 complex of the evoked response, and much lower values outside this complex. The spatial extent of the functionally connected channels estimated before the onset of the stimuli (time 0) and at the N100 peak (time 100) is shown in the left and right bottom panels of Figure 4, respectively.

CONCLUSION

Functional brain mapping is a procedure that attempts to establish the relationship between brain structures and their functions. It has a wide range of potential applications as it can reliably identify cortical areas that mediate sensorimotor and higher cognitive brain functions, such as receptive and expressive language, on an individual-participant basis.

Clinically, it is currently used in the diagnosis of disease and the assessment of disease progression, and for preoperative surgical planning in functional neurosurgery, which is a rapidly advancing field that offers minimally invasive and highly effective treatment options for many difficult neurological disorders. Future clinical applications of mapping can be extended to include brain injury and stroke assessment, dementias, developmental disorders, as well as further characterization of higher cortical areas involved in attention, memory, and cognition. Functional brain mapping is also an active area of research and has rapidly developed as a powerful tool in cognitive neuroscience and, in recent years, has seen widespread application in psychiatry.

Recent technological advances in neuroimaging techniques, the development of larger sensor arrays, the use of sophisticated computer hardware and superior graphics, and the development of new mathematical tools for modeling the head and the intracranial sources underlying the externally recorded neurophysiological signals gradually make more apparent the relevance of this technique by providing answers to complex questions about the structural and functional connectivity of the brain, and the way it represents and processes information.

REFERENCES

Binder, J. R., Frost, J. A., Hammeke, T. A., Cox, R. W., Rao, S. M., & Prieto, T. (1997). Human brain areas identified by functional magnetic resonance imaging. *Journal of Neuroscience, 17*, 353-362.

Ebersole, J. S., & Wade, P. B. (1990). Spike voltage topography and equivalent dipole localization in complex partial epilepsy. *Brain Topography, 3*, 21-34.

Fender, D. H. (1991). Models of the human brain and the surrounding media: Their influence on the reliability of source localization. *Journal of Clinical Neurophysiology, 8*(4), 381-390.

Friberg, L. (1993). Brain mapping in thinking and language function. *Acta Neurochirurgia, 56*(Suppl.), 34-39.

Gomez-Tortosa, E., Martin, E. M., Sychra, J. J., & Dujovny, M. (1994). Language-activated single-photon emission tomography imaging in the evaluation of language lateralization-evidence from a case of crossed aphasia: Case report. *Neurosurgery, 35*, 515-519.

Iyer, D., & Zouridakis, G. (2004). Single-trial EP analysis improves separation of normal and schizophrenia subjects. *Proceedings of the First Joint Conference of the EEG & Clini-*

cal Neuroscience Society (ECNS) & the International Society for NeuroImaging in Psychiatry (ISNP), Irvine, CA.

Ojemann, G., Ojemann, J., Lettich, E., & Burger, M. (1989). Cortical language localization in left, dominant hemisphere: An electrical stimulation mapping investigation in 117 patients. *Journal of Neurosurgery, 71*, 316-326.

Papanicolaou, A. C., Simos, P. G., Breier, J. I., Zouridakis, G., Willmore, L. J., Wheless, J. W., et al. (1999). Magnetoencephalographic mapping of the language-specific cortex. *Journal of Neurosurgery, 90*, 85-93.

Peterson, S. E., Fox, P. T., Posner, M. I., Mintun, M., & Raichle, M. E. (1988). Positron emission tomographic studies of cortical anatomy of single-word processing. *Nature, 331*, 585-589.

Zouridakis, G., & Iyer, D. (2003). Functional brain mapping through intracranial source imaging. In J. E. Moore, Jr. & G. Zouridakis (Eds.), *Biomedical technology and devices handbook.* Boca Raton: CRC Press.

Zouridakis, G., & Iyer, D. (2004). Improved estimation of evoked potentials using an iterative independent component analysis procedure. *WSEAS Transactions on Signal Processing, Robotics and Automation, 2*(1), 288-291.

Zouridakis, G., & Iyer, D. (2005a). Phase aspects and localization analysis of the auditory N100 component. *Proceedings of the Joint Meeting of the Fifth International Conference on Bioelectromagnetism and the Fifth International Symposium on Noninvasive Functional Source Imaging within the Human Brain and Heart,* Minneapolis, MN.

Zouridakis, G., & Iyer, D. (2005b). Single-trial analysis of the auditory N100 component. *Pro-ceedings of the 27th IEEE EMBS Annual International Conference,* Shanghai, China.

Zouridakis, G., Simos, P. G., Breier, J. I., & Papanicolaou, A. C. (1998). Functional hemispheric asymmetry assessment in a visual language task using MEG. *Brain Topography, 11*, 57-65.

Zouridakis, G., Simos, P. G., & Papanicolaou, A. C. (1998). Multiple bilaterally asymmetric cortical sources account for the auditory N1m component. *Brain Topography, 10*, 183-189.

KEY TERMS

Coherence: A measure of the dependence (or similarity) of two random processes.

Correlation: A measure of the strength of the linear relationship between two random processes.

Electroencephalogram (EEG): Tracings representing the spontaneous electrical activity of the brain (brain waves).

Electroencephalography (EEG): The measurement of the electrical activity of the brain by placing electrodes on the scalp.

Epilepsy: A chronic neurological condition characterized by recurrent seizures.

Evoked Potential: Electrical potential recorded on the scalp following the presentation of a sensory stimulus.

Functional Imaging: The use of imaging techniques to localize brain areas that mediate specific sensorimotor and cognitive brain functions.

Functional Magnetic Resonance Imaging (fMRI): The use of MRI to measure the hemodynamic response related to neural activity in the brain.

Magnetoencephalography (MEG): The measurement of the magnetic activity of the brain by placing cryogenic equipment with coils close to the scalp.

Positron-Emission Tomography (PET): Measures emissions from radioactive chemicals injected into the bloodstream to produce functional images of the brain.

Chapter XVIII
ECG Diagnosis Using Decision Support Systems

Themis P. Exarchos
University of Ioannina, Greece

Costas Papaloukas
University of Ioannina, Greece

Markos G. Tsipouras
University of Ioannina, Greece

Yorgos Goletsis
University of Ioannina, Greece

Dimitrios I. Fotiadis
University of Ioannina, Greece
Biomedical Research Institute—FORTH, Greece
Michaelideion Cardiology Center, Greece

Lampros K. Michalis
Michaelideion Cardiology Center, Greece
University of Ioannina, Greece

ABSTRACT

ECG is one of the most common signals used in medical practice due to its noninvasive nature and the information it contains. Several systems and various automated approaches have been developed that use computer technology to provide ECG diagnosis. These systems detect abnormalities and other features in the ECG signal and produce a decision which helps the physician when performing diagnosis. ECG decision support systems can serve as a diagnostic tool for specific cardiac anomalies such as myocardial ischaemia and arrhythmia.

ELECTROCARDIOGRAM

The electrocardiogram (ECG) is a clinical test that records the electrical activity of the heart. ECG is used to measure the rate and regularity of heartbeats as well as the size and position of the chambers, the effects of drugs or devices used to regulate the heart, and the presence of any damage to the heart. An ECG is useful in determining whether a person suffers from a heart disease. If a person has chest pain or palpitations, an ECG will determine if the heart is beating normally. If a person is under medications that affect the heart or if the patient is on a pacemaker, an ECG can provide information on the immediate effects of changes in activity or medication levels. An ECG may be included as part of a routine examination in patients over 40 years old.

ECG ANALYSIS

Automated ECG analysis consists of a series of procedures that can be utilized in order to produce useful clinical information to help the physician to reach a diagnosis concerning the pathophysiological condition of the patient's heart faster and safer. ECG analysis consists of four stages: (a) signal acquisition, (b) processing, (c) feature extraction, and (d) diagnosis. Signal acquisition should fulfill certain specifications concerning the sampling frequency (100Hz to 1 KHz), the resolution (number of bits for each sample, 6 to 16), and the sensitivity, which expresses the signal's amplitude range (usually 5 mV or 6 mV). The digital ECG signal is then processed and filtered to suppress noise and enhance the relevant ECG characteristics.

In the feature-extraction stage, all the relevant ECG characteristics are recognized and some of their features are computed. The extracted features vary from simple ones like the duration and amplitude to the more complex like slopes, intervals, frequencies, or other discriminating indices. These are used in the diagnosis stage since the values of certain features are indicators of the existence of an underlying disease. Apparently, the measurement accuracy (Acc) is vital at this stage, and computerized methods are used to address it efficiently.

The last stage in the ECG analysis is the diagnosis, where explicit medical knowledge is utilized. Collaboration with medical experts is necessary, and the individual characteristics of each patient complicate the decision-making task. Various automated approaches have been proposed. These systems detect the abnormalities in the ECG and some of them can also produce interpretations for the decisions made. ECG analysis can help diagnose specific cardiac anomalies such as myocardial ischaemia and arrhythmia.

MYOCARDIAL ISCHAEMIA DIAGNOSIS

Myocardial ischaemia is the condition in which oxygen deprivation to the heart muscle is accompanied by the inadequate removal of metabolites due to reduced blood flow or perfusion. This reduced blood supply to the myocardium causes alterations in the ECG signal, such as deviations in the ST segment and changes in the T wave (Goldman, 1982). The detection and assessment of those alterations in long-duration ECGs is a simple and noninvasive method to diagnose ischaemia. In Figure 1, some of the typical ECG features employed for the diagnosis of myocardial ischaemia are shown.

Myocardial-ischaemia diagnosis using the ECG signal can be described as a sequence of two tasks: ischaemic beat detection and ischaemic episode definition. The first is related to the classification of beats as normal or ischaemic. Several techniques have been pro-

Figure 1. Typical ECG features extracted for myocardial-ischaemia diagnosis: (a) ST-segment deviation, (b) ST-segment slope, (c) ST-segment area, and (d) T-wave amplitude

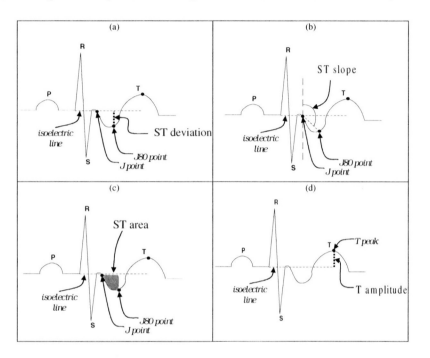

posed for ischaemic beat classification, which evaluate the ST-segment changes and the T-wave alterations using different methodological approaches. More specifically, they use parametric modeling (Papaloukas, Fotiadis, Likas, & Michalis, 2002a; Pitas, Strintzis, Grippas, & Xerostylides, 1983), wavelet theory (Senhadji, Carrault, Bellanger, & Passariello, 1995), a set of rules (Papaloukas, Fotiadis, Liavas, Likas, & Michalis, 2001; Papaloukas, Fotiadis, Likas, Stroumbis, & Michalis, 2002), artificial neural networks (Maglaveras, Stamkopoulos, Pappas, & Strintzis, 1998; Papadimitriou, Mavroudi, Vladutu, & Bezerianos, 2001; Papaloukas, Fotiadis, Likas, & Michalis, 2002b; Stamkopoulos, Diamantaras, Maglaveras, & Stintzis, 1998), multicriteria decision analysis (Goletsis, Papaloukas, Fotiadis, Likas, & Michalis, 2003), genetic algorithms (Goletsis, Papaloukas, Fotiadis, Likas, &

Michalis, 2004), and classification using association rules (Exarchos, Papaloukas, Fotiadis, & Michalis, in press).

Cardiac beat detection and classification is a key process in the definition of the ischaemic episodes in the ECG signal. The accuracy of the beat classification influences ischaemic episode definition, in which sequences of ischaemic beats need to be identified. Various methods have been proposed for ischaemic episode detection based on a set of rules (Papaloukas, Fotiadis, Liavas, et al., 2001; Silipo, Taddei, & Marchesi, 1994), artificial neural networks (Papadimitriou et al., 2001; Papaloukas, Fotiadis, Likas, & Michalis, 2002b; Silipo & Marchesi, 1998), fuzzy logic (Vila, Presedo, Delgado, Barro, Ruiz, & Palacios, 1997), and other signal-analysis techniques (Jager, Mark, Moody, & Divjak, 1992; Lemire, Pharand, Rajaonah, Dube, & LeBlanc, 2000;

Taddei, Costantino, Silipo, Edmin, & Marchesi, 1995).

The most common techniques for the beat-classification problem are neural- and rule-based approaches. Neural-based approaches have resulted in high performance but exhibit an important drawback due to their inability to provide explanations for the classification decisions. Rule-based approaches exhibit the highly desirable feature of interpreting the decisions, but their performance is not equally satisfactory in terms of accuracy.

A recent knowledge-based system analyzes the ECG signal using a four-stage algorithm (Papaloukas, Fotiadis, Liavas, et al., 2001). The four stages correspond to noise handling and ECG feature extraction, beat classification, window classification, and the identification of ischaemic episode duration. In the first stage, the preprocessing of the ECG recording is performed to achieve noise removal and the extraction of the signal features to be used for beat characterization. In the second stage, each beat is classified as normal, abnormal (ischaemic), or artefact. This information is used in the third stage (the window-characterization stage), where each 30-second ECG window is classified as ischaemic or not. In the fourth stage, the identification of start and end points of each ischaemic episode is performed. The above system is used to detect the overall episodes of ischaemia, but to distinguish also the ST episodes from the T episodes (Papaloukas, Fotiadis, Likas, Stroumbis, et al., 2002). The latter is of great clinical importance since the prognosis of ischaemic episodes with ST-segment changes is worse than those with T-wave alterations only.

Another methodology, which is based on ANNs, has been developed for the detection of ischaemic episodes in long-duration ECG recordings (Papaloukas, Fotiadis, Likas, & Michalis, 2002b). The raw ECG signal contain-ing the ST segment and the T wave of each beat is the input to the beat-classification system, and the output is the classification of the beat. The input to the network is produced using principal component analysis to reduce dimensionality. The network performance in beat classification was tested on a subset of the European Society of Cardiology ST-T Database (*European ST-T Database Directory*, 1991), providing 90% sensitivity (Se) and 90% specificity (Sp). The neural beat classifier is integrated in a four-stage procedure for ischaemic episode detection.

Another technique employs a similar approach as fuzzy logic, multicriteria decision analysis, for ischaemic beat recognition (Goletsis et al., 2003). It deals with assigning objects, namely the cardiac beats, into predefined categories. In order to characterize each beat as ischaemic or not, the beat is compared to already assigned category prototypes. Similarity between each beat and the prototype is computed, and each beat is assigned to the category to which the most similar prototype belongs. The fuzzy pairwise comparison is made for a number of criteria that employ the ST-segment deviation and slope, the T-wave amplitude and polarity, and the patient's age. For each criterion, two parameters are estimated, the similarity and the dissimilarity, while the comparison outcome is aggregated into an indifference index with the use of criterion weights. All the parameters of the method, thresholds and weights, were adjusted using medical experience. A more recent approach uses genetic algorithms for the automatic calculation of the thresholds and the weights (Goletsis et al., 2004).

The latest developed approach for ECG beat classification employs data-mining techniques and especially algorithms that use association rules for the classification (Exarchos et al., in press). A methodology based on a three-

Table 1. Comparison of the performance of several methods for myocardial-Ischaemia diagnosis

Method	Se^1 (%)	Sp^2 (%)	Acc^3 (%)
ANN & parametric modelling (Papaloukas et. al., 2002)	81	84	
Rule-based (Papaloukas et. al., 2001)	70	63	
Feed forward ANN and nonlinear principal components analysis (Stamkopoulos et. al., 1998).	79	75	
Bidirectional associative memories ANN (Maglaveras et. al.,1998)			56
ANN (Classification partitioning-Self organising map) (Papadimitriou et. al., 2001)			74
ANN (Classification partitioning-Self organising map & radial basis function) (Papadimitriou et. al., 2001)			77
ANN (Classification partitioning-Self organising map & support vector machine) (Papadimitriou et. al., 2001)			80
ANN & principal components analysis (Papaloukas et. al., 2002a)	90	90	
Multicriteria decision analysis (Goletsis et. al., 2003)	90	89	
Genetic algorithms & multicriteria decision analysis (Goletsis et. al., 2004)	91	91	
Association rule mining (Exarchos et. al., 2005)	87	93	90

[1]*Se: Sensitivity*
[2]*Sp: Specificity*
[3]*Acc: Accuracy*

stage schema was developed. The three stages correspond to noise handling and ECG feature extraction, feature discretization, rule mining, and beat classification. In the first stage, the preprocessing of the ECG recording is performed to achieve noise removal and the extraction of the signal features that are used for beat characterization. In the second stage, every continuous valued feature is discretized (it is transformed to categorical) in order to be utilized in the next stage. In the third stage, association-rule mining algorithms are applied to generate association rules, which are used to establish the beat-classification model. The methodology was evaluated using data from the European Society of Cardiology ST-T Database, and the obtained sensitivity and specificity were 87% and 93%, respectively.

Other approaches for beat classification are based on the combination of an auto-associative, nonlinear ANN and a radial basis function ANN (Stamkopoulos et al., 1998), ANNs and

parametric modeling (Papaloukas, Fotiadis, Likas, & Michalis, 2002a), bidirectional associative memories (Maglaveras et al., 1998), and the Kohonen self-organizing map algorithm combined with radial basis functions or support vector machines (Papadimitriou et al., 2001).

In order to evaluate the performance of automated systems for myocardial-ischaemia diagnosis, a standard reference database has been developed: the European Society of Cardiology ST-T Database (*European ST-T Database Directory*, 1991).

In Table 1, we can see the performance of several systems designed for beat classification.

ARRHYTHMIA DIAGNOSIS

Arrhythmia can be defined as either an irregular single heartbeat (arrhythmic beat), or as an irregular group of heartbeats (arrhythmic episode). Arrhythmias can affect the heart rate, causing irregular rhythms, such as slow or fast heartbeat. Arrhythmias can take place in a healthy heart and be of minimal consequence (e.g., respiratory sinus arrhythmia, which is a natural periodic variation in heart rate, corresponding to respiratory activity), but they may also indicate a serious problem that may lead to stroke or sudden cardiac death (Sandoe & Sigurd, 1991).

Several researchers have addressed the problem of the automatic detection and classification of cardiac rhythms. Some techniques are based on the detection of a single arrhythmia type and its discrimination from normal sinus rhythm, or the discrimination between two different types of arrhythmia utilizing time-domain analysis (Throne, Jenkins, & DiCarlo, 1991), the sequential hypothesis-testing algorithm (Thakor, Zhu, & Pan, 1990), threshold-crossing intervals (Clayton, Murray, & Campbell, 1993), artificial neural networks (Clayton, Murray, & Campbell, 1994; Yang, Device, & Macarlane, 1994), time-frequency analysis (Afonso & Tompkins, 1995; Tsipouras & Fotiadis, 2004), fuzzy adaptive resonance theory mapping (Ham & Han, 1996), and the sequential detection algorithm (Chen, Clarkson, & Fan, 1996). Another category of methods for arrhythmia detection and classification is based on the detection of different heart rhythms and their classification in two or three arrhythmia types, and the normal sinus rhythm. Techniques belonging to this category include multiway sequential-hypothesis testing (Thakor, Natarajan, & Tomaselli, 1994), wavelet analysis (Khadra, Al-Fahoum, & Al-Nashash, 1997), artificial neural networks (Minami, Nakajima, & Toyoshima, 1999), complexity measure (Zhang, Zhu, Thakor, & Wang, 1999), multifractal analysis (Wang, Zhu, Thakor, & Xu, 2001), wavelet analysis combined with radial basis function neural networks (Al-Fahoum & Howitt, 1999), and nonlinear dy-

namical modeling (Owis, Abou-Zied, Youssef, & Kadah, 2002). It is noticeable that all methods address the detection of only a few types of arrhythmia (atrial tachycardia, ventricular tachycardia, atrial fibrillation, and ventricular fibrillation). ECG beat-by-beat classification is another field of interest, where each beat is classified into several different rhythm types utilizing artificial neural networks (Dokur & Olmez, 2001), fuzzy neural networks (Osowski & Linh, 2001), the "mixture of experts approach" (Hu, Palreddy, & Tompkins, 1997), hermite functions combined with self-organizing maps (Lagerholm, Peterson, Braccini, Ebendrandt, & Sornmo, 2000), and time-frequency analysis combined with knowledge-based systems (Tsipouras, Fotiadis, & Sideris, 2002). These methods classify more arrhythmic beat types, but they focus on single-beat classification and not arrhythmic episode detection.

Most of the studies are based on the analysis of the ECG signal. In these methods, ECG features are extracted and used for the detection and/or classification of arrhythmias. However, the presence of noise makes feature extraction difficult and in some cases impossible. Also, most of the methods are time consuming and ineffective for real-time analysis. An alternative would be to use only the RR-interval signal. In this case, it is expected that certain types of arrhythmias can be detected and classified.

A recent work for an arrhythmia-detection method based on time and time-frequency analysis (Tsipouras & Fotiadis, 2004) utilizes only the RR-interval signal and heart-rate features. Initially, the RR-interval duration signal is extracted from ECG recordings and segmented into small intervals. The analysis is based on both time and time-frequency features. Time-domain measurements are extracted and several combinations between the obtained fea-

Table 2. Comparison of several research attempts for arrhythmic beat classification

Method	Signal	Dataset					Acc[1] (%)
Feature extraction: cumulants of the second, third and fourth order Classification: fuzzy hybrid neural network (Osowski, & Linh, 2001)	ECG	7,185 beats from MIT-BIH 4,035 training – 3,150 testing	N : 2,250 L : 1,200 R : 1,000	A : 658 V : 1,500 I : 472 E : 105			96.06%
Feature extraction: discrete wavelet transform Classification: intersecting Spheres network (Dokur, & Olmez, 2001)	ECG	3,000 beats from MIT-BIH N, L, R, P, p, a, E, V, F, f: 300 from each category 1,500 training – 1,500 testing					95.7%
Feature extraction: PCA in 29 points from QRS, instantaneous and average RR-interval, QRS complex width Classification: mixture of experts (SOM, LVQ) (Hu et. al., 1997).	ECG	25 min from each record in MIT-BIH 200 series excluding records 212, 217, 220, 222 and 232 N : 43897	V : 5363				95.52%
Feature extraction: hermite functions, RR-interval Clustering: self organizing maps (Lagerholm et. al., 2000)	ECG	108,963 beats from MIT-BIH N : 74053 L : 8074 R : 7259 A : 2544 a : 150 J : 83 S : 2 V : 7129	F : 803 b : 472 e : 16 j : 229 E : 106 P : 7028 f : 982 Q : 33				98.49%
Feature extraction: RR-interval Classification: knowledge-based system (Tsipouras et. al., 2002)	RR-interval signal	30,000 beats from MIT-BIH N, P, f, p, Q, L, R : 25,188 A, a, J, S : 1,213	V, F : 2,950 e,j,n,E : 265 [, !,] : 384				95.85%
Feature extraction: RR-interval Classification: knowledge-based system (Tsipouras et. al., 2005)	RR-interval signal	93,349 beats from MIT-BIH N, P, f, p, L, R, Q : 86,262 [, !,] : 484	V : 6,183 BII : 420				98.20%
		109,880 beats from MIT-BIH N, P, f, p, L, R, Q : 102,793 [, !,] : 484	V : 6,183 BII : 420				94.26%

[1]*Acc: Accuracy*

tures are used to train a set of neural networks. Short-time Fourier transform, and several time-frequency distributions are used in the time-frequency analysis. The final decision is made using a set of rules. The proposed approach is tested using the *MIT-BIH Arrhythmia Database* (Harvard-MIT Division of Health Sciences and Technology, 1997), and satisfactory results are obtained for both sensitivity and specificity for arrhythmic segment detection (87.5% and 89.5% respectively for time-domain analysis, and 90% and 93% respectively for time-frequency-domain analysis).

Another approach for arrhythmic beat classification and arrhythmic episode detection and classification (Tsipouras, Fotiadis, & Sideris, in press) is also based only on the RR-interval signal. A three RR-interval sliding window is used in the arrhythmic beat classification algorithm. Classification is performed for four categories of beats: normal, premature ventricular contractions, ventricular flutter and fibrillation, and 2° heart block. The beat classification is used as the input of a knowledge-based, deterministic automaton to achieve arrhythmic episode detection and classification. Six rhythm types are classified: ventricular bigeminy, ventricular trigeminy, ventricular couplet, ventricular tachycardia, ventricular flutter and fibrillation, and 2° heart block. The achieved scores for the *MIT-BIH Arrhythmia Database* indicate high performance: 98% accuracy for arrhythmic beat classification and 94% accuracy for arrhythmic episode detection and classification.

In Table 2, several systems and methodologies that address the problem of arrhythmic beat classification are presented.

CONCLUSION

We presented a general review of ECG diagnosis using decision-support systems. Computerized ECG processing can be divided into several stages. The most important ones are the analysis and the diagnosis. The variety of the systems developed in order to address the automation of these two tasks shows the great interest for this scientific area and its clinical importance. The developed methods differ in terms of accuracy, but each one of them has unique advantages. A proper combination of the above techniques can improve the results of ECG analysis and diagnosis. The physician, however, remains responsible to evaluate the systems' output and make the final diagnosis.

REFERENCES

Afonso, V. X., & Tompkins, W. J. (1995). Detecting ventricular fibrillation. *IEEE Engineering in Medicine and Biology, 14*, 152-159.

Al-Fahoum, A. S., & Howitt, I. (1999). Combined wavelet transformation and radial basis neural networks for classifying life-threatening cardiac arrhythmias. *Medical & Biological Engineering and Computing, 37*, 566-573.

Chen, S. W., Clarkson, P. M., & Fan, Q. (1996). A robust sequential detection algorithm for cardiac arrhythmia classification. *IEEE Transactions on Biomedical Engineering, 43*, 1120-1125.

Clayton, R. H., Murray, A., & Campbell, R. W. F. (1993). Comparison of four techniques for recognition of ventricular fibrillation of the surface ECG. *Medical & Biological Engineering and Computing, 31*, 111-117.

Clayton, R. H., Murray, A., & Campbell, R. W. F. (1994). Recognition of ventricular fibrillation using neural networks. *Medical & Biological Engineering and Computing, 32*, 217-220.

Dokur, Z., & Olmez, T. (2001). ECG beat classification by a hybrid neural network. *Computer Methods and Programs in Biomedicine, 66*, 167-181.

European Society of Cardiology. (1991). *European ST-T database directory*. Pisa: S.T.A.R.

Exarchos, T. P., Papaloukas, C., Fotiadis, D. I., & Michalis, L. K. (in press). An association rule mining based methodology for automatic diagnosis of myocardial ischemia using ECGs. *IEEE Transactions on Biomedical Engineering*.

Goldman, M. J. (1982). *Principles of clinical electrocardiography* (11th ed.). Los Altos, CA: LANGE Medical Publications.

Goletsis, Y., Papaloukas, C., Fotiadis, D. I., Likas, A., & Michalis, L. K. (2003). A multicriteria decision based approach for ischemia detection in long duration ECGs. *Proceedings of IEEE EMBS Fourth International Conference of Information Technology and Applications in Biomedicine (ITAB 2003)* (pp. 230-233).

Goletsis, Y., Papaloukas, C., Fotiadis, D. I., Likas, A., & Michalis, L. K. (2004). Automatic ischemic beat classification using genetic algorithms and multicriteria decision analysis. *IEEE Transactions on Biomedical Engineering, 51*, 1717- 1725.

Ham, F. M., & Han, S. (1996). Classification of cardiac arrhythmias using fuzzy ARTMAP. *IEEE Transactions on Biomedical Engineering, 43*, 425-430.

Hu, Y. Z., Palreddy, S., & Tompkins, W. J. (1997). A patient-adaptable ECG beat classifier using a mixture of experts approach. *IEEE Transactions on Biomedical Engineering, 44*, 891-900.

Jager, F., Mark, R. G., Moody, G. B., & Divjak, S. (1992). Analysis of transient ST segment changes during ambulatory monitoring using the Karhunen-Loève transform. *Proceedings of the IEEE Computers in Cardiology* (pp. 691-694).

Khadra, L., Al-Fahoum, A. S., & Al-Nashash, H. (1997). Detection of life-threatening cardiac arrhythmias using wavelet transformation. *Medical & Biological Engineering and Computing, 35*, 626-632.

Lagerholm, M., Peterson, C., Braccini, G., Ebendrandt, L., & Sornmo, L. (2000). Clustering ECG complexes using hermite functions and self-organizing maps. *IEEE Transactions on Biomedical Engineering, 47*, 838-848.

Lemire, D., Pharand, C., Rajaonah, J.-C., Dube, B., & LeBlanc, A. R. (2000). Wavelet time entropy, T wave morphology and myocardial ischemia. *IEEE Transactions on Biomedical Engineering, 47*, 967-970.

Maglaveras, N., Stamkopoulos, T., Pappas, C., & Strintzis, M. (1998). ECG processing techniques based on neural networks and bidirectional associative memories. *Journal of Medical Engineering in Technology, 22*, 106-111.

Minami, K., Nakajima, H., & Toyoshima, T. (1999). Real-time discrimination of ventricular tachyarrhythmia with Fourier-transform neural network. *IEEE Transactions on Biomedical Engineering, 46*, 179-185.

Harvard-MIT Division of Health Sciences and Technology. (1997). *MIT-BIH arrhythmia database* (3rd ed.) [CD-ROM]. Cambridge, MA.

Osowski, S., & Linh, T. H. (2001). ECG beat recognition using fuzzy hybrid neural network. *IEEE Transactions on Biomedical Engineering, 48*, 1265-1271.

Owis, M. I., Abou-Zied, A. H., Youssef, A. M., & Kadah, Y. M. (2002). Study of features based on nonlinear dynamical modelling in ECG arrhythmia detection and classification. *IEEE Transactions on Biomedical Engineering, 49*, 733-736.

Papadimitriou, S., Mavroudi, S., Vladutu, L., & Bezerianos, A. (2001). Ischemia detection with a self-organizing map supplemented by supervised learning. *IEEE Transactions on Neural Networks, 12*, 503-515.

Papaloukas, C., Fotiadis, D. I., Liavas, A. P., Likas, A., & Michalis, L. K. (2001). A knowledge-based technique for automated detection of ischemic episodes in long duration electrocardiograms. *Medical and Biological Engineering and Computing, 39,* 105-112.

Papaloukas, C., Fotiadis, D. I., Likas, A., & Michalis, L. K. (2002a). An expert system for ischemia detection based on parametric modeling and artificial neural networks. *Proceedings of the European Medical Biological Engineering Conference* (pp. 742-743).

Papaloukas, C., Fotiadis, D. I., Likas, A., & Michalis, L. K. (2002b). An ischemia detection method based on artificial neural networks. *Artificial Intelligence in Medicine, 24,* 167-178.

Papaloukas, C., Fotiadis, D. I., Likas, A., Stroumbis, C. S., & Michalis, L. K. (2002). Use of a novel rule-based expert system in the detection of changes in the ST segment and the T wave in long duration ECGs. *Journal of Electrocardiology, 35,* 27-34.

Pitas, I., Strintzis, M. G., Grippas, S., & Xerostylides, C. (1983). *Machine classification of ischemic electrocardiograms.* Proceedings *of the IEEE Mediterranean Electrotechnical Conference (MELECON),* Athens, Greece.

Sandoe, E., & Sigurd, B. (1991). *Arrhythmia: A guide to clinical electrocardiology.* Bingen, Germany: Publishing Partners Verlags GmbH.

Senhadji, L., Carrault, G., Bellanger, J. J., & Passariello, G. (1995). Comparing wavelet transforms for recognizing cardiac patterns. *IEEE Engineering in Medicine and Biology Magazine, 14,* 167-173.

Silipo, R., & Marchesi, C. (1998). Artificial neural networks for automatic ECG analysis. *IEEE Transactions on Signal Processing, 46,* 1417-1425.

Silipo, R., Taddei, A., & Marchesi, C. (1994). Continuous monitoring and detection of ST-T

changes in ischemic patients. *Proceedings of the IEEE Computers in Cardiology* (pp. 225-228).

Stamkopoulos, T., Diamantaras, K., Maglaveras, N., & Strintzis, M. (1998). ECG analysis using nonlinear PCA neural networks for ischemia detection. *IEEE Transactions on Signal Processing, 46,* 3058-3067.

Taddei, A., Costantino, G., Silipo, R., Edmin, M., & Marchesi, C. (1995). A system for the detection of ischemic episodes in ambulatory ECG. *Proceedings of the IEEE Computers in Cardiology* (pp. 705-708).

Thakor, N. V., Natarajan, A., & Tomaselli, G. (1994). Multiway sequential hypothesis testing for tachyarrhythmia discrimination. *IEEE Transactions on Biomedical Engineering, 41,* 480-487.

Thakor, N. V., Zhu, Y. S., & Pan, K. Y. (1990). Ventricular tachycardia and fibrillation detection by a sequential hypothesis testing algorithm. *IEEE Transactions on Biomedical Engineering, 37,* 837-843.

Throne, R. D., Jenkins, J. M., & DiCarlo, L. A. (1991). A comparison of four new time-domain techniques for discriminating monomorphic ventricular tachycardia from sinus rhythm using ventricular waveform morphology. *IEEE Transactions on Biomedical Engineering, 38,* 561-570.

Tsipouras, M. G., & Fotiadis, D. I. (2004). Automatic arrhythmia detection based on time and time-frequency analysis of heart rate variability. *Computer Methods and Programs in Biomedicine, 74,* 95-108.

Tsipouras, M. G., Fotiadis, D. I., & Sideris, D. (2002). Arrhythmia classification using the RR-interval duration signal. In A. Murray (Ed.), *Computers in cardiology* (pp. 485-488). Piscataway: IEEE.

Tsipouras, M. G., Fotiadis, D. I., & Sideris, D. (in press). An arrhythmia classification system based on the RR-interval signal. *Artificial Intelligence in Medicine.*

Vila, J., Presedo, J., Delgado, M., Barro, S., Ruiz, R., & Palacios, F. (1997). SUTIL: Intelligent ischemia monitoring system. *International Journal of Medical Informatics, 47,* 193-214.

Wang, Y., Zhu, Y. S., Thakor, N. V., & Xu, Y. H. (2001). A short-time multifractal approach for arrhythmia detection based on fuzzy neural network. *IEEE Transactions on Biomedical Engineering, 48,* 989-995.

Yang, T. F. Device, B., & Macarlane, P. W. (1994). Artificial neural networks for the diagnosis of atrial fibrillation. *Medical & Biological Engineering and Computing, 32,* 615-619.

Zhang, X. S., Zhu, Y. S., Thakor, N. V., & Wang, Z. Z. (1999). Detecting ventricular tachycardia and fibrillation by complexity measure. *IEEE Transactions on Biomedical Engineering, 45,* 548-555.

KEY TERMS

Artificial Neural Network: An artificial neural network is a massive parallel, distributed processor made up of simple processing units. It has the ability to learn from knowledge, which is expressed through interunit connection strengths, and can make this knowledge available for use.

Data-Mining Association Rules: The process of discovering valuable information from large amounts of data stored in databases, data warehouses, or other information repositories is called data mining. Association-rule mining is the discovery of association relationships or correlations among a set of items.

Genetic Algorithm: Genetic algorithms are derivative-free, stochastic optimization methods based loosely on the concepts of natural selection and evolutionary processes.

Heart-Rate Variability: The alterations of the heart rate between consecutive heartbeats.

Ischaemic Episode: An ischaemic episode is defined as a time period of no less than 30 seconds containing ischaemic beats.

RR-Interval Signal: The signal produced from the durations between consecutive R waves.

Sensitivity: The sensitivity of a test defines the probability that the test will be positive (pathologic) when the outcome is positive (pathologic).

Specificity: The specificity of a test defines the probability that the test will be negative (normal) when the outcome is negative (normal).

Section VI
Data Mining and Medical Decision Making

The process of extracting useful information from a set of data is called data mining. Data-mining techniques have been used as a recent trend for gaining diagnostics results, especially in medical fields such as kidney dialysis, skin cancer and breast cancer detection, and also biological sequence classification. Various data-mining techniques for medical decision making are presented in this section.

Chapter XIX
Information Processing in Clinical Decision Making

Vitali Sintchenko
University of New South Wales, Sydney, Australia

ABSTRACT

This chapter outlines an information-processing model of clinical decision-making which is described as a function of the task, *the* decision maker, *and the* context. *Attributes of the task, the decision maker, and the decision environment are highly interrelated and often interdependent. They directly affect the use of clinical evidence. We argue that information processing is modified significantly by the decision-making context and decision task characteristics. Knowledge of clinical decision-making is therefore becoming increasingly important when designing an intervention that will produce sustained behavioural change. An exploration of the context and information seeking aspects of prescribing is emerging as a first step towards building the concept of task-specific decision support design.*

BACKGROUND

The information-processing approach focuses on information seeking and use as the key attribute in any decision making. It describes decision making as a process of information inputs and outputs, and identifies parts of decision making that may benefit from decision support (Elson, Faughnan, & Connelly, 1997).

An information-processing model of clinical decision making explaining the information flow during a clinical encounter is shown in Figure 1.

First, the decision maker must seek information cues from the environment, such as clinical signs and symptoms, medical history, or results of diagnostic investigations. Selective attention based on beliefs of the individual clinician plays a critical role in the filtering of which cues to process and which to ignore (Wickens & Hollands, 1999).

The information cues selected form the basis for the situation assessment, which includes the identification of decision goals, an assessment of how critical the problem is, and

Figure 1. An information-processing model of decision making (Modified from Wickens & Hollands, 1999)

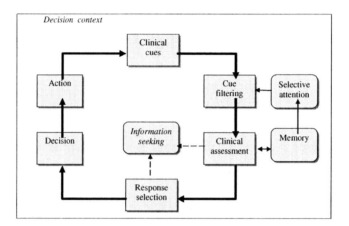

the risks associated with possible outcomes, as well as a comparison of the result of this assessment with previous experience.

It is believed that clinical assessment or problem solving is based on external information cues and knowledge stored in working and long-term memories, and that medical expertise is based more on knowledge than on expert reasoning. The concept of the mental schema, or clusters of related information that can be accessed rapidly and then utilised for decision making, has been introduced to explain how humans acquire and store information. The number, size, and range of mental schemas or illness scripts, and the ability to retrieve and apply this information correctly form the foundation on which expertise resides.

Research from a number of domains has demonstrated the importance of situation assessment as it assists in matching the type of reasoning used by a decision maker to the characteristics of the task. A medical practitioner, for example, uses different decision-making strategies to manage a patient depending on the clinical problem and the urgency of the task. For instance, the assessment of every impor-

tant possible outcome and their implicit utilities is more likely to occur for nonurgent healthcare decisions, but resource-saving reasoning heuristics are often applied by a clinician who is examining an acutely ill person in an emergency department where there is time pressure on the staff (Kushniruk, 2001; Patel & Kaufman, 1998).

During clinical problem solving, a number of diagnostic hypotheses and management options are generated. This number is limited by a person's short-term memory. Relevant mental schemas or clusters of related information available are reviewed and matched. The matching of schemas seems to be more rapid than hypothetico-deductive reasoning as it imposes less of a cognitive load than reasoning (Schmidt, Norman, & Boshuizen, 1990). However, when there is no acceptable match between selected cues and mental schemas, more cognitively demanding reasoning strategies are applied. If data gathering and processing steps of clinical assessment provide insufficient information for selecting a response, then the decision maker may seek additional information cues and use decision-support tools. The alternative options are then considered and assessed according to their values and cost, and the one with the highest value-cost ratio is usually selected.

CLINICAL DECISION MAKING

Information seeking is one of the most important aspects of information processing. It consists of uncertainty-resolution stages as the decision maker moves from problem recognition and assessment to the generation of alternatives and action (Wilson, 1997). Evidence suggests that information seeking can be characterised by personal information-seeking styles reflecting personal attitudes and beliefs. For example, it has been shown that clinicians actively pursue only about a third of the clinical questions they have (Wyatt, 2000). These styles are embedded in the activity that generates information seeking and are responsive to information needs (Wilson, 1997). The information-seeking style may be viewed as an intermediary variable that integrates different attributes of a decision maker and determines his or her information-seeking behaviour.

Decision makers often opt to seek additional information as a part of their decision making. Evidence suggests that information seeking is an integral part of a particular decision strategy. Tasks that require the processing of large amounts of information in a very short period of time tend to induce less analytical processing (Kushniruk, 2001). The main objective of any decision strategy chosen is to ensure the optimal choice and solution of the problem. Several factors may open the problem-solving process to error, such as the uncertain nature of a task, lack of information to match correct schema, insufficient knowledge, or cognitive biases (Elstein, 1999). Cognitive errors (i.e., decisions that are inconsistent with people's own preferences) and communication interruptions have

also been identified as potential contributors to suboptimal decision making (Elstein, 1999). The information-processing model describes decision making as a function of the task, the decision maker, and the context. Each of these can be characterised by a range of variables that potentially can modify their relative impact on the decision making. Specifically:

- Problem or task attributes include differences in decision variables (e.g., number of decision alternatives) and information cues,
- Decision maker attributes represent differences in skills associated with different levels of task knowledge and cognitive abilities, and
- Context attributes recognise variations in the decision environment that could influence decision making.

The interaction of these attributes influences the choice of the strategy used for making decisions. This interaction can also affect the information-seeking behaviour employed for the task. Therefore, these attributes and their potential impact on clinical decisions need to be reviewed in more detail.

Patient- and Disease-Specific Task Attributes

Clinical decisions are shaped by multiple factors and can be associated with variables related to a patient and his or her disease. Several patient-specific task attributes determine the selection of a particular management strategy, such as the patient's age, the duration and progression of symptoms, findings at examinations, concerns about adverse outcomes if treatment is withheld, the prognosis, and the patient's and/or relatives' expectations.

Disease-specific attributes also have an impact on clinical decisions. For example, clinicians adjust the intensity of care in response to a patient's condition and prognosis to assure the longest possible survival time even when the prognosis is poor. As Connors (1999, p. 5) has put it, "we are so afraid of not doing enough that we often do too much." In this context, the opportunity for errors in decision making is high.

Diagnostic uncertainty caused by the non-specific presentations of many life-threatening but treatable conditions is another significant modifier of clinical decisions. Second, the risk of potential adverse drug events, malpractice litigation concerns, and sociocultural and economic pressures are usually considered (Bradley, 1991). All these factors may potentially affect the associated information seeking.

Important Attributes of a Clinician

Personal attributes of clinicians also shape their decisions. Two phenomena that are of importance to any intervention that aims to optimise clinicians' decision making are the variability of clinicians' practice styles and information overload.

Practice Styles Contribute to the Variation in Decision Making

Clinicians do not always behave in accordance with normative principles of decision analysis. They do not make their decisions on a purely rational basis but often deviate from the ideal decisions in a number of ways and show distinct decision-making styles (McKinlay, Lin, Freund, & Moskowitz, 2002). Evidence suggests that clinical decisions depend more on a clinician's behaviour than on the clinical picture because of personal differences in the evidence-evaluation stage of the decision process (Connors,

1999). For example, two clinicians with different risk-taking attitudes may manage the same patient with a suspected infection with or without antibiotics. Importantly, an individual's practice style shapes the content, sequence, and format of information usage and persists over time (Davis, Gribben, Scott, & Lay-Yee, 2000; Long, 2002).

A large and systematic variation in clinical decision making between different countries and healthcare systems, between and within different clinical specialties, and between different decision makers has been documented (Metlay, Shea, & Asch, 2002). This may reflect variations in clinical training and decision making (Long, 2002; Metlay et al.), continuous subspecialisation in healthcare, and differences in information sources used and/or beliefs (Gosling, Westbrook, & Coiera, 2003). Differences in an individual clinician's practice style, risk handling, and the intensity of care, as well as a lack of consensus on the best practice and definitive studies identifying truly beneficial interventions contribute to this problem. For example, risk-averse physicians are more likely to seek additional information before deciding to treat or to do nothing, which increases the use of resources. Evidence also suggests that thresholds for adopting new therapies differ between clinical specialties (Metlay et al.). Existing variations also create challenges for evaluators of healthcare improvement interventions.

There have been suggestions that these variations are due to the differences in clinicians' knowledge and experience in evidence evaluation (Kushniruk, 2001), and, therefore, access to specific knowledge may improve clinical decision making (Elstein, 1999; Long, 2002). However, this view has been challenged by research observations that better knowledge in a specific domain did not ensure better decision making.

Information Overload Challenges Decision Quality

As in many other areas of modern medicine, evidence and knowledge are constantly being reexamined, and the half-life of the truth of evidence is limited. A mismatch between the increasing amount of information available to clinicians and human cognitive resources has led to information overload.

Information overload is one of the most pronounced phenomena of current clinical practice in general and prescribing in particular. For an individual, information overload means a perception that the information associated with a task is greater than that which can be managed effectively. This overload creates a degree of stress for which the individual's coping strategies are ineffective (Coiera, 2000; Yu & Chiang, 2002). For the healthcare system, information overload reduces the overall effectiveness of routine healthcare procedures. Taken together, information overload leads to decision makers' thought patterns becoming more complex, diverse, and less predictable (Yu & Chiang). Importantly, decision quality suffers under situations of information overload as it makes doctors' reasoning vulnerable to a number of cognitive biases (Ayton & Pascoe, 1995; Elstein, 1999); clinicians may have problems with the effective integration of complex information, even if all the necessary information is available upon which to make a valid decision.

Context of Decision

While the different types of information-processing strategies used by people when making decisions have been extensively studied (Wickens & Hollands, 1999), the role of the decision context has only recently received some attention.

Context Attributes

Background context (e.g., time pressure, body of knowledge available about different clinical syndromes, diagnostic procedures, etc.) makes each clinical episode unique. Contextual factors also include specific clinical roles of healthcare decision makers, the number of decisions they are working on simultaneously, the perceived importance of each decision, the established interaction patterns in a healthcare team, and the existing information environment.

Decision context includes both the physical and the social context of decision making. Each decision setting presents a particular mix of resources such as people, tools, and events that can be used to help to solve a problem and determine the way in which such resources are used. It has been suggested, based on simulation analyses, that context variables may have a larger effect on decision making than task variables (Chu & Spires, 2000). There is a perception among many clinicians that they have less time available than in the past because of increased patient volumes, a greater demand for documentation, and the increasing complexity of modern practice. For example, in the critical-care setting, the prescribing task is performed under significant time pressure because of the severity of patients' conditions and the possible impact of delayed actions (Elstein, 1999).

Context as a Decision Modifier

There are three important aspects of decision context that may affect clinical decision making. First, every clinical decision occurs in a patient-specific context. Essentially, decision making is a judgment task in which a clinician makes judgments about the value of different criteria (e.g., positive pathology report) based on the value of information sources in a particular environment. The clinician must make judgments and take actions in a fast-paced, dynamic environment with information that is often incomplete or uncertain.

Lastly, evidence suggests that the social structures of healthcare teams are important contributors to the uptake of information technology (Coiera, 2004; Gosling et al., 2003). It seems that participants playing different roles in an organization have different information requirements. Within a functional group such as consultant physicians, or across roles within a subspecialty, different teams such as intensive-care, cardiology, or infectious-disease communities may develop, each having its own shared understanding of events and ideas, shared vocabulary, and shared knowledge. Each group looks at a process from a different perspective, has different skill requirements, and defines the context by their own interest in the process. For example, a consultant may be interested in high-level information like the clinical unit's performance indicators while a registrar or resident in training needs information support for his or her basic prescribing decisions. Such contextual specifications should be included in system requirements.

CONCLUSION

Attributes of the task, the decision maker, and the decision environment are highly interrelated and often interdependent. Their interaction can only be assessed in the context of a specific decision. The decision maker's concepts and use of evidence are very dynamic and can also depend on the user's knowledge and personal beliefs. Observed practice variation may also be indicative of undesirable treatment preferences. Furthermore, variation in practice pat-

terns and the association of nonclinical factors with decision choice suggest opportunities to improve clinical decision making.

We argue that information processing is modified significantly by the decision-making context and decision task characteristics. Knowledge of clinical decision making is therefore becoming increasingly important when designing an intervention that will produce sustained behavioural change. An exploration of the context and information-seeking aspects of prescribing is emerging as a first step toward building the concept of task-specific decision-support design.

REFERENCES

Ayton, P., & Pascoe, E. (1995). Bias in human judgment under uncertainty? *The Knowledge Engineering Review, 10*(1), 21-41.

Bradley, C. P. (1991). Decision making and prescribing patterns: A literature review. *Family Practice, 8*(3), 276-287.

Chu, P. C., & Spires, E. E. (2000). The joint effect of effort and quality on decision strategy choice with computerised decision aids. *Decision Sciences, 31*, 259-292.

Coiera, E. (2000). When conversation is better than computation. *Journal of American Medical Informatics Association, 7*(2), 277-286.

Coiera, E. (2004). Four rules for the reinvention of health care. *British Journal of Medicine, 328*, 1197-1199.

Connors, A. F. (1999). The influence of prognosis on care decisions in the critically ill. *Critical Care Medicine, 27*(1), 5-6.

Davis, P., Gribben, B., Scott, A., & Lay-Yee, R. (2000). Do physician practice styles persist over time? Continuities in patterns of clinical decision-making among general practitioners. *Journal of Health Service Research Policies, 5*(4), 200-207.

Elson, R. B., Faughnan, J. G., & Connelly, D. P. (1997). An information process view of information delivery to support clinical decision making: Implications for system design and process measures. *Journal of American Medical Informatics Association, 4*(3), 266-278.

Elstein, A. S. (1999). Heuristics and biases: Selected errors in clinical reasoning. *Academic Medicine, 74*, 791-794.

Gosling, A. S., Westbrook, J. I., & Coiera, E. W. (2003). Variation in the use of online clinical evidence: A qualitative analysis. *International Journal of Medical Informatics, 69*(1), 1-16.

Kushniruk, A. W. (2001). Analysis of complex decision-making processes in health care: Cognitive approaches to health informatics. *Journal of Biomedical Informatics, 34*(5), 365-376.

Long, M. J. (2002). An explanatory model of medical practice variation: A physician resource demand perspective. *Journal of Evaluation in Clinical Practice, 8*(2), 167-174.

McKinlay, J. B., Lin, T., Freund, K., & Moskowitz, M. (2002). The unexpected influence of physician attributes on clinical decisions: Results of an experiment. *Journal of Health and Social Behavior, 43*, 92-106.

Metlay, J. P., Shea, J. A., & Asch, D. A. (2002). Antibiotic prescribing decisions of generalists and infectious disease specialists: Thresholds for adopting new drug therapies. *Medical Decision Making, 22*(6), 498-505.

Patel, V., & Kaufman, D. (1998). Medical informatics and the science of cognition. *Journal of American Medical Informatics Association, 5*(6), 493-502.

Schmidt, H. G., Norman, G. R., & Boshuizen, H. P. (1990). A cognitive perspective on medical expertise: Theory and implications. *Academic Medicine, 65*, 611-621.

Wickens, C. D., & Hollands, J. G. (1999). *Engineering psychology and human performance* (3rd ed.). Upper Saddle River, NJ: Prentice Hall.

Wilson, T. (1997). Information behaviour: An interdisciplinary perspective. In P. Vakkari, R. Savolainen, & B. Dervin (Eds.), *Information seeking in context* (pp. 39-52). London: Graham Taylor.

Wyatt, J. C. (2000). Clinical questions and information needs. *Journal of Royal Society of Medicine, 93*(2), 168-171.

Yu, P. L., & Chiang, C. I. (2002). Decision making, habitual domains and information technology. *International Journal of Information Technology and Decision Making, 1*(1), 5-26.

KEY TERMS

Context of a Decision: The context of any decision task can be defined as the collection of surrounding influences that make a situation unique and comprehensible.

Information Impact: Modifications in a practice or protocol.

Information Utilisation: Applying information to make a difference in the thoughts and actions of users.

Information Utility: The relevance of information to a policy or protocol.

Situation Assessment: The process of the identification and clarification, by the decision maker, of the decision problem.

Chapter XX
Data Mining Techniques and Medical Decision Making for Urological Dysfunction

N. Sriraam
Multimedia University, Malaysia

V. Natasha
Multimedia University, Malaysia

H. Kaur
Multimedia University, Malaysia

ABSTRACT

Data mining has been emerging recently as a viable computational tool for autonomous decision making especially in the field of medical applications. It has provided diagnostic solutions for skin and breast cancer detection, brain tumor detection, and also for other classification problems. In this chapter, we explore two data mining techniques, namely, association mining and decision tree mining, for predicting the life span of the kidney failure patients who have undergone routine dialysis. The total parameters used for this study were 28 attributes. The optimal prioritized parameters that decide the survival rate are reported and it can be concluded from the experimental results that the decision tree approach yields promising results.

INTRODUCTION

The process of extracting useful information from a set of data is called data mining. Data mining techniques have been used as a recent trend for gaining diagnostics results, especially in medical fields such as kidney dialysis, skin cancer and breast cancer detection, and also biological sequence classification (Fernando, Juan, & Angel, 2002; Krzysztof & William, 2002; Kusiak, Dixon, & Shah, 2005; Linhua et al., 2004). It is well known that the primary problem for urological dysfunction is acute and chronic renal failure, which can be treated through dialysis. This chapter describes the data mining techniques for predicting the life span of a kidney dialysis patient. Since we are interested in predicting the output for each individual, data mining tools have been opted as the decision making tools due to their individual-based functionality compared to other analysis tools, which are population based. They offer a valid, novel, and helpful solution for the identification of patterns of data, and also develop high-confidence predictions for each individual. Given the predicted outcome, more and better treatments can be made available for every individual. Furthermore, the resulting output serves as a major contribution to medical-care centres in providing enhanced treatment to kidney-dialysis patients to prolong their life spans. Therefore, it is hoped that the application of these techniques could provide us a rough estimation for the survival prediction of dialysis patients based on certain weighed parameters. About 29 parameters were considered as data from the database of kidney patients to provide an effective estimate of one's survival length after kidney failure.

KIDNEY FAILURE AND DIALYSIS

The kidney plays an important role in the body due to its basic functionality of processing all toxic waste together with excess water and salt. Generally, it is an organ that filters about 189 liters of liquid from the blood (1% original filtrate, which appears in the final urine as waste product and water). These waste products that are produced from food tissue are urea and creatinine. However, its main ability is to retain a proper stability of extra cellular fluid (ECF) and electrolyte homeostasis. This process can be done by maintaining the secretion of water and electrolytes to balance the changes (Sherwood, 1993). For a person with kidney failure, waste products that are produced from food tissue, namely, urea and creatinine, start accumulating in the body, and hence the fluid level and water homeostasis will be imbalanced. This eventually leads to endocrine failure and results in death.

Dialysis refers to any medical treatment that aims at replacing normal kidney function by artificial means. The treatment is prescribed for patients with end-stage renal failure (ESRF). Dialysis is an effective life-saving treatment. Without dialysis, the life expectancy for a patient with ESRF is less than a year. Life expectancy on treatment may be as long as 16 years, depending on the age and health status of the patients. There are about 370,000 kidney patients who are undergoing treatment for dialysis, and its annual cost is $11.1 billion in the United States of America (Kusiak, Dixon, et al., 2005; U.S. Renal Data System [USRDS], 2002). Even though the number of kidney patients has been rising yearly with a growth rate of 6%, little attention is given to kidney health. Out of the figure mentioned above, the total number of patients suffering from chronic renal failure is 260,000, and about 50,000 patients die yearly (Cooper, 1999; Kusiak, 2004; USRDS). When the kidney is functioning at less than 50% of its normal capacity, it eventually leads to chronic renal failure. In the end stage of renal failure, kidney function is at less than 10 to 15% of normal capacity. In Malaysia at the end of 2002, a total of 2,223 patients were accepted for dialysis compared to 43 patients in 1980, and prevalent dialysis patients increased rapidly from a total 59 in 1980 to 8,954 in 2002 (Zaki et al., 2003). The acceptance rate for dialysis increased very rapidly from 3 per 1 million to 91 per 1 million in 2002. Death rates for haemodialysis have remained at 10% or lower per year throughout the years from 1980 to

Figure 1. Schematics diagram for data-mining techniques for predicting the survival period of kidney-failure patients

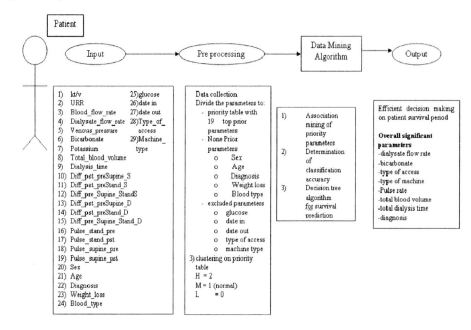

2003; CAPD death rates were higher at 10 to 20% (Zaki et al.). Based on research, it has been found that Malaysian patients who have undergone kidney transplants have a better chance of survival compared to patients who just undergo dialysis.

DATA MINING TECHNIQUES

Data mining, also called knowledge discovery in databases, is defined as the nontrivial extraction of implicit, previously unknown, and potentially useful information from data. It involves the identification of patterns or relationships in data. There are several data mining techniques available in the literature (Antonie, Zaïane, & Coman, 2001; DeClaris, Shalvi, Duong, & Luu, 1996; Hogl et al., 2001; Inanda & Terano, 2002; Kusiak, Dixon, et al., 2005; Kusiak, Kern, Kernstine, & Tseng, 2000) such as decision

trees (DTs), association rules, neural networks, classification rules, and the *k*-nearest algorithm for handling medical and nonmedical applications. The main objective of this research chapter is to develop an automatic decision making tool through data mining to predict the survival period of the kidney failure patient undergoing dialysis. Survival analysis that uses standard statistical tools, for example, logistic regression, Cox's model, and factorial designs, were found to be population-based models whereas data mining tools provide decision making for individual patient predictions, which are obtained from the probability of or the distance from the population estimates (Kusiak, Dixon, et al., 2005). For survival prediction problems, decision trees and rough-set trees have been used with limited parameters (Kusiak, Dixon, et al.; Shah, Kusiak, & Dixon, 2003). In our experimental work, we have used more parameters for evaluation purposes using association

Table 1. Parameter priority

No	Parameter
1.	Kt/V
2.	URR
3.	Blood Flow Rate
4.	Dialysate Flow rate
5.	Venous Pressure
6.	Bicarbonate
7.	Potassium
8.	Total Blood Volume
9.	Time Dialysis
10.	Diff_Pst_PreSupines
11.	Diff_Pst_PreStands
12.	Diff_PreSupine_Stand_S
13.	Diff_Pst_PreSupine_D
14.	Diff_Pst_PreStand_D
15.	Diff_PreSupineStand_D
16.	Pulse_Stand_Pre
17.	Pulse_Stand_Post
18.	Pulse_Supine_Pre
19.	Pulse_Supine_Post

mining and decision tree mining. Figure 1 shows the overview of our work.

DATA CLUSTERING

In order to evaluate the effectiveness of the data mining algorithm, 182 dialysis data sets were used for training and 66 data sets for testing. The test data belonged to new patients who had not undergone dialysis. The preprocessing steps start with the classification of dialysis parameters into three modes based on clinical condition, namely, priority mode, nonpriority mode, and excluded parameter. Data collection is based on known as well as unknown indicators (parameters). Dialysis patients received the treatment three times a week, and readings were listed before and after the dialysis. The priority mode contains the parameter that had more influence on making an effective decision on the survival period of the patient. Table 1 shows the details, in which the higher the number, the lower the parameter priority (as defined by clinicians). Nonpriority parameters consist of age, sex, diagnosis, weight

loss, and blood type as they have less influence on the survival length prediction. Due to inconsistent readings, parameters such as type of access, type of machine, data transfer in, data transfer out, and glucose were excluded for this experimental study.

Clustering is a method with the objective to find natural groupings called clusters. The natural groupings should be in a large dimensional set. Clustering plays a major role in data mining applications such as text mining, medical diagnosis, and computational biology (Aslandogan et al., 2004; Dandekar et al., 2001; Krzysztof & William, 2002). The objects are clustered together if they are similar to one another according to certain measures, and further clustering is done with dissimilar objects. The parameters that were obtained from the medical centre had some loops in which some data were not filled in as the data were missing in the centre itself. Such parameters included standing blood pressure, supine blood pressure, venous pressure, blood type, date of transfer into the medical centre, and date of the transfer out. As only certain data were left in a loop, clustering was applied to these parameters to decide their values. The values that have been clustered fall under three categories, namely, high, low, and medium (normal), which have the values 2, 0, and 1, respectively. Clustered data have these significant values to represent them for decision making. High and low values are defined as:

$$Low < Normal < High, \qquad (1)$$

where a low value is below the average normal value, and a high value is the above the average normal value. The range of values that are categorized into low, medium, and high levels for the dialysis parameters is shown in Table 2. These values have been derived based on medical experts' feedback.

Table 2. Clinical ranges of dialysis parameters

Parameters	Low	Medium	High
Blood pressure (systolic)	<120	120 - 140	> 140
Blood pressure (diastolic)	< 70	70 – 90	> 90
Pulse rate	<60	60 – 90	> 90
Time of dialysis (hour)	< 4	4 (3 x 52)	> 4
Blood flow rate (ml)	< 250	250 – 300	> 300
Venous Pressure	< 100	100 – 150	> 150
Bicarbonate (g)	< 66.0	66.0 – 66.08	> 66.08
Potassium (g)	<5.20	5.20 – 5.228	> 5.228
Total blood volume	< 70 %	70 % - 74%	> 74%
Kt/v	< 1.4	1.4 – 1.6	> 1.6
URR	< 72	72 – 73	> 73
Dialysate flow rate	< 500	500	> 500

It can be observed from Table 1 that certain parameter (10- to 15) values are framed based on certain measures. For example, consider the parameter Diff_Pst_PreSupine_S.

This parameter is based on the difference between the postreading for systolic supine (sitting) and the prereading for systolic supine (sitting). By using the simple operators, H – H = H,

M- M = M, and L – L = L, the data can be clustered. After clustering, the prioritised parameters are combined as shown in Table 3 in order to evaluate the effectiveness of the esti-

mate of the survival period for the kidney dialysis patient.

After all the data have been clustered to significant values of H, M, and L, or 2, 1, and 0, the parameters are framed into a table. Once the parameters are framed, the decision is calculated. Decisions are determined as such:

$$Decision\ (D) = X\ and\ Y, \qquad (2)$$

where X and Y are prioritised dialysis parameters.

The preprocessed data sets are further applied to the data mining algorithm.

EVALUATION

In order to determine the survival period of the kidney failure patient using the training data sets, the following processes are carried out.

1. Association mining of the data sets
2. Determination of classification accuracy
3. Prediction of survival length by decision tree mining
4. Testing the mining algorithms with the available test data (66 data sets)

Association rules are applied to the data sets belonging to Table 3 describing the events that tend to occur together. They provide information about the *if-then* statement, which can be computed directly from the data that are

Table 3. Combinational prioritised dialysis parameters

	Parameters (Total Parameters)
Case A	Kt/V, Venous Pressure, Blood Flow Rate, Dialysate Flow Rate, URR (5)
Case B	Bicarbonate, Potassium, Total Blood Volume, Time dialysis (4)
Case C	Diff_Pst_PreSupine_S, Diff_Pst_PreStand_S, Diff_PreSupineStand_S, Diff_PstSupineStand_S (4)
Case D	Diff_Pst_PreSupine_D, Diff_Pst_PreStand_D, Diff_PreSupineStand_D, Diff_Pst_SupineStand_D (4)
Case E	Pulse_Supine_Pre, Pulse_Supine_Post (2)

probabilistic in nature. In association analysis, the *if-then* statements are sets of items that are disjoint. The effectiveness of the association rule is relatively based on two indicators, namely, support and confidence. Support is simply the number of transactions that include all parameters in the *if-then* statement of the rule (i.e., probability that a randomly selected transaction from the database will contain all the items in the *if-then* part). Confidence is the ratio of the number of transactions that include all parameters in the *if-then* statement to the number of transactions that include all the parameters in the *if* statement. After the association mining of all possible cases, it was found that only 10 combinational cases yielded clinically useful information. Rules obtained from these cases are considered for further investigation. Some of the rules obtained from association mining are shown in the following sections.

Case A_B

Rule 1

IF Kt/V, URR, Blood flow rate, Dialysate flow rate, Venous pressure **AND** Diff_Pst_PreSupine_D, Diff_Pst_PreStand_D, Diff_Pre_Supine_Stand_D, Diff_Pst_Supine_Stand_D IS (>=77.78%) **THEN** CONSEQUENCES IS H (support(a)9; support(c)38; 7; 0.839181)

Case A_C

Rule 1

IF Kt/V, URR, Blood flow rate, Dialysate flow rate, Venous pressure **AND** Diff_Pst_PreSupine_D, Diff_Pst_PreStand_D, Diff_Pre_Supine_Stand_D, Diff_Pst_Supine_Stand_D IS (>=81.25%) **THEN** CONSEQUENCES IS H (support(a)16; support(c)35; 13; 0.951786)

Rule 2

IF Kt/V, URR, Blood flow rate, Dialysate flow rate, Venous pressure **AND** Diff_Pst_PreSupine_D, Diff_Pst_PreStand_D, Diff_Pre_Supine_Stand_D, Diff_Pst_Supine_Stand_D IS (>=76.47%) **THEN** CONSEQUENCES IS H (support(a)17; support(c)35; 13; 0.895798)

Case C_D_E

Rule 1

IF Diff_Pst_PreSupine_D, Diff_Pst_PreStand_D, Diff_Pre_Supine_Stand_D, Diff_Pst_Supine_Stand_D **AND** Diff_Pst_PreSupine_D, Diff_Pst_PreStand_D, Diff_Pre_Supine_Stand_D, Diff_Pst_Supine_Stand_D **AND** Pulse_Supine_Pre, Pulse_Supine_Post IS (>=76.67%) **THEN** CONSEQUENCES IS H (support(a)30; support(c)33; 23; 0.952525)

Rule 2

IF Diff_Pst_PreSupine_D, Diff_Pst_PreStand_D, Diff_Pre_Supine_Stand_D, Diff_Pst_Supine_Stand_D **AND** Diff_Pst_PreSupine_D, Diff_Pst_PreStand_D, Diff_Pre_Supine_Stand_D, Diff_Pst_Supine_Stand_D **AND** Pulse_Supine_Pre, Pulse_Supine_Post IS (>=66.67%) **THEN** CONSEQUENCES IS M (support(a)12; support(c)30; 8; 0.911111)

Case A_B_C_D_E

Rule 1

*IF Kt/V, URR, Blood flow rate, Dialysate flow rate, Venous pressure **AND** Bicarbonate, Potassium, Total blood volume, time*

Table 4. Classification accuracy obtained for dialysis-parameter combinations

Priority group	Total parameters	Below Median	Above Median
CASEA_B	9	65.22	50
CASEA_C	9	76.47	-
CASEA_D	9	-	76.47
CASEB_C	8	62.5	52.82
CASEB_D	8	-	58.33
CASEC_D	8	50	-
CASEC_D_E	10	58.33	66.67
CASEA_B_C_D	17	94.44	76.92
CASEA_B_C_D_E	19	97.44	88.89

dialysis **AND** Diff_Pst_PreSupine_S, Diff_Pst_PreStand_S, Diff_Pre_Supine_Stand_S, Diff_Pst_Supine_Stand_S **AND** Diff_Pst_PreSupine_D, Diff_Pst_PreStand_D, Diff_Pre_Supine_Stand_D, Diff_Pst_Supine_Stand_D **AND** Pulse_ Supine_Pre, Pulse_Supine_Post IS (>=94.44%) **THEN** CONSEQUENCES IS M (support(a)18; support(c)39; 17; 0.992877)

Rule 2

IF Kt/V, URR, Blood flow rate, Dialysate flow rate, Venous pressure **AND** Bicarbonate, Potassium, Total blood volume, Time dialysis **AND** Diff_Pst_PreSupine_S, Diff_Pst_PreStand_S, Diff_Pre_Supine_Stand_S, Diff_Pst_Supine_Stand_S **AND** Diff_Pst_PreSupine_D, Diff_Pst_PreStand_D, Diff_Pre_Supine_Stand_D, Diff_Pst_Supine_Stand_D **AND** Pulse_Supine_Pre, Pulse_Supine_Post IS (>=94.12%) **THEN** CONSEQUENCES IS H (support(a)17; support(c)39; 16; 0.989442)

The mining process resulted in a list of rules whereby specific rules with good confidence intervals were selected first according to the maximum occurrence and the minimum occurrence. The rules with the maximum and minimum occurrence are used to get the classification accuracy. A good confidence interval is essential for this clinical study. Classification accuracy requires a good confidence interval to obtain the number of correctly classified objects from the test set. The results of classification accuracy are shown in Table 4

The DT is one of the most popular classification algorithms in current use for data mining and machine learning. The DT algorithm creates decision trees or sets of decision rules based on the concept of the information gained. A decision tree takes as input an object or situation described by a set of properties, and as outputs a yes-no decision, thereby representing Boolean functions. The basis of a decision tree is that the outcome will be 50-50. Predictions for the survival length of kidney failure patient are made using the decision tree algorithm.

Figure 2. Decision-tree mining for kidney dialysis

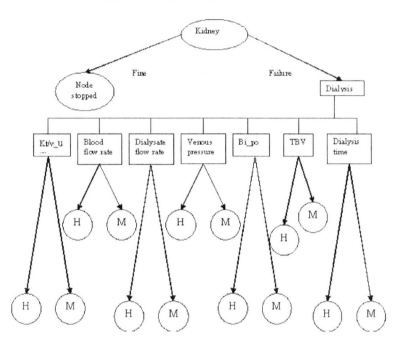

Thirty-two rules were generated by the DT algorithm based on two conditions: the survival length above the median (H) and below the median (M). Figure 2 shows the structure of a DT for kidney-dialysis parameters.

H represents the low risk factor of survival, and M indicates the high risk factor. The following are the exemplary rules generated by DT mining (only a few are given).

Survival Rules Generated by the Decision-Tree Algorithm

Rule 1

IF (Kt/V_URR>=1.6; 73) **AND** (Blood_flow_rate>=300) **AND** (Dialysate_flow_rate>=500) **AND** (Venous_pressure>=150) **AND** (Bi_Po>=66.08; 5.228) **AND** (Total_blood_volume>=74.0%) **AND** (Time_dialysis>= 4) **THEN** (Survival_length=Below_med); [16.667%]

Rule 2

IF (Kt/V_URR>=1.6; 73) **AND** (Blood_flow_rate>= 300) **AND** (Dialysate_flow_rate>=500) **AND** (Venous_pressure>= 150) **AND** (Bi_Po<66.0 ; 5.20) **AND** (Total_blood_ volume<70.0%) **AND** (Time_dialysis<4) **THEN** (Survival_length=Below_med); [83.33%]

Rule 3

IF (Kt/V_URR>=1.6; 73) **AND** (Blood_flow_rate>=300) **AND** (Dialysate_flow_rate>=500) **AND** (Venous_pressure>=150) **AND** (Bi_Po>=66.08; 5.228) **AND** (Total_blood_volume>=74.0%) **AND** (Time_dialysis>=4) **AND** (Diff_Pst_PreSupine_S>0.0) **AND** (Diff_Pst_PreStand_S>0.00) **AND** (Diff_Pre_Supine_Stand_S>0.0) **AND** (Diff_Pst_Supine_Stand_S>0.0) **AND** (Diff_Pst_PreSupine_D>0.0) **AND** (Diff_Pst_PreStand_D>0.00)

AND (Diff_Pre_Supine_Stand_D>0.0) **AND** (Diff_Pst_Supine_Stand_D>0.0) **THEN** (Survival_length=Below_med); [3.5714%]

Rule 4

IF (Kt/V_URR>=1.6; 73) **AND** (Blood_flow_rate>=300) **AND** (Dialysate_flow_rate>=500) **AND** (Venous_pressure>=150) **AND** (Bi_Po>=66.08; 5.228) **AND** (Total_blood_volume>=74.0%) **AND** (Time_dialysis>=4) **AND** (Diff_Pst_PreSupine_S>0.0) **AND** (Diff_Pst_PreStand_S>0.00) **AND** (Diff_Pre_Supine_Stand_S>0.0) **AND** (Diff_Pst_Supine_Stand_S>0.0) **AND** (Diff_Pst_PreSupine_D<=0.0) **AND** (Diff_Pst_PreStand_D<=0.00) **AND** (Diff_Pre_Supine_Stand_D<=0.0) **AND** (Diff_Pst_Supine_Stand_D<=0.0) **THEN** (Survival_length=Below_med); [96.4286%]

Rule 5

IF (Kt/V_URR>=1.6; 73) **AND** (Blood_flow_rate>=300) **AND** (Dialysate_flow_rate>=500) **AND** (Venous_pressure>=150) **AND** (Bi_Po>=66.08; 5.228) **AND** (Total_blood_volume>=74.0%) **AND** (Time_dialysis>=4) **AND** (Diff_Pst_PreSupine_S>0.0) **AND** (Diff_Pst_PreStand_S>0.00) **AND** (Diff_Pre_Supine_Stand_S>0.0) **AND** (Diff_Pst_Supine_Stand_S>0.0) **AND** (Diff_Pst_PreSupine_D<=0.0) **AND** (Diff_Pst_PreStand_D<=0.00) **AND** (Diff_Pre_Supine_Stand_D<=0.0) **AND** (Diff_Pst_Supine_Stand_D<=0.0) **AND** (Pulse_Supine_Pre<=60) **AND** (Pulse_Supine_Post<=60) **THEN** (Survival_length=Below_med); [96.6667%]

Rule 6

IF (Kt/V_URR>=1.6; 73) **AND** (Blood_flow_rate>=300) **AND** (Dialysate_flow_

rate>=500) **AND** (Venous_pressure>=150) **AND** (Bi_Po<66.0; 5.20) **AND** (Total_blood_volume<70.0%) **AND** (Time_dialysis<4) **AND** (Diff_Pst_PreSupine_S>0.0) **AND** (Diff_Pst_PreStand_S>0.00) **AND** (Diff_Pre_Supine_Stand_S>0.0) **AND** (Diff_Pst_Supine_Stand_S>0.0) **AND** (Diff_Pst_PreSupine_D<=0.0) **AND** (Diff_Pst_PreStand_D<=0.00) **AND** (Diff_Pre_Supine_Stand_D<=0.0) **AND** (Diff_Pst_Supine_Stand_D<=0.0) **AND** (Pulse_Supine_Pre<=60) **AND** (Pulse_Supine_Post<=60) **THEN** (Survival_length=Below_med); [4.1667%]

The rules generated by the DT predict the survival length of the kidney failure patient in two modes based on the combination of prioritised dialysis parameters.

- **Survival length=Above_median.** This means the dialysis patient does not need much attention from the clinician, and his or her level of dialysis is sufficient for survival.
- **Survival length=Below_median.** This indicates that the patient needs special attention as he or she is at a high risk level. Furthermore, the DT rules predict the survival period based on a threshold level of the parameters.

Rule 1 indicates that the survival length is below median with a low chance of survival: 16.6667%. Meanwhile, Rule 2 indicates that the patient is also below median but does not need much attention as his or her survival chance is 83.33%, which is a fairly high percentage of survival. It can be concluded from the above two rules that the impact of parameters such as bicarbonate, potassium, total blood volume, and time dialysis decides the survival length and the level of risk. This holds good for the rest of the rules obtained by DT mining

CLINICAL IMPORTANCE

To further confirm the effectiveness of our evaluation scheme, we also used the test data to predict the survival length, and 88.5% of our results match with the clinician opinion. From a clinical point of view, it can be concluded that there are certain values that are significant in deciding the survival prediction. The significant parameters found from the prioritised parameters are the following:

- Bicarbonate
- Potassium
- Total blood volume
- Time of dialysis
- Difference of post- and prereading in supine systolic
- Difference of post- and prereading in standing systolic
- Difference of prereading in supine and standing systolic
- Difference of postreading in supine and standing systolic
- Difference of post- and prereading in supine diastolic
- Difference of post- and prereading in standing diastolic
- Difference of prereading in supine and standing diastolic
- Difference of postreading in supine and standing diastolic
- Pulse rate

The survival length rule generated was mined using data mining algorithms on priority data. When all the data were mined using the data mining algorithm, the significance parameters were found, as shown here:

- Dialysate flow rate
- Bicarbonate

Example 1.

$$\frac{Priority - overall = 13 - 8}{Overall \quad\quad\quad 8}$$
$$= 0.625 \times 100\,\%$$
$$= \underline{\textbf{62.5 \%}}$$

- Type of access
- Type of machine
- Pulse rate
- Total blood volume
- Total dialysis time
- Diagnosis

The final trade-off of the significant parameter is calculated as such (see Example 1).

CONCLUSION

The most significant result obtained from this research was demonstrating that data mining, data transformation, data partitioning, and decision making algorithms were useful for the survival prediction of dialysis patients. Analyzing and comparing the data mining rules produced a list of significant parameters such as bicarbonate, potassium, total blood volume, time of dialysis, difference of post- and prereading in supine systolic, difference of post- and prereading in standing systolic, difference of prereading in supine and standing systolic, difference of post- and prereading in supine diastolic, difference of prereading in supine and standing diastolic, difference of postreading in supine and standing diastolic, and pulse rate. A conservative approach was applied while handling these cases, whereby the outcome below median was assigned to patients who had a shorter survival time compared to patients who were above median. Below median patients were those who had been placed on the transplant list, whose condition was deteriorating, and whose chances of surviving were small. H and M represented patients with a higher chance of survival and patients who had a lower chance of survival, respectively. The outcome resulted in the conclusion that DT-generated rules contain more significant parameters than the rules produced by association rules. Therefore, DTs produce higher trade-offs compared to the latter. The medical relevance of significant parameters was established. The final trade-off of the significant parameter was 62.5%.

REFERENCES

Antonie, M. L., Zaïane, O. R., & Coman, A. (2001). Application of data mining techniques for medical image classification. *Proceedings of the Second International Workshop on Multimedia Data Mining* (pp. 94-101).

Cooper, J. (1999). US incidence of kidney failure is the highest in the world. *The medical reporter*. Retrieved from http://medicalreporter.health.org/tmr0799/kidney.html

DeClaris, N., Shalvi, D., Duong, T., & Luu, T. (1996). Computational intelligence-based methodologies for population studies and laboratory medicine decision aids. *Proceedings of the International Neural Network Society*.

Fernando, A., Juan, P. C., & Angel, L. (2002). Combining expert knowledge and data mining in a medical diagnosis domain. *Expert Systems with Applications, 23*, 367-375.

Inada, M., & Terano, T. (2002). Interactive data mining from clinical inspection data. *IEEE Conf Sys Man and Cyber, 4*, 6.

Krzysztof, J. C., & William, M. G. (2002). Uniqueness of medical data mining. *Artificial Intelligence in Medicine, 26*, 1-24.

Kusiak, A., Dixon, B., & Shah, S. (2005). Predicting survival time for kidney dialysis patients: A data mining approach. *Computers in Biology and Medicine, 35*(4), 311-327.

Kusiak, A., Kern, J. A., Kernstine, K. H., & Tseng, B. T. L. (2000). Autonomous decision-making: A data mining approach. *IEEE Transactions on Information Technology Biomedicine, 4*(4), 274-284.

Lihua, L., Tang, H., Wu, Z., Gong, J., Gruidl, M., Zou, J., et al. (2004). Data mining techniques for cancer detection using serum proteomic profiling. *Artificial Intelligence in Medicine, 32*, 71-83.

Shah, S., Kusiak, A., & Dixon, B. (2003). Data mining in predicting survival of kidney dialysis patients. *Proceedings of Photonics West - Bios, Lasers in Surgery: Advanced Characterization, Therapeutics, and Systems XIII, 4949* (pp. 1-8).

Sherwood, L. (1993). *Human physiology: From cells to systems* (3rd ed.). Wadsworth Publishing Company.

U.S. Renal Data System (USRDS). (2002). *USRD 2002 annual data report: Atlas of end stage renal disease in the United States.* Bethesda, MA: National Institutes of Health, National Institutes of Diabetes and Digestive and Kidney Diseases.

Zaki, M., Shaariah, W., Liu, W. j., Hooi, L. S., Goh, B. L., Philip, N. J., et al. (2003). *Eleventh report of the Malaysian Dialysis & Transplant Registry*.

KEY TERMS

Association Mining: Association rule mining determines the correlation relationships among large sets of data and shows attribute value conditions that occur frequently together in a given data set.

Clustering: Clustering is the classification of similar objects into different groups, or distributing data sets into clusters or subsets.

Data Mining: The process of analyzing data to identify patterns or relationships.

Decision Tree: A decision tree partitions data into smaller segments called terminal nodes or leaves that are homogeneous with respect to a target variable.

Dialysis: Dialysis is a method of removing toxic substances (wastes) from the blood when the kidneys are unable to function properly.

Renal Failure: Sudden and often temporary loss of kidney function.

Chapter XXI
Spline Fitting

Michael Wodny
Ernst-Moritz-Arndt-University, Germany

ABSTRACT

Given are the m points (x_i, y_i), i=1,2,...,m. Spline functions are introduced, and it is noticed that the interpolation task in the case of natural splines has a unique solution. The interpolating natural cubic spline is constructed. For the construction of smoothing splines, different optimization problems are formulated. A selected problem is looked at in detail. The construction of the solution is carried out in two steps. In the first step the unknown $D_i = s(x_i)$ are calculated via a linear system of equations. The second step is the construction of the interpolating natural cubic spline with respect to these (x_i, D_i), i=1,2,...,m. Every optimization problem contains a smoothing parameter. A method of estimation of the smoothing parameter from the given data is motivated briefly.

INTRODUCTION

Model fitting in data mining requires the attention of at least three aspects: the data, the model to be fitted, and the optimization criterion. This general situation is specified for simplicity as follows. The data are a two-dimensional set of real numbers (x_i, y_i), i = 1, 2, ..., m, and the model is a class of spline functions. Selected optimization criteria are subsequently explained.

Spline functions are a class of functions that is characterized by general mathematical properties, instead of data-driven or problem-driven properties. Their application is widespread. There are multidimensional splines and many mathematical generalizations, too, especially on Hilbert spaces.

Spline fitting involves the calculation of the parameters of the chosen spline function from the given data. The data, the class of the functions, and the optimization criterion determined the calculation method for the parameters of the spline function.

Let (x_i, y_i), i = 1, 2, ..., m be given. We assume that $x_1 < x_2 < x_3 < ... < x_m$.

DEFINITION

A spline function s(x) of degree n is a function defined on ○. s(x) is given by some polynomial of degree n or less in each of the intervals $(-\infty, x_1]$, $[x_i, x_{i+1}]$, i = 1, 2, ..., m-1, and $[x_m, +\infty)$. All derivatives of s(x) up to order n-1 are supposed to be continuous everywhere. s(x) is called a natural spline if n = 2k-1 is odd and s(x) is given in each of the intervals $(-\infty, x_1]$ and $[x_m, +\infty)$ by polynomials of degree k-1 or less.

For example, the class of all splines of degree n with the knots x_i includes all polynomials of degree n or less.

INTERPOLATION

A special task of curve fitting is the interpolation problem. One looks for a function f(x) satisfying the strong conditions $f(x_i) = y_i$ for all i from 1 to m.

The interpolation problem has a unique solution for natural splines s(x). The main property of natural splines is proved by deBoor (2001) and Schoenberg and deBoor. In the case n = 3, the result was given already by Holladay (1957).

THEOREM

Let s(x) be the interpolating natural spline of degree n = 2k-1, with respect to (x_i, y_i), i = 1, 2, ..., m, and f(x) any interpolating function with continuous derivatives up to order k. Then

$$\int_a^b s^{(k)}(x)^2\,dx \le \int_a^b f^{(k)}(x)^2\,dx \text{ for all } a \le x_1 \text{ and } b \ge x_m.$$

In the case where k > 1, the strong inequality is valid.

We furthermore refer to natural cubic splines because they are widely used. It is possible to generalize the afterward-derived calculation procedure of the parameters of a natural cubic spline to arbitrary natural splines.

Looking at the definition, a cubic spline can be written in the interval $[x_i, x_{i+1}]$ as:

$$s(x) = A_i(x-x_i)^3 + B_i(x-x_i)^3 + C_i(x-x_i) + D_i.$$

Obviously,

$$s(x_i) = D_i = y_i, \quad i=1, 2, ..., m-1. \tag{1}$$

Furthermore, it follows that $s''(x_i) = 2B_i$, and so:

$$B_i = s''(x_i)/2. \tag{2}$$

The second derivation s''(x) is a straight line with the slope $(s''(x_{i+1})-s''(x_i))/(x_{i+1}-x_i)$. Consequently, one obtains:

$$A_i = 1/3(B_{i+1}-B_i))/(x_{i+1}-x_i) \tag{3}$$

for all i = 1, 2, ..., m-1.

The C_i can be represented with the data and the B_i as:

$$C_i=(y_{i+1}-y_i)/(x_{i+1}-x_i) - 1/3(x_{i+1}-x_i)(2\,B_{i+1}+B_i) \tag{4}$$

as seen in Equations (1), (2), and (3).

From these considerations it follows that an interpolating cubic spline is uniquely determined and completely represented by $(x_i, s(x_i))$ and B_i (especially $B_m = s''(x_m)/2$). One uses the continuity of s'(x) in the x_i, i=1, 2, ..., m to calculate the unknown B_i. Consequently:

$$s'(x_i) = 3A_{i-1}(x_i-x_{i-1})^2 + 2B_{i-1}(x_i-x_{i-1}) + C_{i-1} = C_i, \quad i = 2, 3, ..., m-1$$

holds true. Short remodeling together with the specifications $\Delta x_i := x_{i+1}-x_i$ and $\Delta y_i := y_{i+1}-y_i$, i = 1, 2, ..., m-1 leads to:

Figure 1. An example of an interpolating natural cubic spline

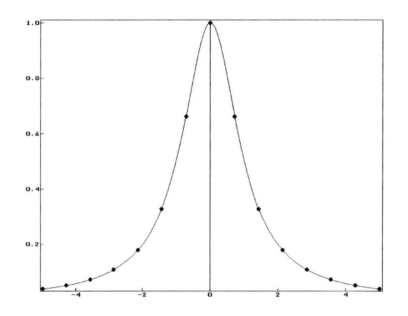

$$\Delta x_{i-1} B_{i-1} + 2(\Delta x_{i-1} + \Delta x_i) B_i + \Delta x_i B_{i+1} = 3\left(\frac{\Delta y_i}{\Delta x_i} - \frac{\Delta y_{i-1}}{\Delta x_{i-1}}\right)$$

$$(5)$$

These are only m-2 equations (i = 2, 3, ..., m-1) for the determination of the m unknown B_i. Additionally, from the definition it follows that $s''(x_1)$ = B_1 = 0 and $s''(x_m)$ = B_m = 0 because $s''(x)$ is continuous everywhere.

Summarizing, the calculation of an interpolating natural cubic spline requires the solution of a linear system of equations.

SMOOTHING SPLINES

Interpolation methods are not suitable when the data are influenced by measurement errors. Smoothing splines can be constructed in this situation. For this, several optimization problems are explained subsequently:

(OP1).

Minimize $\mu \int_{x_1}^{x_m} f''(x)^2 dx + \sum_{i=1}^{m}(y_i - f(x_i))^2$ for all over the interval $[x_1, x_m]$ twice continuous differentiable functions f(x), f 0 $C^2[x_1,x_m]$ and fixed $\mu \exists 0$.

$C^2[x_1,x_m]$ denotes the set of all over $[x_1,x_m]$ twice continuous differentiable real funtions. The parameter μ controls the trade-off between the "roughness", as measured by $\int_{x_1}^{x_m} f''(x)^2 dx$, and the coincidence of the data and the function f(x) as measured by $\sum_{i=1}^{m}((y_i - f(x_i))^2$. It must be chosen in advance.

The interpolating spline results when the object function of (OP1) is reduced to the least squares criterion.

Another problem was formulated and solved by Reinsch (1967):

(OP2).
Minimize $\int_{x_1}^{x_m} f''(x)^2 dx$ for all f0$C^2[x_1,x_m]$ satisfying the condition $\sum_{i=1}^{m}((y_i - f(x_i))^2 \leq S$.

A third criterion follows:

(OP3).

Find the minimum of $\sum_{i=1}^{m}((y_i - f(x_i))^2$ for

$f0C^2[x_1,x_m]$ where $\int_{x_1}^{x_m} f''(x)^2 dx \, dx \leq T$.

Due to Holladay's theorem (1957), each of the problems (OP1), (OP2), and (OP3) is uniquely solved by a natural cubic spline. The problems OP1, OP2, and OP3 can be reformulated as quadratic optimization problems in the $\circ^m$ with regard to Equations 1 to 5.

The construction of the solution s(x) of OP1 will be demonstrated now.

In the first step, the unknown $D_i=s(x_i)$ will be calculated via the uniquely solvable linear-system of equations

$$[I + 2\mu Q^T ÐZ^{-1}ÐQ]ÐD = Y.$$

In Equation 6, I denote the m-dimensional identity matrix:

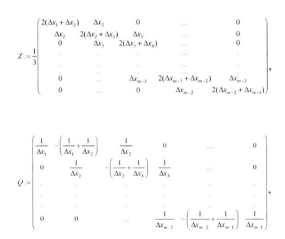

$\Delta x_i := x_{i+1} - x_i$, $D = (D_1, D_2, \ldots D_m)^T$ and $Y = (y_1, y_2, \ldots, y_m)^T$.

In the second step, the interpolation problem $s(x_i) = D_i$, i=1, 2, ..., m is solved. μ is the smoothing parameter.

In (OP2) and (OP3), smoothing parameters are S and T, respectively. The interpolating spline results for $\mu = 0$. The straight line is the consequence of $\mu \rightarrow \infty$.

Estimation of μ

The estimation of μ requires statistical context. Suppose $y_i = g(x_i) + e_i$. The e_i are stochastically independent realizations of a random variable e with expectation E[e] = 0 and variance V(e) = σ^2.

Let $\mu \geq 0$ be arbitrary but fixed. Let $s_\mu(x)$ denote the uniquely determined solution to (OP1). Furthermore:

$$MSE(\mu) = \tfrac{1}{m}\sum_{i=1}^{m} E[(s_\mu(x_i) - g(x_i))^2]$$

defines the average mean-squared error, and

$$PSE(\mu) = \tfrac{1}{m}\sum_{i=1}^{m} E[(s_\mu(x_i) - y_i^*)^2]$$

defines the average predictive squared error with new, unused y_i^*.

The parameter μ can be estimated by the well-known cross-validation method. It works as follows. Remove exactly one observation (x_i, y_i) from the data. Calculate the smoothing spline $s_\mu^{-i}(x)$ with regard to the remaining m-1 observations with the given μ. The response of the separated single point is measured by $(y_i - s_\mu^{-i}(x_i))^2$. Do so for all observations and calculate $CV(\mu) = \tfrac{1}{m}\sum_{i=1}^{m}(y_i - s_\mu^{-i}(x_i))^2$.

It can be shown that $PSE(\mu) = MSE(\mu) + \sigma$ and $E[CV(\mu)]$ is approximately $PSE(\mu)$. This is motivation to use the minimum μ^* of $CV(\mu)$ as an estimator for μ and $s_{\mu^*}(x)$ as an estimator for g(x).

At first glance, the calculation of $CV(\mu)$ is very expensive.

Figure 2. A smoothing spline and noisy data

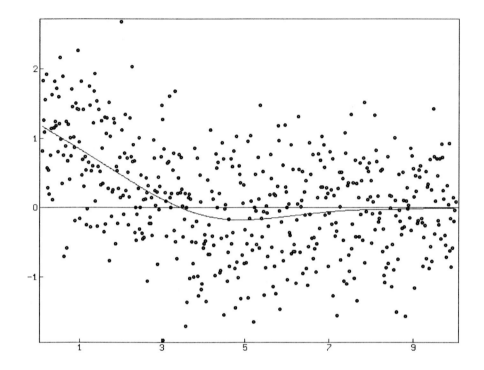

Define $H = (h_{ij})_{i,j=1\ldots m} := [I + 2\mu Q^T \text{Đ} Z^{-1} \text{Đ} Q]^{-1}$.

Hastie and Tibshirani (1990, pp. 46-48) proved the equation

$$CV(\mu) = \tfrac{1}{m}\sum_{i=1}^{m}\left(\frac{y_i - s_\mu(x_i)}{1 - h_{ii}}\right)^2 .$$

The generalized cross-validation method GCV(μ) of Craven and Wahba (1979) replaces each h_{ii} by the mean of the h_{ii}. In the past, it was easier to calculate the trace of H. Currently available algorithms compute h_{ii} in O(m) operations. So, the original motivation for GCV is no longer valid.

REFERENCES

Ansalone, P. M., & Laurent, P. J. (1968). A general method for the construction of interpolating or smoothing spline functions. *Numerische Mathematik, 12,* 66-82.

Craven, P., & Wahba, G. (1979). Smoothing noisy data with spline functions: Estimating the correct degree of smoothing by the method of generalized cross-validation. *Numerische Mathematik, 31,* 377-403.

De Boor, C. (2001). *A practical guide to splines.* New York: Springer-Verlag.

DeVore, R. A., & Lorentz, G. G. (1993). *Constructive approximation: Polynomials and splines approximation.* Berlin, Germany: Springer.

Eubank, R. L. (1988). *Spline smoothing and nonparametric regression.* New York: Dekker.

Greville, T. N. E. (Ed.). (1969). *Theory and*

applications of spline functions. New York: Academic Press.

Hastie, T. J., & Tibshirani, R. J. (1990). Generalized additive models. In *Monographs on statistics and applied probability* (No. 43). London: Chapman and Hall.

Holladay, J. C. (1957). A smoothest curve approximation. *Mathmeatical Tables and other Aids to Computation, 11,* 233-243.

Hutchinson, M. F., & de Hoog, F. R. (1985). Smoothing noisy data with spline functions. *Numerische Mathematik, 47,* 99-105.

Knott, G. D. (2000). *Interpolating cubic splines.* Boston: Birkhäuser.

Reinsch, C. H. (1967). Smoothing by spline functions. *Numerische Mathematik, 10,* 177-183.

Wodny, M. (1998). Ausgewählte probleme der kurvenanpassung. *Greifswalder Seminarberichte Heft 5, Gutzkow, GinkgoPark Mediengesellschaft.*

KEY TERMS

Cross-Validation Method: Cross-validation is a model-evaluation method. Holdout cross-validation is the simplest kind. Observations are randomly chosen from the given data set to form the validation data. The remaining observations are retained as the training data and allow for the determination of the model parameters. So, it is possible to give predictions via the model and compare it with the validation data that have not already been seen. This provides the background of model validation. A special case of holdout cross-validation is the so-called leave-one-out method. Exactly one observation is removed. The rest serve as a training sample.

Interpolating Spline: Let m points (x_i, y_i), i=1, 2, ..., m, $x_1 < x_2 < x_3 < ... < x_m$ be given. An interpolating spline s(x) is a spline function satisfying the so-called interpolating conditions $s(x_i) = y_i$ for all i=1, 2, ..., m.

Natural Cubic Spline: This function is a natural spline of degree n=3. This means k=1.

Natural Spline Function: Spline s(x) is called a natural spline if the degree of s(x) is n=2k-1 (odd) and s(x) is given in each of the intervals $(-\infty, x_1]$ and $[x_m, +\infty)$ by polynomials of degree k-1 or less.

Smoothing Spline: A smoothing spline does not satisfy the interpolating conditions. The starting point of its construction is an optimization problem. For example:

$$\text{minimize } \mu \int_{x_1}^{x_m} f''(x)^2 \, dx + \sum_{i=1}^{m} (y_i - f(x_i))^2 \quad \text{(OP1)}$$

for all in the interval $[x_1, x_m]$ twice continuous differentiable functions f(x). $\mu \geq 0$ is a given smoothing parameter. The optimization problem (OP1) has a unique solution, and this solution is a natural cubic spline s(x). For $\mu=0$ s(x) it is the interpolating spline, and for $\mu \rightarrow \infty$ we get the straight line.

Spline Function of Degree n: Let m real numbers $x_1 < x_2 < x_3 < ... < x_m$ be given. A spline function s(x) of degree n is a function defined on °. s(x) is given by some polynomial of degree n or less in each of the intervals $(-\infty, x_1]$, $[x_i, x_{i+1}]$, i = 1, 2, ..., m-1, and $[x_m, +\infty)$. All derivatives of s(x) up to order n-1 are continuous everywhere.

Chapter XXII
Parameter Estimation

Karl-Ernst Biebler
Ernst-Moritz-Arndt-University, Germany

ABSTRACT

Parameters are numbers which characterize random variables. They make possible the summarizing description of the observations, serve as the basis of statistical decisions and are calculated from the data. Point estimations and confidence estimations are introduced. Samples of the observed random variable are a starting point. The maximum-likelihood method for the construction of parameter estimations is introduced here. Examples concern the normal distributions and the binomial distributions. Approximate methods of the parameter estimation also can be too inaccurate at large sample sizes. This is demonstrated in an example from genetics.

INTRODUCTION

Statistical parameter estimation is a standard task in most data-mining procedures. It is presupposed that the data are a sample of the interesting random variable.

Parameters, unknown values of characterizing numbers concerning the observed random variable, can be calculated from the data. Such a calculation is called an estimate if it is carried out following statistical principles.

Examples of parameters are the expectation, the standard deviation, the median, quantiles, and so forth of a random variable. Furthermore, parameters can be components of data models, for example, the numbers α and β in the simple model $Y = \alpha X + \beta$.

The calculation of an approximate value for the interesting parameter from the observed data is called point estimation. A confidence estimation delivers a certain region in which the interesting parameter is contained with given (high) probability. It reflects the information content of the data with respect to the parameter and the sample size better than point estimation.

Parameter-estimation procedures are developed following special principles and considering the distribution of the random variables. They should fulfill quality requirements.

POINT ESTIMATION

Definition: Let X be a random variable, $F_{X,a}(x)$ its distribution function, and $(X_1, ..., X_N)$ a sample of size N. A point estimator $\hat{\alpha}_N$ of the parameter α is a function $\hat{\alpha}_N = \hat{\alpha}_N(x_1,...,x_N)$ of the sample. A point estimation is the value of $\hat{\alpha}_N$ at given data $(x_1, ..., x_N)$.

The most essential methods for the construction of point estimators are based on the maximum-likelihood principle, the Bayesian principle, the moments principle, the minimum-chi-square principle, or the least squares principle. The last named is not a statistical principle but a geometric one. Its relation to the maximum-likelihood principle is the clue of the Gausss-Markov theorem in mathematical statistics. Only one method is introduced here.

Maximum-Likelihood Estimation

The idea of the maximum-likelihood principle consists in the choice of the parameter value so that the observation gets maximal probability.

Definition: Let the parameter be $\forall 0 A \phi|^m$, X be a continuous random variable with probability density $f_{X,\forall}(x)$ depending on $\forall$ and $(x_1, ..., x_N)$ be the sample data. Then:

$$L(x_1,...x_N,\alpha) = \prod_{i=1}^{N} f_{X,a}(x_i)$$

is called the likelihood function of $(x_1, ..., x_N)$ and $\forall$.

For a discrete random variable, the input is:

$$L(x_1,...x_N,\alpha) = \prod_{i=1}^{N} P(X = x_i).$$

The maximum-likelihood estimator MLE $\hat{\alpha}_{MLE}$ calculates α_{MLE} from the given data so that $L(x_1,...,x_N, \alpha_{MLE})$ is a maximum of the likelihood function.

Examples

Normal Distribution

Let X be a normal distribution $X \approx N(:, \Phi^2)$ with expectation $E(X) = \mu$ and variance $V(X) = \sigma^2$. Then the parameter $\alpha = (:, \Phi^2)$ is an element of a two-dimensional set. The MLE of the expectation is the sample mean:

$$\bar{x} = \frac{1}{N} \sum_{i=1}^{N} x_i,$$

and the MLE of the variance is:

$$s_{MLE}^2 = \frac{1}{N} \sum_{i=1}^{N} (x_i - \bar{x})^2.$$

Binomial Distribution

For a binomial-distributed random variable, the relative frequency of the event in a sample of size N is an MLE of its unknown probability.

The One-Locus-Two-Allele Model in Population Genetics

A two-allele model regarding the alleles A_1 and A_2, and $P(A_1) = p$ and $P(A_2) = 1 - p$, without any dominance relations, is described by the probabilistic model

$$M_1 = \begin{bmatrix} \{(A_1 A_1),(A_1 A_2),(A_2 A_2)\}; \\ P(A_1 A_1) = p^2, P(A_1 A_2) = 2p(1-p), P(A_2 A_2) = (1-p)^2 \end{bmatrix}$$

The phenotypes observed are exactly the genotypes $A_i A_j$. The maximum-likelihood estimator for p based on a sample of size N with observed genotype frequencies $N(A_i A_j)$ related to M_1 is the so-called gene-counting method:

$$\hat{p}_{M1} = (2N(A_1 A_1) + N(A_1 A_2)) / (2N).$$

If A_1 is the dominating allele, you obtain:

$$M_2 = \begin{bmatrix} \{(A_1 A_1, A_1 A_2),(A_2 A_2)\}; \\ P(A_1 A_1, A_1 A_2) = 1-(1-p)^2, P(A_2 A_2) = (1-p)^2 \end{bmatrix}$$

and the MLE:

$$\hat{p}_{M2} = 1 - \sqrt{\frac{N(A_2 A_2)}{N}}.$$

If A_2 is the dominating allele, the probabilistic model:

$$M_3 = \begin{bmatrix} \{(A_1 A_1),(A_1 A_2, A_2 A_2)\}; \\ P(A_1 A_1) = p^2, P(A_1 A_2, A_2 A_2) = 1-p^2 \end{bmatrix}$$

gives the MLE:

$$\hat{p}_{M3} = \sqrt{\frac{N(A_1 A_1)}{N}}.$$

Properties of Point Estimators

The characterization of the quality is also necessary for the point estimators. Since estimators are random variables, concepts are used for this from the probability calculus.

Definition: A point estimator $\hat{\alpha}_N$ is called unbiased if its expectation is $E(\hat{\alpha}_N) = \alpha$ for all $\alpha \in A$. The bias $B_N(\hat{\alpha}_N)$ of the point estimator $\hat{\alpha}_N$ is $B_N(\hat{\alpha}_N) = E_N(\hat{\alpha}_N) - \alpha$. An unbiased point estimator $\hat{\alpha}_N{}^*$ is called effective if its variance is minimal in the class of all unbiased estimators of α.

Examples

Normal Distribution

The sample mean is an unbiased and effective estimator for the expectation of a normally distributed random variable. The point estimator $s_{MLE}{}^2$ is not unbiased for:

$$E(s_{MLE}{}^2) = \frac{N-1}{N}\alpha.$$

Consequently, the usual sample variance:

$$s^2 = \frac{N}{N-1} s_{MLE}{}^2 = \frac{1}{N-1}\sum_{i=1}^{N}(x_i - \bar{x})^2$$

is an unbiased estimator. It is also an effective estimator of the variance.

Binomial Distribution

The relative frequency of the event in a sample of size N is an unbiased and effective estimator of its unknown probability.

The One-Locus-Two-Allele Model in Population Genetics

The random variable $2N \, \hat{p}_{M1}$ describes the number of alleles of type A_1 in a sample of size $2N$. It is binomially distributed with parameters $2N$ and p. The estimator $\hat{p}_{M1}$ is unbiased for:

$$E(\hat{p}_{M1}) = \frac{1}{2N} E(2N \, \hat{p}_{M1}) = \frac{1}{2N} 2Np = p.$$

Its variance:

$$V(\hat{p}_{M1}) = \frac{1}{(2N)^2} V(2N \, \hat{p}_{M1}) = \frac{1}{(2N)^2} 2Np(1-p) = \frac{p(1-p)}{2N}$$

coincides with the inverse of the Fisher information. Due to the Rao-Cramer inequality, the maximum-likelihood estimator $\hat{p}_{M1}$ is efficient.

Both $\hat{p}_{M2}$ and $\hat{p}_{M3}$ are neither unbiased nor effective estimators of p.

The random variables $N(1-\hat{p}_{M2})^2$ and $N(\hat{p}_{M3})^2$ are binomially distributed with parameters N, $(1-p)^2$ and N, p^2, respectively. The estimators $\hat{p}_{M2}$ and $\hat{p}_{M3}$ are both asymptotically efficient and asymptotically unbiased according to the theory of estimation. Their asymptotic variances (Rao-Cramer inequalities) are calculated from the related Fisher information as:

$$V_{asymp}(\hat{p}_{M2}) = \frac{2p - p^2}{4N}$$

and

$$V_{asymp}(\hat{p}_{M3}) = \frac{1 - p^2}{4N} \ .$$

(Biebler, Jäger, & Wodny, 2003)

CONFIDENCE ESTIMATION

A point estimation from sample data gives only an approximate value of the unknown parameter. It was the idea of Neyman (1935) to calculate an interval of parameter values consistent with the data.

Definition: A set $CI \subset A \subseteq I^m$ is called the confidence interval for the parameter α at the confidence level $\varepsilon > 0$ if $P(\alpha \in CI) \geq 1 - \varepsilon$.

Examples

Normal Distribution

Let $X \approx N(:, \Phi^2)$. Then $\bar{X} \approx N(:, \Phi^2 / N)$ and

$$\frac{\bar{X} - \mu}{\sigma / \sqrt{N}} \approx N(0, 1).$$

Set $\dfrac{\bar{X} - \mu}{\sigma / \sqrt{N}} = u_{1-\varepsilon/2}$

with $u_{1-\varepsilon/2}$ the $(1 - \varepsilon/2)$ – quantile of the standard normal distribution. Consequently:

$$P(\bar{X} - u_{1-\varepsilon/2} \cdot \sigma / \sqrt{N} \leq \mu \leq \bar{X} + u_{1-\varepsilon/2} \cdot \sigma / \sqrt{N}) = 1 - \varepsilon.$$

This means:

$$\left[\bar{X} - u_{1-\varepsilon/2} \cdot \sigma / \sqrt{N} \ ; \ \bar{X} + u_{1-\varepsilon/2} \cdot \sigma / \sqrt{N} \right]$$

is a $(1 - \varepsilon)$ – confidence interval for the expectation.

The quantile $u_{1-\varepsilon/2}$ must be replaced by the quantile $t_{N-1; 1-\varepsilon/2}$ of the t-distribution if the variance of the random variable X is unknown and estimated by the sample variance s^2.

The $(1 - \varepsilon)$ – confidence interval now reads:

$$\left[\bar{X} - t_{N-1; 1-\varepsilon/2} \cdot s / \sqrt{N} \ ; \ \bar{X} + t_{N-1; 1-\varepsilon/2} \cdot s / \sqrt{N} \right].$$

Binomial Distribution

Let X be binomially distributed with the parameters N and p, where $X \approx B(N, p)$. There are three possibilities for the calculation of a confidence interval CI of p.

Method 1: Calculate CI exactly with respect to the binomial distribution with the parameters N and p.

A $(1 - \varepsilon)$ – confidence interval for p is $CI = [p_l; p_u]$, where the interval bounds are solutions of the equations:

$$\sum_{m=k}^{N} \binom{N}{m} p_l^m (1 - p_l)^{N-m} = \frac{\varepsilon}{2}$$

and

Figure 1. Exact width of the 0.95 confidence interval as a function of p, where N = 50

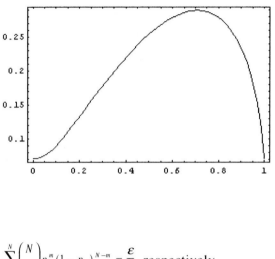

Figure 2. Difference between the width of the exact and the width of the asymptotic due to maximum-likelihood-calculated 0.95 confidence intervals as a function of p, where N = 50

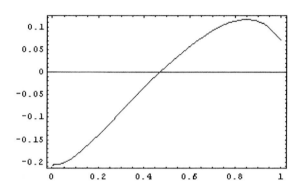

$$\sum_{m=k}^{N} \binom{N}{m} p_u^m (1 - p_u)^{N-m} = \frac{\varepsilon}{2},\ \text{respectively.}$$

The solution of these equations is not simple. Calculation problems occur for large values of N. The exact calculation of confidence intervals for the parameter p of a binomial distribution for arbitrary N is possible with the help of incomplete Beta functions I_p (Johnson, Kotz, & Kemp, 1992):

$$I_p(k, N - k + 1) = \frac{\int_0^p t^k (1 - t)^{N-k} dt}{\int_0^1 t^k (1 - t)^{N-k} dt} = P(X \geq k) \quad,$$

and

$$P(X \geq k) = \sum_{j=k}^{N} \binom{N}{j} p^k (1 - p)^{N-k}.$$

Calculation tools are available in MATHEMATICA and in SAS (e.g., Daly, 1992).

Method 2: Calculate *CI* asymptotically according to the central-limit theorem of Laplace under reference to the normal distribution with the expectation Np and the variance $Np(1-p)$.

This method is most frequently used.

Method 3: Calculate *CI* asymptotically according to the limit theorem from the theory of maximum-likelihood estimations under reference to the normal distribution with the expectation value p and the variance V_{asymp}.

The One-Locus-Two-Allele Model in Population Genetics

It shall be demonstrated that approximate methods to noteworthy faults can lead to the simple example of the calculation of phenotype probabilities for phenylketonuria (PKU) from population data. The model of inheritance of PKU is M_3 because the available tests of herozygocity are applied only in special situations. The data-mining operation $N(\hat{p}_{M3})^2$ is a binomially distributed random variable with parameters N and p^2. This allows for the confidence estimation for p.

The calculation methods yield different confidence intervals for p. Figures 1, 2, and 3 illustrate these differences for an example.

Figure 3. Difference between the width of the exact and the width of the asymptotic due to the Laplace central-limit-theorem-calculated 0.95 confidence intervals as a function of p, where N = 50

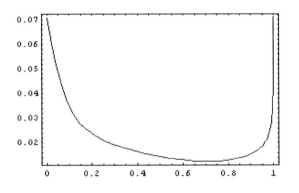

Figure 4. Exact width B = p² of the 0.95 confidence interval of p² as a function of sample size N, calculated in the neighbourhood of p² = 0.0001

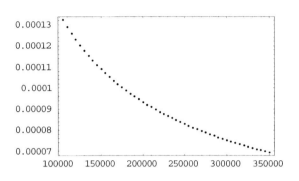

The differences between the methods of confidence-interval calculation will be illustrated also in the context of the sample-size calculation.

The confidence level is 0.05 in the following; the width B of the confidence interval has to be fixed. For given values of p, necessary sample sizes are calculable from the probability distributions of $\hat{p}_{M3}$.

PKU is one of the most frequent hereditary diseases. For a certain population, the allele probability of PKU is supposed as $p = 0.01$. This is a realistic order of magnitude. The incidence (phenotype probability) for someone having the disease is $p^2 = 0.0001$.

Figure 4 shows the width $B = p^2$ of the 0.95 confidence interval of the phenotype probabilities p^2 as a function of the sample size N.

For $B = p^2 = 0.0001$, the necessary sample size is $N = 173,146$ (Method 1). The approximate Method 2 yields $N = 153,649$.

Consider now the estimation of the allele probability p. For $p = 0.01$ and the same width B of the 0.95 confidence interval, you get a

necessary sample size of $N = 38,413$ with Method 3. The exact Method 1 yields $N = 45,865$ here.

The information content has to be carefully judged also for large-population genetic data sets. Already, for the very simple model of inheritance M_3 for PKU, there are considerable differences between the approximate and the exact calculated sample sizes. Consequently, the approximate calculation methods should not be used any longer.

REFERENCES

Bickel, P. J., & Doksum, K. A. (1977). *Mathematical statistics: Basic ideas and selected topics.* NJ: Prentice Hall.

Biebler, K. E., Jäger, B., & Wodny, M. (2003). How exactly do we know inheritance parameters? In P. Perner, R. Brause, & H. G. Holzhütter (Eds.), *Medical data analysis* (pp. 9-14). Berlin, Germany: Springer.

Cox, D. R., & Hinkley, D. V. (1974). *Theoretical statistics.* London: Chapman & Hall.

Daly, L. (1992). Simple SAS macros for the calculation of exact binomial and Poisson confidence limits. *Comput. Biol. Med., 22,* 351-361.

Efron, B., & Tibshirani, R. J. (1993). *An introduction to the bootstrap.* London: Chapman & Hall.

Encyclopedia of Biostatistics. (1998). Chichester: Wiley.

Johnson, N. L., Kotz, S., & Kemp, A. W. (1992). *Univariate discrete distributions* (2nd ed.). New York: John Wiley & Sons.

Lachin, J. M. (2000). *Biostatistical methods: The assessment of relative risks.* New York: John Wiley & Sons.

Lehmann, E. L. (1983). *Theory of point estimation.* New York: John Wiley & Sons.

Neyman, J. (1935). On the problem of confidence intervals. *Annals of Mathematical Statistics, 6,* 111-116.

Neyman, J. (1937). Outline of a theory of statistical estimation based on the classical theory of probability. *Philosophical Transaction of Royal Society of London (Series A), 236,* 333-380.

Vogel, F., & Motulsky, A. G. (1979). *Human genetics.* Berlin, Germany: Springer.

KEY TERMS

Asymptotically Efficient: The property of efficiency almost applies to large sample sizes.

Asymptotically Unbiased: The property of being unbiased almost applies to large sample sizes.

Bayesian Principle: Statistical calculation principle founded on Bayes' theorem. The prob-ability of a sample may be expressed via the conditional probability of the random variable given the parameter values of its distribution (a priori distribution). Following Bayes, the a posteriori distribution of the parameters given the sample data can be expressed. The parameters can be calculated so that the given sample data becomes more probable according to the a posteriori distribution.

Beta Functions: The function $B(p,q) = \int_0^1 t^{p-1}(1-t)^{q-1}\,dt$, $p > 0$, $q > 0$, is called a Beta function. An incomplete Beta function is defined as $B(p,q) = \int_0^{\alpha} t^{p-1}(1-t)^{q-1}\,dt$, $0 < \forall < 1$. Beta functions and their inverses are applied in statistics, for example, for tail probability calculations of binomial distributions.

Binomial Distribution: The observation of the occurrence vs. the nonoccurrence of an event in a random experiment. When the random experiment is repeated, the number k of occurrences in n trials is a random variable. Its probability distribution is the binomial distribution with the parameters n and the probability p for the occurrence of the event.

Confidence Interval: From sample data, an interval is calculated that contains the desired parameter of a random variable at a predefined level of confidence. Confidence levels are probabilities, for example, 0.95 or 0.99.

Effective Point Estimator: A point estimator is the statistical method to calculate a parameter value from sample data. Effectiveness is one of its most desired properties. It is the best exploitation of the information contained in the data for the purpose of parameter calculation.

Fisher Information: Consider a sample of size n of a random variable. The Fisher information is calculated via the probability distribution of the random variable and the sample size *n*. It can be understood as a measure for the information content of the sample and is closely related to the minimal variance of a statistical point estimator due to the Rao-Cramer inequality.

Gauss-Markov Theorem: Linear models of random variables are of importance in regression analysis, for example. The Gauss-Markov theorem describes the special way to get point estimates of the parameters of linear models.

Least Squares Principle: This principle concerns curve fitting and is of geometric nature. Neither random variables nor samples are required. Curve parameters are calculated so that the sum of squared differences between function values and data values becomes minimal.

Likelihood Function: The likelihood function expresses the likelihood (simply, the probability) of a sample of the random variable in observation. It is derived from the related probability function (in case of a discrete random variable) or the related probability density (in case of a continuous random variable).

Maximum-Likelihood Estimator: It is a calculation procedure and the result of the application of the maximum-likelihood principle to a parameter-estimation problem.

Maximum-Likelihood Principle: It concerns random variables and their parameters. These parameters are calculated from the data so that the likelihood (simply, the probability) of the sample at hand becomes a maximum.

Minimum-Chi-Square Principle: The unknown parameters of a random variable are calculated so that the difference (measured by Pearson's chi-square formula) between ex-

pected and observed values of that random variable becomes minimal.

Moments Principle: Probability distributions are characterized by parameters and, on the other hand, by moments. One can calculate from the given sample data the moments, and from these the desired parameters.

Normal Distribution: The normal distributions are a special type of probability distributions for continuous random variables. They are completely characterized by the two parameters mean and variance. The standard normal distribution has a mean of zero, a variance of one, and the well-known Gaussian bell-shape density function. The normal distributions play an important role in applied statistics.

Parameter: A characterizing quantity, especially in statistics. Examples are the mean and the variance of a random variable, or the coefficients in a linear regression model. It is a standard task of statistics to calculate parameters from data.

Point Estimation: When a point estimator is applied to given data, the calculation result is called a point estimation.

Point Estimator: This is a statistical method to calculate a parameter value from sample data.

Population Genetics: Population genetics studies processes of heredity in populations. It concerns biology and medicine first, but also fields from history to ethnology. Most of its methods come from biometry. The effects of evolution, migration, selection, and mutation on the genetic constitution of populations are especially investigated.

Rao-Cramer Inequality: A statistical point estimator is a random variable. Its variance has a lower bound (Rao-Cramer bound) under certain suppositions concerning the probability distribution of the observed random variable. The Rao-Cramer bound depends only on this distribution and the sample size, but not on the sample data.

Unbiased Point Estimator: A point estimator is the statistical method to calculate a parameter value from sample data. Being unbiased is one of its most desired properties. This means there is the absence of any systematic failure in the sense of statistics.

Chapter XXIII
The Method of Least Squares

Bernd Jaeger

Ernst-Moritz-Arndt-University, Germany

ABSTRACT

The method of least squares is a geometric principle of curve fitting. The unknown parameters of a function are calculated in such a way that the sum of squared differences between function values and measurements gets minimal. Examples are given for a linear and a nonlinear curve fitting problem. Consequences of model linearizations are explained.

INTRODUCTION

Model fit is a general task in data mining. It is a basic component of general problems like optimization, statistical data evaluation, data imaging, and so forth. The method of least squares (MLS) is a widely used principle of geometric character to fit a model to given data. The method goes back to the work of C. F. Gauss and A. M. Legendre.

Suppositions concern merely the model to be adapted: The data must be numbers. Many data-related optimization criteria are extensions of the classic least squares method. Statistical parameter estimation and the method of least squares are closely connected in linear statistical models (e.g., the Gauss-Markov theorem in mathematical statistics).

The method of least squares is explained at its simplest examples in the following paragraphs. In addition, difficulties occurring in the model linearization are demonstrated.

The so-called method of least squares is a universal method for the calculation of the parameters $\alpha_1, ..., \alpha_k$ of a model function $y = f_{\alpha_1,...\alpha_l}(x)$, which in the best possible way goes through a given set of points (x_i, y_i), $i = 1, ..., n$. The basic idea is to minimize the sum of the squared distances between the function $f_{\alpha_1,...,\alpha_k}(x_i)$ and the measurement y_i:

$$g(\alpha_1,...,\alpha_k) = \sum_{i=1}^{n} \left(f_{\alpha_1,...\alpha_k}(x_i) - y_i \right)^2 .$$

For that, the equations

$$\frac{\partial g(\alpha_1,...,\alpha_k)}{\partial \alpha_j} = 0, \quad j = 1, ..., k$$

formulate the necessary conditions. These k equations are the system for the determination of the unknown parameters α_1, ..., α_k. The solutions must still be examined to determine whether they satisfy the sufficient conditions for a minimum.

EXAMPLE 1

A linear function $y = f(x) = ax + b$ shall be fitted to the set of points. The function:

$$g(a,b) = \sum_{i=1}^{n} \left((ax_i + b) - y_i\right)^2$$

depends on the unknown a and b and shall be minimized.

The necessary conditions for the existence of a minimum are:

$$\frac{\partial g(a,b)}{\partial a} = \sum_{i=1}^{n} 2\left((ax_i + b) - y_i\right)x_i = 0 \text{ and}$$

$$\frac{\partial g(a,b)}{\partial b} = \sum_{i=1}^{n} 2\left((ax_i + b) - y_i\right) = 0.$$

The conditions lead to a linear system of equations:

$$(I) \quad \left(\sum_{i=1}^{n} x_i^2\right)a + \left(\sum_{i=1}^{n} x_i\right)b = \left(\sum_{i=1}^{n} x_i y_i\right)$$

$$(II) \quad \left(\sum_{i=1}^{n} x_i\right)a + nb = \left(\sum_{i=1}^{n} y_i\right).$$

The solution (a_0, b_0) of this system of equations is uniquely determined in case the deter-minant of the coefficients of the linear system is different from zero.

Unfortunately, there are only a few model functions that lead to such an easily solvable system of equations. Nonlinear systems of equations result mostly. In these cases, one must be content with iterative approximate solutions.

EXAMPLE 2

The model function $y = f(x) = c \cdot \exp(dx)$ leads to nonlinear equations for the determination of the parameters c and d. It is calculated from:

$$g_1(c,d) = \sum_{i=1}^{n} \left((c \cdot \exp(dx_i)) - y_i\right)^2 \quad (*),$$

$$\frac{\partial g_1(c,d)}{\partial c} = \sum_{i=1}^{n} 2\left((c \cdot \exp(dx_i)) - y_i\right)\exp(dx_i) = 0, \text{ and}$$

$$\frac{\partial g_1(c,d)}{\partial d} = \sum_{i=1}^{n} 2\left((c \cdot \exp(dx_i)) - y_i\right)(c \cdot \exp(dx_i))x_i = 0.$$

The resulting system of nonlinear equations follows:

$$(I) \quad \left(\sum_{i=1}^{n} (\exp(dx_i))^2\right)c - \sum_{i=1}^{n} y_i \exp(dx_i) = 0$$

$$(II) \quad \left(\sum_{i=1}^{n} (\exp(dx_i))^2\right)c^2 - \left(\sum_{i=1}^{n} x_i y_i \exp(dx_i)\right)c = 0$$

One can get the solution using a numeric approximation method, for example, the Gauss-Newton method. Most iterative procedures need a start value (c_s, d_s). This start value shall be contained in a close neighbourhood of the solution. However, this is not a sufficient condition for the convergence of the algorithm toward the desired solution.

Figure 1. Measurements (x_i, y_i) and the MLS fitted function $y = f_1(x) = 3.3139 \cdot \exp(-0.4263x)$

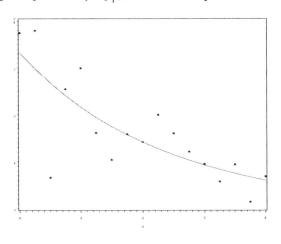

The following procedure seems seductive: Transform the original problem into a problem that is linear dependent on the searched parameters and fit it to the transformed data without the use of an approximation method. You get for the problem (*) of Example 2:

$$Log(f_1(x)) = Log(c) + dx = h + dx$$

and, with $(x_i, Log(y_i))$, the new minimum problem:

$$g_2(h,d) = \sum_{i=1}^{n}\left((dx_i + h) - Log(y_i)\right)^2 \qquad (**)$$

with an explicit solution.

The inverse transformation $(\exp(h_0), d_0)$ of the solution (h_0, d_0) into the original space of parameters does not yield any solution of the original problem (*). This has been known already for a long time (Wittstein, 1882). Today, this is nevertheless still frequently misunderstood, too.

The data in Table 1 are concentrations y_i of an active agent of a medication measured x_i times in the serum of a patient. The concentration-time function is supposed to be $y = f_1(x) = c \cdot \exp(dx)$.

The parameters $c = 3.3139$ and $d = -0.4263$ are calculated via MLS. Figure 1 represents the measurements and the fitted function.

The linear function $Log(y) = 1.13948017 - 0.45372974*x$ is fitted to the log measurements in Figure 2. With the inverse transform of the parameters, $f_2(x) = 3.12514\exp(-0.45372974x)$ results. The squares of differences between the measurements and the model functions are indicated in Columns 4 and 6 of Table 1.

Figure 2. Transformed model $Log(y) = 1.13948017 - 0.45372974*x$ and the log measurements

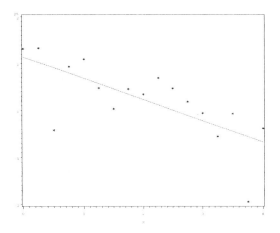

Table 1. Measurements $f_1(x)$ and $f_2(x)$

x_i	y_i	exact (MLS) $f_1(x) = 3.3139 * \exp(-0.4263x)$		transformation $f_2(x) = 3.1251 *\exp(-0.4537x)$	
		$f_1(x)$	$(f_1(x_i) - y_i)^2$	$f_2(x)$	$(f_2(x_i) - y_i)^2$
0.00	3.74184	3.31300	0.18390	3.12514	0.38032
0.25	3.79231	2.97808	0.66296	2.79001	1.00459
0.50	0.65957	2.67702	4.07011	2.49083	3.35350
0.75	2.54683	2.40639	0.01972	2.22372	0.10440
1.00	2.99364	2.16313	0.68975	1.98526	1.01683
1.25	1.61417	1.94445	0.10909	1.77237	0.02503
1.50	1.03785	1.74788	0.50414	1.58231	0.29643
1.75	1.58489	1.57118	0.00019	1.41263	0.02967
2.00	1.41626	1.41235	0.00002	1.26114	0.02406
2.25	1.99844	1.26957	0.53124	1.12591	0.76131
2.50	1.60539	1.14123	0.21544	1.00517	0.36026
2.75	1.20958	1.02586	0.03375	0.89738	0.09747
3.00	0.94700	0.92215	0.00062	0.80115	0.02127
3.25	0.57369	0.82893	0.06515	0.71524	0.02004
3.50	0.93629	0.74513	0.03654	0.63854	0.08866
3.75	0.14282	0.66980	0.27771	0.57006	0.18253
4.00	0.68264	0.60209	0.00649	0.50893	0.03017
		Σ	7.40682	Σ	7.79655

The function $f_2(x)$ does not solve the minimal problem (*) as can be seen from the sums of the deviation squares in Column 4 (7.40682) and in Column 6 (7.79655).

REFERENCES

Armitage, P., & Berry, G. (1991). *Statistical methods in medical research.* Oxford: Blackwell Sc. Pub.

Fisher, R. A. (1973). *Statistical methods and scientific inference.* New York: Hafner.

Hartung, J. (1984). *Statistik, lehr: Und handbuch der angewandten statistik.* München: Oldenbourg Verlag.

Lachin, J. M. (2000). *Biostatistical methods.* New York: John Wiley & Sons.

Rosner, B. (1989). *Fundamentals of biostatistics.* Boston: PWS-Kent Publishing Company.

Wittstein, T. (1882). Ein zusatz zur methode der kleinsten quadrate. *Z. Math. Phys., 27*, 315-317.

KEY TERMS

Gauss-Markov Theorem: The theorem says that in a linear model in which the errors are independent and identically normally distributed with expectation zero and with equal variances, the best linear unbiased estimators and the least squares estimators are the same. Even with weaker conditions, the theorem holds true: The errors need to have expectation zero, and need to be uncorrelated with equal variances.

Gauss-Newton Algorithm: It is an iterative algorithm to solve a nonlinear system of equations or to find the minimum of a function. In a line-search version of the Gauss-Newton algorithm, the search direction and the following point of iteration $(x_1^{(n+1)}, ..., x_m^{(n+1)})$ is calculated by an approximated linear system on the point $(x_1^{(n)}, ..., x_m^{(n)})$.

Method of Least Squares (MLS): Least squares problems appear in data-fitting applications. Suppose that the function f(x) depends on a parameter vector $(p_1, ..., p_m)$, and y_i is the actual observation (including errors) of the system at x_i. Then $g = \sum (f(x_i)-y_i)^2$ is the sum of the squares of the residuals between the function and the observations. Methods for the calculation of the minimum of g are methods of least squares.

System of Linear or Nonlinear Equations: A system with m linear equations (being valid simultaneously), n unknown variables x_1, x_2, ..., x_n, fixed variables a_{ij} (i = 1, ..., m; j = 1, ..., n) and b_i (i = 1,...,m), and can be written as:

$$a_{11} x_1 + a_{12} x_2 + ... + a_{1n} x_n = b_1$$
$$a_{21} x_1 + a_{22} x_2 + ... + a_{2n} x_n = b_2$$
$$.......$$
$$a_{m1} x_1 + a_{m2} x_2 + ... + a_{mn} x_n = b_m;$$

otherwise, it is a nonlinear system. A simple method to solve the system for a small number of equations is the Gauss algorithm. Gauss-Jordan elimination and Cholesky decomposition are the methods for larger systems of linear equations.

Section VII
Current Aspects of Knowledge Management in Medicine

Knowledge management is a basic tool for all those working in the health field and for hospitals. It helps in sending the right information to the right person at the right time so that the right decisions can be made depending on the existing problems. It is certain that with the help of knowledge management, effectiveness in the health field will be increased through unified systems, processes, and methods; the cultivation of exchanging knowledge; and the promotion of the effective use of available information. In this section, basic principles and theoretical aspects of the use of knowledge management in medicine are clearly presented.

Chapter XXIV
The Data–Information–Knowledge Model

Andrew Georgiou
University of New South Wales, Australia

ABSTRACT

The generation and transformation of data into information and knowledge is a basic formula in health informatics. This process is often represented in a model that portrays each component hierarchically with data at the bottom followed by an intermediary layer of information and topped by the knowledge layer. This model is a simple way to conceptualize important components of the informatics process, but it also has major limitations. The capture of data does not lead seamlessly to information or knowledge. The process is much more complex involving a multi-faceted web of interactions and issues.

INTRODUCTION

Health informatics is still an emerging and rapidly expanding academic discipline (Greenes & Shortliffe, 1990), located at the intersection of ICT and the many areas of healthcare. Its growth is a direct consequence of the dramatic expansion of ICT across health services over the last two decades. More than just the study of computers within medicine and its related fields, health informatics embraces a number of different fields and activities including patient care, healthcare research, education, and organizational planning and management (Peel, 1994; Shortliffe, 1991).

The heterogenous nature of the discipline means that it finds itself enmeshed in the many methodological and epistemological issues involved in the practice of healthcare (Georgiou, 2002). Indeed, even health informatics' most basic formula—the generation and transformation of data into information and knowledge—invites divergent opinions about the assumptions that underpin its claims (Hirschheim et al., 1995).

THE HEALTH-INFORMATICS MODEL

The process of distinguishing different forms and objects, and naming and categorizing them is an essential part of our ability to interact and communicate. This process is no less important to medical science and its need for communication channels to describe illnesses and share treatment options (Coiera, 2003). Models form an important element to the way we perceive and interpret the world (NHS Executive, 1996). Not only do they help us to describe and communicate aspects of the world, they also assist in understanding what is going on, perhaps even helping us to change and manage a part of reality.

The model often referenced within health informatics is the data-information-knowledge model. It is used to help identify and understand the different components and interrelationships within healthcare (Abdelhak et al., 1996; Coiera, 2003; Degoulet & Fieschi, 1997; Sheaff & Peel, 1995). The origin of this basic model can be traced back to the 19th century and the development of the functions of taxonomy and classification. Early statisticians used and developed classification systems as knowledge repositories developed from data and information (Desrosieres, 1998). Their model involved three essential parts arranged hierarchically, with data at the bottom and an intermediary layer of information topped by the knowledge layer.

Within this model (see Figure 1), data take on the character of facts or observations, which, in and of themselves, have little or no meaning. They take on significance only when they are provided with a contextual framework to manage and make sense of them. Information is assumed to be the product of processed data. The generation of knowledge then proceeds through a complex process involving deduction

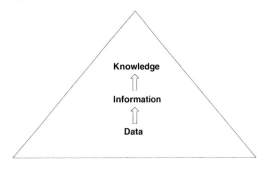

Figure 1. The informatics model

(based on principles of logical implication, e.g., statements of certainty), abduction (which aims to establish links between observations such as cause and effect, e.g., statements of possibility), and induction (whereby generalizations are generated from specific examples to formulate general rules; Coiera, 2003; Degoulet & Fieschi, 1997).

This hierarchical model has underpinned many of the information infrastructures within healthcare including the use of disease classification data to help research and plan healthcare. The United Kingdom National Health Service's Information Management and Technology strategy in the 1990s described the process as a "language of health" (NHS Centre for Coding and Classification, 1996). It posited healthcare information as based on clinical terms that could then be transformed into classification systems such as the *International Statistical Classification of Diseases and Related Health Problems* (World Health Organization [WHO], 1993), and from there into casemix groups for cost and resource management.

Even the growth of evidence-based medicine (EBM) with its commitment to using science, research, and evidence to guide decision making (Appleby et al., 1995) envisages information flows that broadly replicate the informatics model. The main tasks involved in EBM can be described as:

- Finding, appraising, and using research-based knowledge in decision making;
- Using systems for managing medical knowledge, and for obtaining, storing, and promoting the use of evidence; and
- Promoting and facilitating evidence-based decision making. (Muir Gray, 1997)

It is relatively easy to conceptualize these tasks using associated informatics functions such as knowledge browsing to assess information from a knowledge base; messaging to communicate records, assessments, and referrals; and counting to generate and analyze data (Benson, 1997). It is not surprising, therefore, that the growth of EBM has been linked to organizational commitments to establishing robust clinical information systems alongside greater attention to health informatics (Muir Gray, 1997).

LIMITATIONS OF THE INFORMATICS MODEL

The data-information-knowledge informatics model is an abstraction: a simple way to conceptualize a complex process. Therein lies its value but also its greatest weakness. The model views the generation of knowledge as a linear process whereby the capture of data from one side of the spectrum can lead seamlessly to information and knowledge on the other side (Georgiou, 2002). The problem with this conception is that the whole process of knowledge management is viewed overwhelmingly as just a matter of capturing, organizing, and retrieving information based on databases, mining, documents, and so forth (Thomas et al., 2001). It is not so simple.

Many of the problems associated with the model are directly applicable to coding and classification systems. These are tools designed for a specific purpose. There is no pure set of codes or terms that can be universally applied in healthcare. This is because they are heavily context dependent and change over time with developments in medical science and understanding (Coiera, 2003). The choice of which classification to use must be determined by the area of investigation (WHO, 1993). In the NHS in the '90s, leading clinicians and health-service commentators questioned the reliance on ICD classification codes that were geared to producing administrative contract data to the detriment of clinical data (Hopkins, 1996; Wyatt, 1995). The capture of classification codes and their transformation into larger aggregate groups was not producing the type of information or knowledge required.

EBM has made dramatic inroads into many levels of healthcare, but it is not a perfect decision-making tool (Cohen et al., 2004). Critics of EBM question the ability of large databases to provide best guidance for clinical practice. There is always the potential for the misapplication of EBM using irrelevant or outdated evidence from randomized and controlled trials, systematic reviews, and expert guidelines (Evans, 1995; Greenhalgh & Worrall, 1997).

The statistical technique of meta-analysis in EBM is based on the belief that trial results from apparently similar interventions (e.g., drugs) can be pooled. This process works best with many trials of a single drug, as in the case of aspirin for diseases in coronary, cerebral, or peripheral arteries (Antiplatelet Trialists Collaboration, 1994). But reality is not always straightforward. Trial registers and the follow-up of nontrial patients demonstrate that inclusion and exclusion criteria lead to the recruitment of younger and more mobile patients who can attend follow-up care, are free from other diseases, and are not being treated with multiple drugs. This leads to an implicit bias against older people (Hampton, 2000). Other criticisms of EBM contend that it has led to an obsession with measurement and accountability, which fosters illusions that complexities in medicine can be reduced to numbers to be manipulated (Charlton & Miles, 1998; Goodman, 1998). As Cohen et al. (2004, p. 40) point out, "There is no 'mean tendency' for a single patient. A therapy is beneficial for a person, or it is not."

Information-system developments and data-modeling enterprises are always underpinned by certain general assumptions that guide their approach. Examining these assumptions is a prerequisite to better understanding the practice of informatics (Hirschheim et al., 1995). The health-informatics model sits within a positivist framework, which has traditionally dominated information-systems research and systems development (Mingers, 2004). Positivism visualizes reality as the sum of sense impressions (Robson, 2002) with a focus on recording and measuring events and then using statistical and mathematical models to capture the patterns that appear in the data (Mingers, 2004). While positivist approaches dominate many fields of scientific enquiry, they have been criticized for their emphasis on superficial facts without providing an understanding of the underlying mechanisms or meanings to individuals (Bowling, 1997).

There are other approaches to knowledge generation that attempt to deal with the apparent restraints of positivism. Phenomenological approaches interpret the world in terms of meanings that construct an individual social reality (Robson, 2002). Knowledge generation is not viewed as a logically ordered accumulation of facts leading to scientific laws, but a process of conflicts and paradigm shifts (Kuhn, 1970). Other approaches include critical real-ism, which recognizes that reality exists independently of our thoughts or beliefs (Robson) and aims to explore the context and inherent mechanisms that generate events (Danermark et al., 1997; Mingers, 2004; Sayer, 2004).

CONCLUSION

The health-informatics model offers a simple and straightforward way to conceptualize important components of the informatics process. Its value lies overwhelmingly in its ability to differentiate the concepts that underpin the process. The model is not new; indeed, it has been associated with the development and use of statistics to help understand, monitor, and even govern society (Desrosieres, 1998; Georgiou, 2001; Georgiou & Pearson, 2002). This probably explains why the model is more closely identified with statistically oriented approaches involving disease classifications and EBM. However, it is very important to understand the limitations of the model. Knowledge generation is not a seamless operation. Understanding the use of information systems and their impact requires one to consider the complex web of interactions that are implicated in the process (Coiera, 2004). It is clearly an involved course of action incorporating social and technical issues, scientific debate, and successes and failures. The traditional health-informatics model offers a start to understanding this process, but it is by no means the finish of the story.

REFERENCES

Abdelhak, M., Grostick, S., Hanken, M., & Jacobs, E. (1996). *Health information: Management of a strategic resource.* Philadelphia: WB Saunders.

Antiplatelet Trialists Collaboration. (1994). Collaborative overview of randomised trials of antiplatelet therapy. I: Prevention of death, myocardial infarction, and stroke by prolonged antiplatelet therapy in various categories of patients. *British Medical Journal, 308*(6921), 81-106.

Appleby, J., Walshe, K., & Ham, C. (1995). *Acting on the evidence of a review of clinical effectiveness: Sources of information, dissemination and implementation.* Birmingham, UK: HSMC.

Benson, T. (1997). The message is the medium. *Health Service Journal, 107*(5538), 4-5.

Bowling, A. (1997). *Research methods in health.* Buckingham, UK: Open University Press.

Charlton, B. G., & Miles, A. (1998). The rise and fall of EBM. *Quarterly Journal of Medicine, 91*(5), 371-374.

Cohen, A. M., Stavri, P. Z., & Hersh, W. R. (2004). A categorization and analysis of the criticisms of evidence-based medicine. *International Journal of Medical Informatics, 73*(1), 35-43.

Coiera, E. (2003). *Guide to health informatics* (2nd ed.). London: Oxford University Press.

Coiera, E. (2004). Four rules for the reinvention of health care. *British Medical Journal, 328*(7449), 1197-1199.

Danermark, B., Ekstrom, M., Jakobsen, L., & Karlsson, J. C. (1997). *Explaining society: Critical realism in the social sciences.* London: Routledge.

Degoulet, P., & Fieschi, M. (1997). *Introduction to clinical informatics.* New York: Springer.

Desrosieres, A. (1998). *The politics of large numbers: A history of statistical reasoning.* Boston: Harvard University Press.

Evans, J. G. (1995). Evidence-based and evidence-biased medicine. *Age & Ageing, 24*(6), 461-463.

Georgiou, A. (2001). Health informatics and evidence based medicine: More than a marriage of convenience? *Health Informatics Journal, 7*(3-4), 127-130.

Georgiou, A. (2002). Data information and knowledge: The health informatics model and its role in evidence-based medicine. *Journal of Evaluation in Clinical Practice, 8*(2), 127-130.

Georgiou, A., & Pearson, M. (2002). The role of health informatics in clinical audit: Part of the problem or key to the solution? *Journal of Evaluation in Clinical Practice, 8*(2), 183-188.

Goodman, N. W. (1998). Clinical governance. *British Medical Journal, 317*(7174), 1725-1727.

Greenes, R., & Shortliffe, E. (1990). Medical informatics: An emerging academic discipline and institutional priority. *Journal of the American Medical Association, 263*, 1114-1120.

Greenhalgh, T., & Worrall, J. G. (1997). From EBM to CSM: The evolution of context-sensitive medicine. *Journal of Evaluation in Clinical Practice, 3*(2), 105-108.

Hampton, J. R. (2000). Evidence, guidelines, audit and cardiology: Principles and problems in secondary and tertiary care. In A. Miles, J. R. Hampton, & H. B. London (Eds.), *NICE, CHI and the NHS reforms* (pp. 65-78). London: Aesculapius Medical Press.

Hirschheim, R., Klein, H. K., & Lyyvtinen, K. (1995). *Information systems development and data modelling: Conceptual and philosophical foundations.* Cambridge, UK: Cambridge University Press.

Hopkins, A. (1996). Clinical audit: Time for a reappraisal? *Journal of the Royal College of Physicians of London, 30*(5), 415-425.

Kuhn, T. (1970). *The structure of scientific revolutions.* Chicago: University of Chicago Press.

Mingers, J. (2004). Re-establishing the real: Critical realism and information systems. In J. Mingers & L. Willcocks (Eds.), *Social theory and philosophy for information systems* (pp. 372-406). Chichester, UK: John Wiley & Sons.

Muir Gray, J. A. (1997). *Evidence-based healthcare.* Edinburgh, UK: Churchill Livingstone.

NHS Centre for Coding and Classification. (1996). *An introduction to the NHS Centre for Coding and Classification Version 4.0 IMG F6163.* Loughborough, UK: Information Management Group, NHS.

NHS Executive. (1996). *Building a bigger picture.* UK.

Peel, V. (1994). Management-focused health informatics research and education at the University of Manchester. *Methods of Information in Medicine, 33*, 273-277.

Robson, C. (2002). *Real world research.* Oxford: Blackwell Publishers Ltd.

Sayer, A. (2004). Foreword: Why critical realism? In S. Fleetwood & S. Ackroyd (Eds.), *Critical realist applications in organisation and management studies* (pp. 6-20). London: Routledge.

Sheaff, R., & Peel, V. (1995). *Managing health service information systems: An introduction.* Buckingham: Open University Press.

Shortliffe, E. H. (1991). Medical informatics and clinical decision making: The science and the pragmatics. *Medical Decision Making, 11*(Suppl. 4), S2-S14.

Thomas, J., Kellogg, W., & Erickson, T. (2001). The knowledge management puzzle: Human and social factors in knowledge management. *IBM Systems Journal, 40*(4), 863-884.

World Health Organization (WHO). (1993). *International statistical classification of diseases and related health problems* (10th revision, Vol. 2). Geneva, Switzerland: Author.

Wyatt, J. C. (1995). Hospital information management: The need for clinical leadership. *British Medical Journal, 311*(6998), 175-178.

KEY TERMS

Classifications: The action of classifying or arranging in classes according to common characteristics or affinities.

Code: The unique numerical identifier associated with a concept, which may be associated with a variety of terms all with the same meaning.

Critical Realism: The view that reality exists independently of our thoughts or beliefs. Research refers to this reality rather than constructing it.

Epistemology: The theory or science of the method or grounds of knowledge.

Models: Representations of real objects or phenomena, or templates for the creation of objects or phenomena.

Paradigm: A set of ideas about the phenomena under enquiry.

Phenomenology: A philosophical belief that interprets and experiences the world in terms of meanings and actively constructs an individual social reality.

Positivism: A philosophical view that aims to discover laws using quantitative methods and emphasizes positive facts.

Term: In medical terminology, it is a recognized name for a medical condition or treatment.

Chapter XXV
Goals and Benefits of Knowledge Management in Healthcare

Odysseas Hirakis
National and Kapodistrian University of Athens, Greece

Spyros Karakounos
National and Kapodistrian University of Athens, Greece

ABSTRACT

The aim of this chapter is to explain the role of knowledge management and how it can be successfully applied in the area of healthcare in order to improve health services and to increase patients' satisfaction. The first part of this chapter is about explaining the theories beyond knowledge management as "what is knowledge" and how it can be transformed and captured across people and organizations. The second part consists of the theory of knowledge management and the benefits of it in the area of healthcare in comparison with the old traditional systems. Knowledge management systems can be used to index and at the same time to spread all that information across people, libraries, and hospitals.

INTRODUCTION

During the last 10 to 15 years, knowledge management (KM) has become more popular day by day. There is a lot of interest in the concept of capturing and sharing knowledge with technology as the enabler. This requires the existence of a knowledge-sharing culture. The KM system stores historical knowledge and knowledge created during exchanges of information among people who are interested in learning. Knowledge management allows everyone to reuse the knowledge (best practice) or to create new ideas (innovation).

According to Syed Sibte Raza Abidi (2001, p. 1), "Knowledge Management (KM) in healthcare can be regarded as the confluence of formal methodologies and techniques to facilitate the creation, identification, acquisition, development, preservation, dissemination and finally the utilisation of the various facets of a healthcare enterprise's knowledge assets."

People in their everyday practice collect massive amounts of data and information that are knowledge poor, a fact that makes their decision about patients' cures more complicated. Knowledge in healthcare is deemed a high-value form of information that is necessary for healthcare professionals to act. For that matter, with the emergence of KM, the raw empirical data can be changed into empirical knowledge and provide professionals with a decision-support tool (Syed Sibte Raza Abidi, 2001).

KM in healthcare presents further interest for all those who are involved in the delivery of health services. KM allows rapid access to a knowledge treasure. The KM model goes beyond the need to manage data or information overload. It satisfies the requirements for implementing best practice and supplying high-quality health services, which increase patient satisfaction. The model aims at greater efficiency, coordination, and cost reduction. It is a portfolio of knowledge that increases ealth-care professionals' effectiveness and productivity. A KM system offers them the opportunity to learn how other colleagues successfully carried out similar problems (De Lusignan, Pritchard, & Chan, 2002).

WHAT IS KNOWLEDGE?

According to ITIL People (http://www.itilpeople.com/Glossary/Glossary_k.htm), "Knowledge is part of the hierarchy made up of data, information and knowledge. Data are raw facts. Information is data with context and perspective. Knowledge is information with guidance for action based upon insight and experience."

Figure 1. Knowledge pyramid (Marco, 2003)

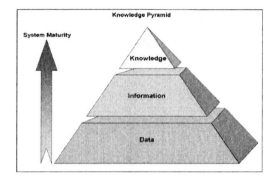

Knowledge is very difficult to define; it is not just a simple document or something that someone told us. In order for a person to gain knowledge, there are three stages to progress through as the pyramid (see Figure 1) indicates. The actual content in each stage becomes smaller, starting with data and finishing with knowledge.

1. **Data:** Documents, unorganized and unprocessed (raw material)
2. **Information:** Selected data ➔ Interpretation of the data (processed data)
3. **Knowledge:** Selected information ➔ Interpretation of the information

Example: In order to complete an academic assignment, some steps need to be taken:

1. Research at libraries and on the Internet; Collect some documents ➔ Data
2. Interpretation of that data ➔ Information
3. Interpretation and evaluation of the information ➔ Knowledge

TYPES OF KNOWLEDGE

Two types of knowledge exist in an organization.

1. **Explicit ("Know that"):** Something that is written down (informative texts) and can be easily understood if read, for example, technical reports and books
2. **Tacit ("Know how"):** Something that is written in the mind and cannot be easily expressed, for example, experience gained from a job

Knowledge management refers to the knowledge of a company as an asset, the same as land, for example (Ahmad, 2001).

TRANSFORMATION OF KNOWLEDGE

The transformation of knowledge is very important. The following explains Nonaka and Takeuchi's (1995) model of the four methods of knowledge conversion:

1. **Socialization:** Convert tacit knowledge into tacit knowledge; share experiences (tacit knowledge)
   Example: Two people discussing
2. **Externalization:** Convert tacit knowledge into explicit knowledge; write it down
   Example: Writing a report
3. **Combination:** Convert explicit knowledge into explicit knowledge; combine explicit knowledge
   Example: Reading two theories and from them creating a new one
4. **Internalization:** Convert explicit knowledge into tacit knowledge; gain experience
   Example: Learning from a book

Figure 2 demonstrates the conversion of knowledge according to Nonaka and Takeuchi's model.

Figure 2. Nonaka and Takeuchi's model

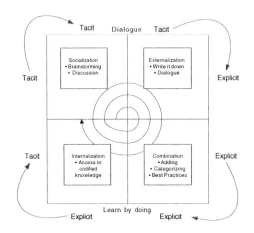

KNOWLEDGE MANAGEMENT

Peter Drucker first introduced the terms knowledge work and knowledge worker in the 1960s. Knowledge management as a term was coined back in the 1990s due to the fact that Japanese companies were at the top compared to other companies globally. Knowledge management is about organizing and managing the knowledge of workers.

To begin with, in order for a company to introduce knowledge management, it should first develop a culture of knowledge sharing within the organization. However, in order to develop a culture of sharing in a company, the employees need to trust each other and the company in advance. After the preparation of the ground, the IT part can take place. Workers then must take a training course on the KM software. Additionally, good management of the knowledge database is vital. This can be achieved by categorizing the knowledge database by subjects and dates, and by means of a search engine (Ahmad, 2003).

Imagine a library (physical) with a list of books that can be traced via computer software that indicates each bookshelf's column code and book details in order for a person to locate and borrow a book. Additionally, there are people (librarians) that make sure that the right book is in the right location. A knowledge-management system without knowledge sharing is like a virtual library that needs librarians to take care of it.

Knowledge management is completely based on a knowledge-sharing culture inside a company or between companies. People, by interacting with each other, create communities of practice. These people have common interests and aims; so, by cooperation, they develop their own kind of communication and rules.

People must share and exchange knowledge in order to find the best practice for a subject orto innovate knowledge. Once the knowledge is in the knowledge base, the knowledge analysts can begin seeking, studying, and analyzing the information in order to pull the quality knowledge. Afterward, the workers or professionals can go through the information, and pull and reuse the knowledge. This avoids the duplication of effort and dramatically reduces decision-making time. Knowledge management supports the requirement that successes and failures have to be recorded. The knowledge can then be accessed by the use of technology (Ahmad, 2003).

Knowledge management refers to knowledge as an asset that the company owns, like, for example, land and machinery. KM supports the fact that the most important resource in an organization is the people's knowledge. As a popular song says, "people have the power..."

A McKinsey survey outlined in the article "Creating a Knowledge Culture" illustrates the importance to create a need for knowledge:

Less successful companies tend to take a top-down approach: pushing knowledge to where it is needed. Successful companies, by contrast, reward employees for seeking,

sharing and creating knowledge. It requires effort to develop what we call "knowledge pull"—a grassroots desire among employees to tap into their company's intellectual resources. (Knowledge Portal, http://www.knowledge-portal.com/people.htm)

KM aims at keeping knowledge up to date and correct, providing knowledge in the right location, applying knowledge of the most suitable type, and providing knowledge at the time at which it is needed.

In other words, KM allows for securing and distributing knowledge in order to assure and optimise its availability (Montani & Bellazzi, 2002).

KNOWLEDGE MANAGEMENT IN HEALTHCARE

According to the Royal College of Surgeons in Ireland (http://www.rcsi.ie), there are 10,000 different diseases and syndromes, 3,000 types of drugs, 1,100 different types of laboratory tests, and finally 400,000 articles added per annum to the biomedical literature.

Furthermore, internal medicine includes 2 million facts (Wyatt, 2003). The growth rate in biomedical literature doubles every 19 years (Wyatt, 1991).

Doctors' decisions determine three quarters of healthcare costs and depend critically on medical knowledge (Tierney, Miller, Overhage, & McDonald, 1993). Once knowledge has been captured in some form such as a guideline, it can be managed (Wyatt, 2001).

Knowledge in medicine arrives from reports, libraries, experience, guidelines, laboratory experiments, protocols, practice, group meetings, and so forth. By adding interaction between these forces, then the outcome can be superior.

Because of the above reasons, the use of knowledge management is critical in the healthcare sector. By having a sharing culture with a common aim—the best possible patient care—and by using an information system, not for data warehousing but instead for interpretation and annotation to create knowledge, then the healthcare sector can be dramatically improved.

Healthcare organizations need to improve the quality of patients' treatment. This includes a decision-support system (best practice) and the reduction of errors in patients' diagnoses and treatment.

Two kinds of healthcare information exist: information about patients and information about cases. In order for professionals to be accurate, both kinds of information are needed. By combining these two kinds of information, professionals are able to come up with the right solution (UCL, http://www.ucl.ac.uk/kmc/resources/top_tips.html).

By using a successful knowledge-management system tool, professionals are able to make conclusions by interpreting and understanding patients' data and by carrying out a successful diagnosis in order for the right actions to be applied.

Furthermore, by using a KM system, professionals are able to access the right information and advice at the right time. However, if there is a difference between a theory in the knowledge base and the related practice, professionals can add comments for later improvement.

By implementing knowledge management, professionals can have access to best practices, and if they are able to understand the importance of a knowledge-sharing culture, then there is also some space for development and innovation. Furthermore, a KM system can improve the decision-making time and so also reduce the costs of a hospital (as a famous slogan says, "time is money").

Professionals can explore and learn faster by going through the knowledge database and studying the cases of other patients and the specific treatments that were applied to them. Furthermore, professionals can apply to evidence-based clinical guidelines.

Besides this, each hospital may be positioned in different places globally, which makes it difficult for a person to access another hospital's knowledge. With KM, research (healthcare) departments that are carrying out experiments can provide other hospitals with knowledge by using a KM system.

Imagine that a conference on a new infection is to take place, but not all doctors across the country are able to attend. By using a knowledge-management system, the doctors that were absent could log in and see a video or a tape on a specific subject and contribute later to that problem by using the KM system.

Moreover, other problems based on the management of the hospital's staff and strategies could be discussed between managers or doctors in order to improve the quality of services offered. Afterward, the amount of information could be written down (explicit) for future reuse by other hospitals.

According to Wyatt (2001, p. 8):

The future of knowledge management in health is bright. We already have adequate technology in the shape of the Internet and a good intellectual framework in evidence-based health, which are being used to improve each other. We also have many health librarians who are knowledge management professionals.

The importance of knowledge management can also be justified by presenting Table 1, which illustrates the differences between the old and the new healthcare elements.

Table 1. Old and new health-care paradigms (Olson, 2004)

Old Health-Care Paradigm	New Health-Care Paradigm
• HIS System • Operations Oriented • Hierarchical Database • Programmer Centric • Silo Based • Character Based • Fragmented Decision Support	• Enterprise-Wide Knowledge-Management System • Analysis Oriented • Relational Database • End-User Centric • Process Based • GUI (Graphical User Interface) and Web Based • Holistic Decision Support

Example: Alerts or recommendations described in literature (McDonald, 1976)

If treatment includes cardiac glycoside
  and last premature ventricular systoles/minute > 2
  then "Consider cardiac glycoside as cause of arrhythmia"

Result: When data matches events, a recommendation is printed out for the doctor.

Impact: The frequency with which doctors responded to target events doubled from 22% to 51%.

GOALS AND BENEFITS OF KNOWLEDGE MANAGEMENT IN HEALTHCARE

- Support in decision making about patients, interference, and the evaluation of research
- Enhanced healthcare system by improving communication between professionals in the decision-making process
- Improved patient healthcare
- Improved quality, access time, and portability of healthcare
- Increased communication between professionals and hospitals

- Improved cost management by reducing the time of patients' hospital treatment
- Reduced time of decision making by using a knowledge database and consequently the reduction of the time of patients' residence in hospitals
- Reduced error rate (defects) in decision making
- Reduced inconvenience
- Increased patient satisfaction

CONCLUSION

Without doubt, the KM model constitutes a hopeful innovation in the health sector with more possibilities and uses. It is about time for a qualitative upgrade of health-services provision to take place. It is obvious that the direct access o all healthcare professionals in KM will minimise medical errors, decrease the medium duration of hospitalisation, reduce the cost of hospitalisation, increase the patient's satisfaction, and have a positive contribution to the relation of cost and effectiveness.

People have to bear in mind that the health-services sector has a specific particularity: Patients are human beings with particular needs, special characters, and different interactions in therapeutic interventions. KM is a tool that helps healthcare professionals to implement the best practices while considering the special needs of each patient, and sometimes to innovate. IT in knowledge management is just the enabler; the idea is for people to start sharing experiences and ideas with a common aim. Finally, healthcare remains a human science with a strong scientific basis; its consultations have such high levels of complexity that they probably can never be completely computerised and automated.

REFERENCES

Abidi, S. S. R. (2001). Knowledge management in healthcare: Towards "knowledge-driven" decision-support services. *International Journal of Medical Informatics, 63,* 5-18.

Ahmad, K. (2001). *The knowledge of organisations and the organisation of knowledge.* UK: University of Surrey.

De Lusignan, S., Pritchard, K., & Chan, T. (2002). A knowledge-management model for clinical practice. *J Postgrad Med, 48,* 297-303.

Godbolt, S. (n.d.). *Moving into knowledge management in the NHS, issue 3.* London: London Library.

Marco, D. (2003). *A meta-data repository is the key to knowledge management.* Brookfiled: Enterprise Warehousing Solutions.

McDonald, C. J. (1976). Protocol-based computer reminders: The quality of care and the non-perfectability of man. *New England Journal of Medicine, 295,* 1351-1355.

Montani, S., & Bellazzi, R. (2002). Supporting decisions in medical applications: The knowledge management perspective. *International Journal of Medical Informatics, 68,* 79-90.

Myers, F. (2003). *Knowledge management in healthcare: Succeeding in spite of technology.* FL: AFSM International.

Nanaka, I., & Takeuchi, H. (1995). *The knowledge-creating company: How Japanese companies create the dynamics of innovation.* New York: Oxford University Press.

Olson, E. (2004). *Knowledge management & business intelligence in healthcare.* Coppell: The Shams Group.

Tierney, W. M., Miller, M. E., Overhage, J. M., & McDonald, C. J. (1993). Physician order writing on microcomputer workstations. *JAMA, 269,* 379-383.

Wyatt, J. (1991). Use and sources of medical knowledge. *Lancet, 338,* 1368-1373.

Wyatt, J. (2001). *Clinical knowledge and practice in the information age: A handbook for health professionals.* London: RSM Press.

Wyatt, J. (2003). *When do we need support systems?* London: National Institute for Clinical Excellence.

KEY TERMS

Best Practice: The distillation of accumulated wisdom about the most effective way to carry out a business activity or process. However, what is best is highly subjective and context dependent, so the term implies that no further improvements are possible.

Community of Practice: A group of people who share and develop their knowledge in pursuit of a common purpose or task, even though they do not necessarily work in the same department or organization.

Explicit Knowledge: Knowledge that is codified and articulated. It appears in the form of documents and procedures and can be found in databases.

IT: Information technology.

Knowledge Analyst: A person or business that interprets the needs of a knowledge seeker and finds the most suitable sources.

Knowledge Base: A computer-held database that records knowledge in an appropriate format for later extraction. It may take various forms depending on whether it supports an expert system or contains documents and textual information for human retrieval.

Knowledge Management: The explicit and systematic management of vital knowledge and its associated processes of creation, gathering, organization, diffusion, use, and exploitation in pursuit of organizational objectives.

Tacit Knowledge: Knowledge that is not codified but held in people's heads. Intuitive, experiential, judgmental, and context sensitive, it may be difficult to articulate.

Chapter XXVI
Knowledge Management in Medicine

Nikolaos Giannakakis
National and Kapodistrian University of Athens, Greece

Efstratios Poravas
National and Kapodistrian University of Athens, Greece

ABSTRACT

In the last decades, the amount of information has risen because of the technology revolution. The need for organizing information, in a way that the staff and the managers of a hospital require, lead to the generation of a new value, the knowledge management. Its benefits are sensible, not only for the staff, but also for the hospital as an entity. Many techniques are applied to solve all the daily problems in the health sector.

INTRODUCTION

During the last three decades of the previous century, there was a revolution in technology and its applications in medicine and the field of information. The promotion of knowledge and its communicability certainly have profited all the scientific sectors, both in the increase of efficiency and productivity, and in the growth of innovations.

Knowledge management is a notion that is difficult to define. A lot of definitions have been formulated, one of which is that knowledge management is an organism that is constituted of small parts that aim to collect, assess, unify, improve, and produce value from intellectual and information-based resources (Association of State and Territorial Health Officials [ASTHO], 2005).

Progress in medicine is essential; there has always been the mass production of knowledge, and those who are related to this science should take it into account, develop it, and apply it. Traditional sources of information are available, but they usually fail to provide answers whenever and wherever they are needed. Thus, roughly two thirds of problems in clinical practice remain unsolved (Gale Group, 2001). Unfortunately, the information and knowledge that are available to doctors nowadays are poorly organized and old.

In the healthcare field, doctors and patients need help with the choice of better actions for a given situation. The rate of growth and change in worldwide biomedical knowledge leads to the fact that no one is able to know the current practices in a sector without any kind of support (Purves & Robinson, 2003). A partial solution to this problem can perhaps be brought by medical knowledge management. Its aim is the regrouping, incorporation, and connection of any medical knowledge that was produced in the past in order for one to reach a reasonable decision in the present and useful study in the future (Quantum Enterprises, Inc., 2003).

Generally, knowledge management in the medical field can ensure the effective growth and dissemination of better practices, and a continuous assessment aiming at their improvement. Knowledge is created within time. All the data that constitute its base become information when they can be summarized and organized under reasonable models. Information becomes knowledge when it can be managed for active decision making, and knowledge can be turned into perspicacity when it is well developed within regular periods of time (Lobodzinski & Criley, n.d.).

USE AND VALUE OF KNOWLEDGE MANAGEMENT

The continuous effort toward efficiency and economic effectiveness creates a balance among the quality of provided services, and it includes costs that lead to the more effective management of medical knowledge that is derived from biomedical research. The need for a

clinical process in the providing of medical care is rather obvious (Stefanelli, 2002). Thus, knowledge management in the field of medicine focuses on the knowledge of technologies used in clinical, administrative, and demographic activity. Today, the pressure of cost also influences the sector of health. The adoption of information technology is considered one of the basic mechanisms for the reduction of cost ("Data and Knowledge Management in Healthcare," 2005).

The society of public health is continuously focused on digital communication for the fulfillment of different kinds of tasks. Although technology has improved for the possibility of the collection, analysis, and dissemination of data, there are still obstacles in the use of information, such as the existence of information that is not well organized and systems that are not complete. The continuous improvement of technology, the lack of resources, the failure to confirm the requirements of data, and complicated data have led experts to the use and exploitation of existing knowledge for the promotion of health (Data and Knowledge Management for Public Health, 2005).

Through knowledge management we can certainly reduce the gap between the lack of data and the lack of systems that develop those data. Starting with the presumption that every problem has a solution, the effective management of knowledge in the health sector can constitute the base of knowledge, which is essential for the presentation of its innovations and distribution in a dynamically regenerative process (Bailey, 2003). Generally, there is a framework in hospitals that can be used as a driver for the management of knowledge. This is a methodology that helps with the designing of a strategy and its processes, and that enriches the transmission of knowledge and tools that support the collection and analysis of knowledge, and the storage and search of informa-

Table 1. Causes of errors (Institute of Medicine [IOM], 2000)

• Technical errors		44%
• Incorrect diagnosis		17%
• Failure in damage prevention		12%
• Errors in pharmaceutical contact ion		10%

Table 2. Most frequent errors (IOM, 2000)

• Incorrect diagnosis		40%
• Incorrect issuing of medicines		28%
• Errors in medical protocols		22%
• Administrative errors		4%

tion. All these occur in collaboration with the personnel, the economic resources, suitable systems that allow communication in all kinds of situations, and the infrastructure so that the maximum effectiveness, efficiency, and creativity are ensured (*Managing Knowledge to Improve Reproductive Health Programs*, 2004).

BENEFITS OF KNOWLEDGE MANAGEMENT

In a hospital, even more than in any other organization, knowledge management becomes a necessity since a vast number of research by global organizations, both in Europe and the USA, has proven that a lot of people have died and a great part of the government budget was spent due to errors, which would probably have been avoided with the use of knowledge management. Even though there has been major

technological and scientific growth, which has been observed during the last few decades in all the scientific sectors, the medical errors, and, generally speaking, all kinds of errors, that occur in hospitals remain frequent and rather expensive. In the year 2000, the Medical Institute reported that medical errors cost the medical industry and the pharmaceutical industry $37 billion annually, and 100,000 people lose their lives each year because of these errors (Detmer, 2001).

Table 1 presents the basic reasons that led to medical errors.

Table 2 presents the types of errors that occur most frequently.

Table 3 presents errors due to the medical personnel.

It is obvious that there are plenty of medical errors, they cost the state a lot of money, they can be dangerous for the lives of patients, and they basically occur due to human factors. About 70% of these errors could have been

Table 3. Errors due to medical personnel (IOM, 2000)

• Negligence/carelessness	29%
• Inexperienced/uneducated personnel	14%
• Communication	12%
• Incorrect diagnosis	8%
• Tiredness of personnel	8%
• Illegible recipe or incorrect issuing of medicines	6%
• Other errors	14%

avoided or even prevented. According to the Medical Company of the USA, in the year 2000, 250,000 deaths were caused due to medical factors (JAMA, 2000). Even though the number seems rather small compared to the entire population of the USA (about the 0.07% of the population), it is very important and should have called to action all experts in the health sector. Knowledge management basically aims to reduce expenses and costs, as well as to increase productivity and efficiency, which will lead indirectly to the reduction of human losses. Each employee should consider his or her knowledge so we can trust him or her when it comes to the resolution of problems, the avoiding of errors, and the assuring of positive results and practices.

OBJECTIVES OF KNOWLEDGE MANAGEMENT: PROBLEM SOLVING

Knowledge management has a very positive impact on all sciences. Its aim is to serve each science separately and minimize the errors derived from the lack of knowledge. Generally, we should choose which information is essential in an organization, such as a hospital, and how we can facilitate the transport of knowledge to it. It is crucial to improve the perception of all the factors involved in the field of health and to support the new methods and technologies, which are not always accepted easily by the personnel of hospitals.

The main objective of knowledge management is to help in the briefing of our knowledge, and to aid its enrichment and exploitation. Today there are systems that aim at improving and promoting knowledge. This can be achieved through the review of practical progress in order to find, develop, disseminate, and use the knowledge for the profit of doctors and patients. Furthermore, these systems achieve an approach among the experts in different kinds of sciences facilitating exchange between the existing and the new techniques in the field of health (*Advances in Clinical Knowledge Management Workshops*, n.d.).

Table 4 presents examples of techniques in knowledge management in the medical field.

From Table 4 comes the conclusion that the main objectives of knowledge management are the isolation and later development of the structures of knowledge, the production of its gradual structures for the description of a future connection, the proposal to create functional systems for the development of medical knowl-

Table 4. Examples of techniques in knowledge management

- Best practices in the management of special medical situations
- Analysis of indications for those situations
- Reports on existing and new medicines
- Development of direct and explicit information regarding complicated medical subjects
- Use of special vocabulary and a common language for names of medicines, illnesses, and so forth
- Determination of the available sources
- Analysis of data, taking into consideration the danger factors
- Ability for direct access to the data anytime, anyplace
- Information regarding actions that should be done in case of emergency
- Creation of protocols under which people in the health field should work
- Research and better practices for the settlement of medical subjects
- Research for new diseases that appear in society
- Finding of information related to the health conditions of a population in a given geographical zone
- Thorough interconnection of information among multiple choices, for example, handbooks and depictions
- Access to descriptions of diseases, practices, and research reports
- Knowledge regarding treatments that can be applied
- Access to informative pages of the hospital, and more important for other hospitals, the acquisition of data and comparison of situations
- Unified communication and informative sending-receiving data systems

(ASTHO, 2005)

edge, better comprehension of problems and decision making, and the application of knowledge management in medical information technology in all clinical departments and health systems.

SAFETY OF KNOWLEDGE MANAGEMENT

The information conveyed to doctors is turned later into knowledge, either through the development of computer-based systems or through the development of tools that will be used by experts in the field of information in collaboration with clinical groups. The knowledge and information by themselves are not in a position to improve clinical practices. The organized and professional management of information is required by all professionals (Sozou, 1998).

Knowledge is undefined, is precious in its acquisition, and can be easily lost or stolen in order to be converted or erased afterward. In the world of technologies nowadays, where everything tends to function digitally, a lot of mechanisms as well as structures are used for the protection of knowledge. A model that can ensure knowledge management should ensure its protection as well. In other words, it is essential in an informative system to ensure the authenticity of knowledge; the safety of data from any kind of involuntary or voluntary modification, destruction, or revelation of its elements; the integrity of data; and the general application of political safety to information (Mundy & Chadwick, n.d.).

Table 5. Advantages of knowledge management for hospital personnel

- To avoid errors that happened in the past
- To reduce the time needed for the detection of information, mainly for urgent incidents
- To assure the best clinical decisions by inexperienced employees
- To find alternative procedures of care in emergency situations
- To identify a lack of information, which can lead to errors
- To encourage the flow of ideas, which leads to innovations
- To avoid unnecessary procedures and increase cohesion and collaboration among employees
- To increase productivity and efficiency

Table 6. Advantages of knowledge management in a hospital

- Improvement of quality of sanitary care through the increased efficiency and productivity of personnel
- Facilitation of communication between medical personnel
- Reduction of expenses mainly from the pointless use of medicines and unnecessary insertion of patients in the hospital
- Creation of strategies for a vast number of data
- Contribution of hospital profits and better use of money, which would be unavailable without knowledge management

ADVANTAGES IN THE USE OF KNOWLEDGE MANAGEMENT

Knowledge management has a lot to offer to a hospital, and even more to its personnel. A technical and organizational infrastructure can be achieved. Table 5 presents its advantages for the personnel of a hospital.

Table 6 presents the major advantages of knowledge management in a hospital.

DISADVANTAGES IN THE USE OF KNOWLEDGE MANAGEMENT

Knowledge management has a lot of advantages, but also presents a lot of disadvantages. If there is not an explicit determination of knowledge and we do not recognize its importance, then we will not be able to achieve its appropriate management. In some cases, we focus on the past and the present and care less

Table 7. Disadvantages presented by knowledge management due to certain reasons

- Knowledge in medicine is incomplete, vague, and inaccurate, and requires many years for its acquisition.
- There is a continuous alteration of knowledge as technology develops.
- There is excessive emphasis on the reserve of knowledge and not on its flux.
- Doctors usually forget the aim of knowledge management and do not realize the complexity of the knowledge that is distributed.

about the future, giving emphasis on counting knowledge and not on its results.

Generally, despite the increasing power of information technology, knowledge management in the form of supporting decisions and information concerning doctors has minimum impact on the results of healthcare. This occurs due to the fact that knowledge management addresses the relationship between patients and personnel; it does not provide harmony between the complexity of individuals and their regular actions that form special practices (Purves & Robinson, 2003).

Usually the efforts toward the medical management of knowledge are underestimated. As far as the systems are concerned, an uncontrolled increase of medical knowledge can lead to disaster (Quantum Enterprises, Inc., 2003). Table 7 presents some of the reasons why knowledge management is not efficient and presents disadvantages.

THE FUTURE OF KNOWLEDGE MANAGEMENT

Through the practices and techniques, doctors can have easier access to new information concerning medicine and their applications, diagnostic tests, and the way diseases are treated,

as well as established policies and processes. This access will decrease the possibility of costly medical errors and will promote healthcare for patients in the hospital (Detmer, 2001).

It is very important to create a network aiming at collaboration among experts and at the improvement of methods for the collection and analysis of data both for the present needs and the forthcoming ones. The future of medical knowledge management is in the present. We should take advantage of the revolution of technologies and information that has begun during the last decades (Gale Group, 2001). In the future, in order to reach the use and application of knowledge, we should analyze the existing aims, the types of knowledge, the users and their sources, the processes, and the technologies (Bouthillier & Shearer, 2002).

CONCLUSION

Knowledge management is a basic tool for all those working in the health field and for hospitals. It helps in sending the right information to the right person at the right time so that the right decisions can be made depending on the existing problems. It is certain that with the help of knowledge management, effectiveness in the health field will be increased through unified systems, processes, and methods; the cultivation of exchanging knowledge; and the promotion of the effective use of available information.

REFERENCES

Advances in clinical knowledge management workshops. (n.d.). Retrieved from http://www.ucl.ac.uk

Association of State and Territorial Health Officials (ASTHO). (2005). *Knowledge management for public health professionals.*

Baily, C. (2003). *Bulleting of the World Health Organization, 81*(11).

Bouthillier, F., & Shearer, K. (2002). Understanding knowledge management and information management: The need for an empirical perspective. *Information Research, 8*(1). Retrieved from http://Information.net/ir/8-1/paper14

Data and knowledge management in healthcare. (2005). *Proceedings of the 38th International Conference on System Sciences.*

Detmer, W. M. (2001). *Medical knowledge management solutions: Revolutionizing the delivery of medical information to the point of need.* Retrieved from http://www.unboundmedicine.com/healthcarereview.htm

Gale Group. (2001). *Healthcare review.* Retrieved April 2005, from http://www.findarticles.com

Institute of Medicine (IOM). (2000). *To err is human: Building a safer health system.* Retrieved from http://www.iom.edu./object.file/Masater/4/117/ToErr-8paper.pdf

Lobodzinski, S. M., & Criley, M. (n.d.). *Medical knowledge management.* Torrance: California State University Long Beach & Harbor UCLA Medical Center.

Managing knowledge to improve reproductive health programs (MAQ Paper No. 5). (2004).

Mercola. (2000). *Journal of the American Medical Association* (JAMA), *284*(4), 483-485.

Mundy, D., & Chadwick, D. W. (n.d.). *Secure knowledge management for health care organizations.* Retrieved from http://sec.isi.salford.ac.uk/download/SecureKM.pdf

Purves, I., & Robinson, P. (2003). Knowledge management for health. *Medical Education, 37,* 429-433.

Purves, I., & Robinson, P. (2004). Knowledge management for health programs. *Medinfo,* 678-682.

Quantum Enterprises, Inc. (2003). Knowledge integration and management. Retrieved from http://www.quantument.com

Sozou, P. (1998). *Advances in clinical knowledge management.* London: University College.

Steffanelli, M. (2002). Knowledge management to support performance-based medicine. *Methods of Information in Medicine, 41*(1), 36-43.

KEY TERMS

Data: The representation of facts, concepts, or instructions in a formalized manner suitable for communication, interpretation, or processing by humans or by automatic means.

They are also any representations such as characters or analog quantities to which meaning is or might be assigned.

Empirical or A Posteriori Knowledge: Prepositional knowledge obtained by experience. It is contrasted with a priori knowledge, or knowledge that is gained through the apprehension of innate ideas, intuition, pure reason, or other nonexperiential sources.

Information System: A system, whether automated or manual, that comprises people, machines, and methods organized to collect, process, transmit, and disseminate data that represent user information.

Knowledge: A fluid mix of framed experience, values, contextual information, and expert insight that provides a framework for evaluating and incorporating new experiences and information. It originates and is applied in the minds of knowers. In organizations, it often becomes embedded not only in documents or repositories, but also in organizational routines, processes, practices, and norms.

Knowledge Base: A special kind of database for knowledge management. It is the base for the collection of knowledge. Normally, the knowledge base consists of the explicit knowledge of an organization, including troubleshooting, articles, white papers, user manuals, and others. A knowledge base should have a carefully designed classification structure, content format, and search engine.

Knowledge-Based System: A program for extending and querying a knowledge base.

Knowledge Management: Caters to the critical issues of organizational adaptation, survival, and competence in the face of increasingly discontinuous environmental change. Essentially, it embodies organizational processes that seek the synergistic combination of data and the information-processing capacity of information technologies, and the creative and innovative capacity of human beings.

Knowledge-Management System: A distributed hypermedia system for managing knowledge in organizations.

Knowledge Relativity: The relation between a form of representation, two sorts of intent (communication and use goals), and three subjects (one who knows, one who is informed, and one who observes and confirms).

Chapter XXVII
Knowledge Management in Telemedicine

Jayanth G. Paraki
Telemedicine Research Laboratory, India

ABSTRACT

Knowledge management (KM) can be defined as the discovery and dissemination of new knowledge. It has also been defined as the efficient utilisation of the existing intangible knowledge-related resources available in every sector of the economy to enhance the productivity of all factors of production. Telemedicine is a tool to enhance equitable distribution of healthcare across the world. In this chapter the author discusses the various aspects of knowledge management and telemedicine and proposes to globalize telemedicine.

INTRODUCTION

Organizations all over the world are adapting to rapid changes in many ways, and an approach that has made significant contributions to the resurrection of postwar Japanese industry is Deming's philosophy of total quality management (TQM). Deming's TQM is indeed applicable to the management of Internet businesses and eminently suitable for telemedicine and data-mining projects in life sciences. The apparent complexity of the system may appear as a deterrent to many, but the inherent simplicity is clear on examination of the Deming charter points. Leaders of Internet business houses will derive rich benefits from applying Deming's TQM to their organization, while investors will find it comfortable to interact with such organizations.

There is an urgent need for healthcare professionals to be multiskilled. Doctors and nurses have to introspect periodically and adopt a plan for self-improvement that should include acquiring new knowledge, developing a positive mental attitude, and learning new skills to meet the rapidly changing health needs of people across the globe.

The methods of diagnosis and treatment of human diseases have altered significantly in the last decade. In the early 1990s, the first signals of change began to surface with patients expressing dissatisfaction and discontent with one or more aspects of their care. Unknown to their primary-care physicians, they began to talk about their experiences with the hope that a degree of attitudinal change would emerge in some physicians, and permanent solutions to chronic health problems would start emerging. Direct patient-doctor communication was not in evidence, and institutions committed to healthcare chose not to encourage free discussions with their clients. This pattern persisted over the best part of that decade and led to strained communications between physicians and patients. This at one time resembled an estranged love affair, with neither party willing to move forward to resolve the conflict. However, before long, the Internet revolution became a phenomenon and made its presence felt in healthcare activities. Curiously, the initial recognition of the value of this phenomenon was made by suffering patients who realized the Internet was a handy tool to share their tales of woe amongst themselves and to obtain a degree of temporary relief and comfort. It was fortunate that some physicians had woken up to this phenomenon simultaneously and had begun to address the different scientific aspects in a proactive manner.

During the period of 1998 to 2000, the undercurrents of rapid information exchange were being felt, with different nations discovering its effects through a variety of experiences. Limiting the discussion on the influence of the Internet phenomenon on healthcare, we begin to see certain common patterns emerging across a wide spectrum of diseases across the globe, making data mining an exciting and profitable activity. The need is to automate:

- The right process,
- To the right population,
- At the right time,
- Through the right channel.

It is obvious that there are many elements of equal importance that have to be brought together in order to succeed at biomedical computing and data mining. What then has to be done to amalgamate these elements into a single whole in order to begin the process of data mining? Simply stated, if we have a foolproof system and the necessary human intelligence, it is possible to build a data warehouse and then mine it into saleable data marts for global consumption. I believe that the global scientific community possesses both the system and the intelligence to do this successfully.

The purpose of this chapter is to highlight the capability of Deming's total quality management to provide the directions and impetus to establish a framework for data mining in life sciences, and to demonstrate through a simple application the different ways to apply Deming's 14 charter points in actual practice (Creech, 1995). The future possibilities are varied and some thoughts will be shared toward creating an international consortium for the research and development of telemedicine applications (Paraki, 2001).

THE CONTEXT

In the last decade, observations of results of treatment with allopathy show it is incomplete and inadequate. This applies to both the outpatient and inpatient care of those with acute and chronic ailments. Patient dissatisfaction is evident in patients with chronic diseases such as arthritis, bronchial asthma, and many functional disorders like migraines, obstinate constipation, and irritable bowel syndrome. Furthermore, extensive interaction with professionals from other disciplines like management, IT, telecommunications, fundamental sciences, psychology, and philosophy has provided a solid basis for the development of holistic medicine as a preferred approach to the prevention and treatment of acute and chronic disease. This is keeping in tune with the current changes in developed nations such as the USA and those in Europe where holistic medicine is gaining popularity.

Management in this context not only implies the way hospitals and health universities function, but also the need for a change in the healthcare systems and processes themselves. Data mining in life sciences will truly and correctly provide the right evidence and direction to nations keen on making holistic medicine a viable, cost-effective alternative to meet their healthcare challenges and needs.

In the year 2000, in a report titled *To Err is Human: Building a Safer Health System*, the Institute of Medicine estimated that as many as 98,000 deaths per year occur in the United States because of medical errors that could have been prevented. The additional cost in pain and suffering as well as in dollars—estimated between $17 billion and $29 billion—as a result of preventable medical errors is unconscionable in an age where the technology exists to virtually eliminate such occurrences. Worse, these studies account only for hospitals. They do not begin to address the errors and their resulting consequences in other healthcare settings such as nursing homes, home care, day surgery, outpatient clinics, and care delivered in doctors' offices.

According to the Institute of Medicine, the majority of medical errors do not result from individual recklessness, but from "basic flaws in the way the health system is organized."

These flaws reach into every aspect of the healthcare enterprise, from illegible, paper-based medical charts to large segmented health systems that fail to provide for adequate communications among caregivers. Medical care today can be a complex combination of therapeutic treatments and sophisticated drug regimens administered by many different healthcare professionals at different sites. Under these conditions and given more than ample opportunity for human error, it is no mystery we have a problem. Long-term solutions require considerable political will and the ability to attract champions who can help craft answers that will not cripple the process with malpractice litigation. The Institute of Medicine has sounded the alarm. Are we prepared to answer it?

WHY DEMING?

The 1994 *Survey on Change Management* published by the AMA and Deloitte & Touche says, "It seems that many organizations have to change in order to change. Their present structures and cultures tend to disallow the successful implementation of change initiatives." I find the same in the healthcare industry, too. This change is of a global dimension, and Deming's TQM (Creech, 1995) will be able to bring many organizations and nations together on a common platform to strive for a higher global cause. Telemedicine technology coupled with Deming's TQM will ensure that change initiatives will meet with success. Networked organizations thrive better than others and are ideal for live projects in life sciences (Woodcock, 2001).

Application of Deming Charter Points

Point 1: The constant improvement of health services is a must. Technology integration speeds up the process. Holistic medicine offers paths to total quality health for those with the following diseases: cancer, AIDS (acquired immunodeficiency syndrome), and mental depression. TQM is ideal for securing global cooperation to fight these diseases with vigor and vitality.

Point 2: The philosophy of holistic medicine is the need of the hour. There are different schools of thought, and each nation has to harmonize their philosophical thinking with scientific temper to allow proven benefits to reach the masses.

Point 3: Dependence on laboratory tests alone is to be avoided, and close personal interaction with patients is a must. Furthermore, the careless repetition of tests, too-frequent tests, and inappropriately timed tests are some of the sources of avoidable drain of financial resources to the individual and the organization. Herein lies one of the values of a robust, correctly designed informational database. Later, we will see its relationship to an operational database, which is a part of a data warehouse and its different uses.

Point 4: I have deliberately left out addressing this point at this stage. I believe that this is a very personal issue at this stage of global telemedicine technology development, and while there are several financial and revenue models that have proved successful, none have evolved fully to become a reference model for global following. Continued learning and mature knowledge sharing is essential to enable unshakeable clarity of perception to be gained in the economics of telemedicine technology,[1] and this may well prove to become a major aspect of global research study in the future.

Point 5: Improve constantly and forever the diagnostic and therapeutic processes. To do this successfully, baseline data have to be recorded, stored, and retrieved at will. Database systems and data-mining methodology will influence the outcome of disease research and hence is of overriding importance.

What is data mining? Data mining, by its simplest definition, automates the detection of relevant patterns in a database. However, data mining is not magic. For many years, statisticians have manually mined databases, looking for statistically significant patterns. In traditional business use, data mining uses well-established statistical and machine-learning techniques to build models that predict customer behavior. When discussing models in life sciences, the definition of a customer undergoes a bit of a modification in the sense that a patient is not viewed as a customer, and a customer need not be a patient. The need for building models in life sciences exists in diverse situations, and when viewed globally, is a healthy exercise physically, mentally, and financially.

Data Mining and Data Warehousing: The Connection

Data mining describes a collection of techniques that aim to find useful but undiscovered patterns in collected data. The goal of data mining is to create models for decision making that predict future behavior based on analyses of past activity. Data mining supports knowledge discovery, defined by William Frawley and Gregory Piatetsky-Shapiro (1991) as "the nontrivial extraction of implicit, previously unknown, and potentially useful information from data" This definition holds the key to the substantial interest in data warehousing and data mining. The method used today in data mining, when it is well thought out and well executed, consists of just a few very important concepts. The first of these is the concept of finding a pattern in the data. In many cases, this just means any collection of data that occurs a surprising number of times. Usually, surprising is better defined, but in general it means any sequence or pattern of data that occurs more often than one would expect it to if it were a random event. For example, the occurrence of breast cancer in unmarried women in the age group 30 to 40 is significantly higher than in married women of the same age group. What is the relationship between marriage and the incidence of breast cancer? The answer lies in the simple fact that in unmarried women, the intended natural function of pregnancy and subsequent child rearing being denied renders them more susceptible to the development of breast cancer. This piece of data makes it easy to suspect early breast cancer in susceptible women in the age group 30 40, and alerts doctors and/or patients to request for further tests to confirm or refute the suspicion. Data mining will throw further light on various subgroups within this larger main group, allowing far greater precision and control in designing breast-cancer screening programs and the clinical evaluation of various treatment protocols including that drawn from alternative and complementary medicines. Another very important concept associated with data mining is that of validating the predictive models that arise out of data-mining algorithms. For example, if lesbian women remain unmarried in their lifetime and if it is proved that the incidence of breast cancer is statistically higher in them, then an intervention program based on alternative and complementary medicines is already available for implementation and may prove valuable in the age group 20 to 30 to ward off future threat from this dreaded disease. There is a growing body of scientific literature attesting to this fact, and multination clinical trials are justified to validate the data. If the four parts of data-mining technology are patterns, sampling, validation, and the choosing of the model, then the study of the incidence of breast cancer in lesbian women and its diagnosis and treatment is warranted and justified, and is suitable for multination trial since the disease is ubiquitous in distribution. Equally suitable is

the use of data-mining technology to gather data from many different breast-cancer centers around the world.

Point 6: Institute training for both vendor and client organizations is of vital importance vital importance if the intended product or service is to be marketed successfuly. Healthcare professionals engaged in telemedicine activity can ill-afford to neglect this vital exercise. The ranges of skills are varied and are determined by functional needs. Training can be as simple as learning how to use Microsoft Word or as complex as learning Oracle Database Management. Nevertheless, training flows seamlessly with the rest of the activities of the organization and does not usually pose a serious problem.

Point 7: Adopt and institute leadership (Adair, 1993). Successful Leaders are those who convert ideas, contexts, and discoveries into practical undertakings. Greater success will be achieved through the optimal use of technology and team functioning. Highly focused efforts with minimal scattering of energies are more likely to produce noticeable results than diverse activities aimed at several goals. Scaleable-systems development is the need of the hour in life sciences, and it is essential to recognize what the ideal fundamental system is.

Point 8: Drive out fear. Fear as an incentive to improve work performance has been explored at length. Universally, it has a finite limit to induce consistent elevation of performance or to produce quality products and services. Deming realized this during his experience in Japan after World War II and stressed the need for leaders to arrive at suitable methods to drive out fear from within their organizations. One of the possible methods is to structure the primary organization with care with attention to minute details as regards the functional abilities of the hired or chosen people, and to put in place a system of reward and punishment that is attitude based rather than incentive based. Team working and collective consciousness also help to minimize and eliminate fear progressively.

Point 9: Break down barriers between staff areas. Academic and research activities are often slow due to several barriers that exist within a group. While some are necessary and healthy, others are simply laborious and energy sapping and are better removed than allowed to exist undetected. In the modern information age, intellectual property rights have assumed greater relevance than ever before and appear to govern conscious and unconscious thinking to a large extent. Nevertheless, it is mandatory for decision makers to be alert to new opportunities in their primary or related disciplines, and one way to do this successfully is to have highly trained and trustworthy team members to function uninhibitedly and spontaneously at all times.

Point 10: Eliminate slogans, exhortations, and targets for the workforce. The workforce looks at patient care as a divine activity and is prepared to go the extra mile. The attitude of the doctors and nurses is crucial in the affairs of a hospital. They are the pillars of strength of any hospital, and active participation at all levels of the workforce is the key to success. This is determined by the nature of the relationship that exists between top management and the lower levels of professional and nonprofessional staff in a hospital. Charter Point 10 is probably the most vexatious issue in any organization and it is true for hospitals also. A practical approach to minimize this problem is to provide the ownership of smaller satellite hospitals and clinics to teams of doctors and nurses and encourage them to independently manage and produce results. The structure of the parent organization is critical to enable such a relationship to be developed with the

workforce, and this reminds us of the statement of Raymond Miles: "The greatest barrier to success will be outmoded views of what an 'organization' must look like and how it must be managed."

Points 11, 12, and 13 are a cohesive interlinked movement of earlier thought processes toward the strong-willed decisive action of the transformation and implementation of a process that has proven benefits in global healthcare. Action at the end will serve to demonstrate the validity of the expressed scientific thinking and stimulate others to follow similar lines of thinking, paving the way for the Internet revolution to make a rapid foray into the domain of life sciences in a convincing and incisive manner.

Point 14: Take action to accomplish the transformation.

Data-Warehouse Architecture for a Data-Mining Project in Life Sciences

Operational and External Data

See Figure 1. Example outputs from a data warehouse include the following:

1. Homeopathic history to maintain transactions
2. Analysis of homeopathic histories to identify patterns
3. Identifying progressive disease patterns to initiate critical treatment measures
4. Mobilizing work-flow processes for emergency and critical situations like natural disasters
5. Recording the evolution of cancers from many patients within a nation and from many nations to create a data background for the comparison and prediction of outcomes of treatment plans, for the study

Figure 1.

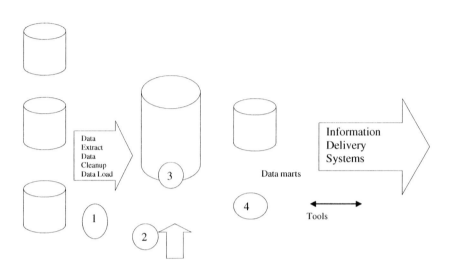

and analysis of demographic patterns, and so forth

6. Creating self-help treatment processes for widespread ailments like chronic nasal allergies

7. Creating products and services for homeopathic students in training

8. To initiate global action against widespread epidemics like gastroenteritis, malnutrition, tuberculosis, and so forth

Relevance of Data Mining to Cancer Research

Models of Human Breast Cancer

The lack of absolute knowledge of the development and progression of cancer has resulted in many empirical and hypothetical treatment models. The number and type of questions that can be answered by controlled trials are limited by logistical and ethical considerations, and it is for this reason that models of human cancer are sought. Cancer is neither a single disease nor a group of diseases. It is a phenomenon of uncon-

trolled and unrestrained biological activity that alters the basic human functions and eventually kills the host. Hitherto, animal models were employed to understand the biology of cancer and extrapolate the results to humans. The animal model has failed to make us fully aware of the origins of human cancer.

Several models of breast cancer are currently in use, each of which embodies some accepted criterion. However, a universal model does not exist simply because the criterion adopted varies enormously from center to center, and also because the nature of the criterion selected is difficult to determine all over the world. Therefore, it is necessary to establish a set of criteria that is fairly universal and fundamental in order to proceed with a meaningful research program involving large numbers of people and many breast-cancer research centers.

Types of Models Available

The following models are commonly employed in many research centers. They are the canine model, rodent model, and human model. Models are necessary to formulate a scheme for obtaining, analyzing, and testing data in appropriate environments in order to apply the results to a larger population.

The Canine Model

Breast tumors occur commonly in dogs, and these tumors represent a close model of human breast cancer in morphology, clinical behavior, and incidence. However, by virtue of its closeness to the human situation, this model includes all the variables encountered clinically and necessitates the same staging of tumors and randomization of subjects as applied in human clinical trials. In addition, the time required for the evaluation of treatment modalities is long, and together these factors make the cost of using the model to obtain statistically significant results too great.

The Rodent Model

Aside from using different methods to study cancer in rodents, the overall results are not significantly different from the canine model and hence are not suitable for incorporating into a data warehouse.

The Human Model

While it is reasonable to assume that the basic mechanisms of hormone action and metastasis may be similar in human and rat breast cancers, it is less probable that they should show similar sensitivities to chemotherapeutic agents. It is for this reason that a model system that enables human material to be used for experimentation would be of value. Significant developments in this direction are taking place in many centers across the world, and a large amount of scattered data is available for incorporating into a central data warehouse.

The nature of experimental data is different from either epidemiological or clinical data. Epidemiological data is easy to collect and should be drawn from many nations to provide a definite and conclusive base to expand on seamlessly. The attributes of this database are a combination of general and peculiar characteristics spread across several age groups. The peculiar characteristics determine how an injurious agent produces its effect over time. Contrary to the traditional allopathic model of cancer causation, in which there is not much emphasis on a continuous cause operating in the background, the holistic integrated model of cancer causation believes in the existence of smaller cause-effect changes occurring all the time, albeit imperceptible to normal human senses. This resembles a chain of events that occurs in all the links of a computer network when the main switch is turned on.

A. M. Neville (1981) has some insights into the developments in research with relevance to human breast cancer. One overriding conclusion is that we must try to escape from viewing breast disease in a conventional sense as this approach to date has failed. It seems more important to detect those factors that are involved intimately in the control of the growth of breast cells, both normal and neoplastic. An understanding of those factors, and how and where they act will allow us to gain a greater appreciation of the progression of this disease and how it may be modulated to the patients' advantage. Growth factors and their receptors draw attention once more to the properties of the cell surface. Increased appreciation of this aspect of cell biology and biochemistry may well have value in the diagnosis and monitoring of the disease. Without such knowledge, it is unlikely that we will be able to devise meaningful and rational approaches to therapy in the coming decade.

Hopefully, with the advent of RAD tools, research time can be reduced and results made more meaningful and of a uniform quality in all the participating centers in a multination clinical trial. There is reason to believe that light can be shed on perplexing and controversial aspects of breast-cancer treatment within 3 years of beginning an accurately designed study.

SOME ISSUES ADDRESSED AT THE TELEMEDICINE RESEARCH LABORATORY

1. Infrastructure development for e-business and e-health
2. Research into health information systems and the development of prototypes
3. Data warehousing and data mining in life sciences
4. E-publishing
5. E-learning
6. E-communications
7. Mobile technologies and healthcare

CONCLUSION

The last few years have seen a growing recognition of information as a key business tool. Those who successfully gather, analyze, understand, and act upon the information are among the winners in this new information age. Translating this to the domain of life sciences, biological organisms obtain information through sensory and extrasensory means and methodically unravel the continuous flow of information for purposeful behavior. With behavior ranging from simple survival to a life of uninhibited and spontaneous activities, human beings are a different class of biological organisms. This is reflected in one's choice of behavior when faced with many conflicting choices. Of all the physical and mental activities we can perform,

there is no other activity as important as decision making in our daily lives. The varied and complex process of decision making is at the soul of all activities in life sciences.

Data mining in life sciences with emphasis on cancer and AIDS will prove to be a profitable e-business opportunity for the current millennium. One of the many interesting business aspects of this opportunity is the profound transformation it can bring about in personal and business relationships, replacing old and worn out ideas with fresh and revolutionary thinking, and paving the way for a new practical approach to the economics of Web businesses. E-business economy will alter the lifestyles of many people, and the only attribute that may leave behind some losers in the bargain is the relative apathy and lethargy of some organizations and an unwillingness to adapt speedily to rapidly changing business processes. "The future allows unlimited and infinite opportunities to those who can discern in the present the mistakes of the past and clearly commit to themselves that they will never again repeat the same or other mistakes in the present or the future." Considering the global epidemic nature of cancer and AIDS, an international consortium for the research and development of telemedicine applications is a distinct reality in the not-too-distant future.

REFERENCES

Belbin, M. (2001). *Team roles at work*. Butter Worth-Heinemann.

Berson, A., Smith, S., & Thearling, K. (2000). *Building data mining applications for CRM*. India: Tata McGraw-Hill.

Creech, B. (1995). *The five pillars of TQM*. Truman Tally Books, Penguin Group.

Paraki, J. G. (2001). Abstract: Telemedicine 2001, 6th International Conference on the Medical Aspects of Telemedicine. *Technology and Health Care, 9*(4), 366.

Woodcock, J. (2002). *Step up to networking.* India: Prentice Hall.

KEY TERMS

Cancer: Is defined as uncontrolled proliferation of cancer cells that impair the function of normal organs by local tissue invasion and metastic spread to distant anatomic sites.

Data Mining: By its simplest definition, means to automate the detection of relevant patterns in a database.

Decision-Making: Is a process through which a correct decision is reached. For a decision to be correct, one must be able to say "yes" or "no" confidently.

Epidemiology: Is the study of the distribution, effects, and causes of diseases in populations and the means by which they may be treated or prevented.

Insight: Is the realization of the relationship of all factors in a given situation to one another.

Knowledge Management: Emerging scientific discipline of new knowledge discovery and dissemination.

Network: Is defined as a set of nodes and connecting lines to describe intricate structures (e.g., neuronal network, computer network, data network).

Telemedicine: Telemedicine is defined as the actual delivery of healthcare using audio, visual, and data communication.

Section VIII
Telemedicine and E–Health Services

Rapidly emerging information and communication technologies have spurred the recent escalation of various telehealth applications. It is true that there is an enormous interest in finding new ways to apply telehealth as much as telemedicine as a special part of telehealth. This section has, along with providing a better understanding of what telehealth is, investigated the ways in which such an avant-garde, advancing, and newly emerging technology could be used in order to be available at the upper healthcare level. This section helps to clarify the issue with regard to the confusion between the terms telehealth and telemedicine, and even telecare and e-health.

Chapter XXVIII
Use of Telemedicine Systems and Devices for Patient Monitoring

Dionisia Damigou
National and Kapodistrian University of Athens, Greece

Fotini Kalogirou
National and Kapodistrian University of Athens, Greece

Georgios Zarras
National and Kapodistrian University of Athens, Greece

ABSTRACT

Today's health standards demand a high quality and efficiency as a major characteristic of every health service provided to the public, even in cases where patients have to be treated from a distance. The combination of medicine and information technology (telecommunications) led to the introduction of the term telemedicine. Telemedicine services are used in assisting remote patients. Interaction and feedback through patient monitoring systems and devices allow the health providers interfere when necessary, so medical maintenance can be guaranteed. This chapter deals with the different kinds of such systems and devices. The contribution of old and new telecommunication technologies is currently being discussed. The individual needs of every remote patient are taken into account, thus, several devices and systems are used for telemonitoring. This chapter indicates characteristics and features of the various kinds of patient monitoring systems and devices.

INTRODUCTION

Due to the technological revolution and the entry of informatics in our everyday lives, the expansion of telecommunications became a reality. Challenging telecommunication applications such as cellular telephony, communications through the intervention of satellites, the Internet, and so forth, support the extensive exchange of information. Several scientific areas have become related to telecommunication applications, including the field of health in which the term telemedicine was first introduced.

Telemedicine involves the transfer of medical information for use in diagnosis, treatment, and education over distances and brings medical services directly to the point of need.

A monitoring system adapts to the needs of each and every patient, care unit, and hospital equipped with hardware and software designed to give maximum functionality, flexibility, and responsiveness. Concerning the monitoring devices, severall types are available, including pulse oximeters, spirometers, glucose monitors, and so forth (Demiris, 2004).

TELEMEDICINE SYSTEMS FOR PATIENT MONITORING

There was a big demand for devices for patient monitoring, especially for people who are far away from health providers. The population is growing old, and the high health standards of nowadays claim that patients should be cared for and rehabilitated at their homes. Several telemonitoring systems were developed. The primary aim of such systems is to maintain the autonomy, independence, and quality of life for the frail elderly, disabled persons, remote patients, and their informal family careers by the application of telematic technology. For ex-

ample, home health tele-assistance systems could provide a large range of services that would permit the user or patient to remain in his or her normal environment:

*   Emergency alarm systems (tele-alarms),
*   Post-hospital treatment monitoring,
*   Social assistance (24-hour tele-assistance) and so forth (Linkous, 2003).

Remote medical services can also be used in other areas as medical care is provided to prisons, on board commercial aircraft and ships, in the military, and even at the South Pole.

TELEMEDICINE SYSTEMS AND TELEHOMECARE

The most common utilization of telemedicine for patients' monitoring is telehomecare. With more technologies moving into home care, and more and sicker patients being treated outside of the hospital environment, the home-care approach to health care is here to stay. Telehomecare is viewed as a method that uses telecommunication and videoconferencing technologies to enable a health-care provider at the clinical site to communicate with patients at their homes. It is one of the brightest examples of the new frontier of health care. These telehomecare solutions are low cost compared to the classic way of monitoring (Linkous, 2003).

TELEMEDICINE SYSTEMS AND INTERACTION

The telemedicine systems permit monitoring devices to interact with doctors' displaying systems. Such an interaction is called a virtual visit. These devices collect information and signs from the patient, and the resulting data can then be transferred through telephone lines (regular, ISDN, DSL, or T1), the Internet, or the wires of a LAN (local area network) or WAN (wide area network) to the doctor or other health scientists (Kyriacou, Voskarides, Pattichis, Istepanian, Pattichis, & Schizas, 2002). Recent technologies such as Bluetooth might also be used (Roke Manor Research Limited, http://www.roke.co.uk). The diffused data, in many cases, has the potential of updating the doctor's displaying devices in real time. Whenever there is a need (urgent case), the medical personnel might immediately interfere and get in contact with the patient.

There are several types of telemonitoring system applications; their purposes differ in proportion to the concerning situation. Examples of telemonitoring systems are provided in the following sections.

Systems for Monitoring Heart Function and Circulation

a. **Systems for Monitoring Cardiac-Rehabilitation Patients:** The first applications that were evaluated concerned systems that monitor cardiac-rehabilitation patients unable to return to a hospital-based program. Devices for these patients could detect arrhythmia and were found to be more effective than ambulatory electrocardiography. The most recent systems are much more complicated and sophisticated.

b. **Systems for Hypertensive Patients:** Other disease-management applications support hypertensive patients, enabling them to control their blood pressure, and are found to be efficient at the evaluation process.

c. **Systems for Chronic Heart Failure:** Studies for home monitoring of chronic

heart failure revealed that there is a need for further investigation (Demiris, 2004).

Systems for Pulmonary Function

a. **Systems for Asthma Patients:** Telemonitoring systems for asthma patients provide assistance in daily routines; the systems alert health-care providers when necessary.

b. **Systems for Lung-Transplant Patients:** Systems for the monitoring of pulmonary function in lung-transplant recipients via the Internet are feasible and accurate.

Systems for the Management of Insulin-Dependent Diabetes

Distributed computer-based systems for the management of insulin-dependent diabetes were developed utilizing Internet technology and monitoring devices to support the normal activities of physicians and diabetic patients by providing a set of automated services enabling data collection, transmission, and analysis, and decision support (Demiris, 2004).

Systems to Assist Post-Transplant Patients

Other Web-based telemonitoring systems were developed to assist post-transplant patients; for example, for lung-transplant recipients, regular spirometry monitoring can be used for the early detection of acute infection and rejection of the allograft. A Web-based telemonitoring system, for these cases, provides direct transmission of home spirometry to the hospital (Demiris, 2004).

Systems for Emergency Response

Telemonitoring systems have also been introduced to provide emergency response to disaster situations. The goal is to offer quality health-care services to persons who are victims of a disaster. Portable telemedicine instrumentation packages can provide a compact, integrated suite of tools such as data-acquisition devices for ear, nose, throat, and skin imaging, lung sound auscultation, and so forth (Demiris, 2004).

Similar system projects were developed in many countries for several purposes.

- **United Kingdom:** In Oxford, a remote physiological-monitoring network was established to evaluate cardiorespiratory function during sleep in a number of infants in their homes for research purposes. The center designed and developed portable monitors for the continuous measurement of vital signs, which allowed downloading data from monitor memory to the hospital. This information was then further analyzed.
- **Israel:** A program was developed to gain access to cardiac patients. In the process of a typical patient call, a health professional collects descriptive information about the patient's condition while simultaneously receiving and recording the 12-lead electrocardiograph (ECG) transmitted by the client-managed portable ECG device. The ECG results are displayed and analyzed, and compared with previous ECGs using proprietary transtelephonic ECG-management software.
- **The Netherlands:** One of the areas that seem to be exceptionally well developed in the Netherlands is the use of handheld computers for electronic case management. After data are collected, they can be immediately transferred, using dial-up networking capacity, from the point of care to the central home-care database. Records are regularly updated and are available to different health professionals within the continuum of care.

- **Germany:** A telemonitoring project was designed in Germany and included extensive home monitoring of the vital parameters of infants at risk for sudden infant death syndrome (SIDS). The project monitored breathing movements, ECG, heart rate, and oxygen saturation. All sensors were noninvasive and integrated with the babies' pajamas. The parents were trained in assessing the physiological status of the children and in emergency intervention measures. Information was also transmitted to the test and research telemedical laboratory for further analysis.
- **A Four-Country Project (Greece, Great Britain, France, Germany):** This project was related to patients with renal failure requiring home hemodialysis. The goal of the project was to develop, apply, and evaluate telematics monitoring and consultation services for enabling the supervision of each hemodialysis session and possible intervention (Demiris, 2004).

TELEMEDICINE DEVICES FOR PATIENT MONITORING

Portable Monitoring Devices

There are several commercially available portable monitoring devices that are approved by the FDA, including pulse oximeters, blood-pressure monitors, weight scales, and glucose monitors. In some cases, data are stored in the device and retrieved at a later point or are displayed on a monitor at the completion of the test session (Demiris, 2004).

Wearable Sensors

There are three kinds of wearable sensors: physical, chemical, and biological. These sensors produce a signal in response to an event, which is then transferred to a circuit and becomes digitised. A physical sensor measures physical parameters such as temperature or pressure, whereas a biological or chemical sensor involves a receptor that binds with an analyte. The resulting digital data can be stored and/or displayed.

The concept of wearable sensors is based on the incorporation of sensors into watches, items of clothing, and eye glasses. Thus, one could argue that wearable sensors can function as noninvasive, in vitro diagnostic tools as they are capable of analyzing, among others, human sweat, tears, stress, strain, and pH increases.

There exists a knee-wearable sensor that is also known as the intelligent knee sleeve, and it was first designed for football players. It monitors knee strain or injury. Originally, this device was strapped to the knees, and its sleeve provided feedback to users by emitting an audio tone. It can be a useful application for homecare patients with mobility impairments or for those at the rehabilitation phase.

Another example of a wearable sensor is a small, portable detector in the form of a wristwatch that provides test results for cystic fibrosis in minutes, rather than the 24 hours that is the typical response time for a laboratory. Another wristwatch device uses an electric field to push pilocarpine nitrate into the skin, thereby dilating the pores. Sweat is absorbed and stored in a duct in the watch. The sample is analyzed by a sensor, and the levels of sodium, chloride, and potassium ions are recorded. Other devices in the form of wristwatches include glucose meters that measure glucose in the interstitial fluid as a low electric current pulls glucose through the skin, and a blood oxygen monitor.

In the last few years, the Smart Shirt was introduced that incorporates technology into the design of clothing to monitor the wearer's heart rate, ECG, respiration, temperature, and vital functions, alerting the wearer or physician if there is a problem. The Smart Shirt also can be used to monitor the vital signs of military personnel, chronically ill patients, firemen, and frail elderly persons living alone (Demiris, 2004).

Also, for military purposes, the U.S. military is developing innovative applications for advanced sensors and smart materials. Devices resembling wristwatches will be worn by all soldiers as part of the combat uniform. These devices will monitor the soldier's vital signs continuously by monitoring parameters such as noninvasive blood pressure, pulse oximetry, and medical imaging (Garshnek & Burkle, 1999).

Robots

It is impressive that robots have started claiming doctors' duties. At present, these robots are navigated by an operator using a joystick at a control station and can perform rounds within the hospital. A camera and microphone are mounted above the computer screen, allowing the operator to see and hear. A similar camera and microphone at the control station transmit the operator's face and voice. It is surprising that a number of doctors perform rounds on their patients with these robots, particularly from their homes. The full potential of robots is beginning to be explored. Future generations of control stations are expected to be portable and operational from virtually anywhere in the world (Norris, 2004).

ADVANTAGES OF TELEMEDICINE

The categories of telemedicine are the following:

- Teleconsultation
- Telediagnosis
- Telecare
- Remote clinical sessions and tele-education
- Remote data access
- Teleradiology
- Home care
- Telemonitoring (Mantas & Hasman, 2002)

Telemedicine's objective is to provide users with an integrated health-information service through an expert system, which gives access to existing information related to health, social care, and other general issues that is now distributed in dispersed databases. After achieving this objective, we expect the following advantages.

1. **Advantages in Monitoring the Patient:** The use of telemedicine is followed by an improvement of the quality of the monitoring of patients and an increase in the number of patients being monitored. Moreover, tools are provided for medical decision support and guided monitoring work is allowed.

2. **Advantages in the Management of Treatment and Training:** Telemedicine improves the communication between doctor and patient, promotes patients' self-management and training, and decreases the response time in the treatment.

3. **Advantages in Telecare:** Telecare reduces the number of visits to hospitals, facilitates patients in finding information regarding their illnesses, allows the patients autonomy, and decreases short-term as well as long-term complications (Mantas, Aguilera, del Pozo Guerrero, Arredondo Waldmeyer, & Martínez Fernández, 2000).

In general, telemedicine offers the following:

- Reduction of health-care costs
- Access to health services in previously unserved or underserved areas
- Easy cooperation between health professionals
- Improved quality of care

CONCLUSION

The development of information-systems technology has led us to an increased number of telemonitoring applications to help with patient health care. These applications enable health professionals to carry out home health visits (virtual visits). Such applications and systems complete the management of data collection and reinforce data analysis. Telemedicine services can be shared among patients and several regional hospitals and other specialized health centers. Thus, patients are allowed to ask for advice, and, as a response, health professionals may interfere when necessary. It appears that the use of telemonitoring systems can cut the cost of medical care for rural and urban areas.

Interesting research and implementations have been developed to evaluate systems delivering assistance to different scientific health fields, contributing to cardiology, neurology, surgery, orthopedics, pediatrics, and so forth. A lot of them were found to be accurate and efficient enough, although the future promises more potent and sophisticated systems for patient monitoring.

However, there are still barriers to the wider adoption of telemedicine, affecting both health-care professionals and their patients. The general public is not mature enough to get involved in such procedures due to the fact that it is not well acquainted with the subject. In the future, a lot of these difficulties will be overcome, and we expect that the public will accept the challenges of telemedicine and telemonitoring.

REFERENCES

Demiris, G. (2004). *Electronic home healthcare: Concepts and challenges.* Columbia: University of Missouri.

Gantenbein, R. (1992). Telehealth technology: Wyoming's efforts to facilitate research and service in a rural state. *American Stroke Association Conference,* Ft. Lauderdale, FL. Center for Rural Health Research and Education.

Garshnek, V., & Burkle, F. (1999). Applications of telemedicine and telecommunications to disaster medicine. *Journal of American Medical Informatics Association, 6,* 26-37.

Kyriacou, E., Voskarides, S., Pattichis, C., Istepanian, R., Pattichis, M., & Schizas, C. (2002). Wireless telemedicine systems: A brief overview. *IEEE Antennas & Propagation Magazine, 44*(2), 143-153.

Linkous, J. (2003). *Advances in telemedicine technology.* Helsinki, Finland: American Telemedicine Association (ATA).

Mantas, J., Aguilera, E. G., del Pozo Guerrero, F., Arredondo Waldmeyer, M. T., & Martínez Fernández, A. (2000). *Health informatics. Textbook in health informatics.* Athens: IOS Press.

Mantas, J., & Hasman, A. (2002). *Textbook in health informatics.* Athens: IOS Press.

Norris, K. (2004). *Medicine and technology: Robot makes the rounds.* Detroit, MI: Detroit Free Press.

KEY TERMS

Home-Care Technology: Any technology used to implement home-care telemedicine services. It can also incorporate any device or instrument for patient monitoring, therapy, or environmental control (Mantas & Hasman, 2002).

Telecare: The use of telecommunication systems to provide remote assistance in therapy to patients (Mantas & Hasman, 2002).

Teleconsultation: Remote access to a specialist's knowledge. This type of service is seen as a particular case of cooperative work or cooperative diagnosis (Mantas & Hasman, 2002).

Telediagnosis: Diagnosis of a patient by a remote physician. This kind of service does not operate directly between the patient and remote doctor (Mantas & Hasman, 2002).

Telehomecare: Uses telecommunication and videoconferencing technologies to enable a health-care provider at the clinical site to communicate with patients at their homes (Demiris, 2004).

Telemedicine: The use of electronic information and communication technologies to provide and support health care when distance separates the participant. It emphasizes applications that link clinician to patient or one clinician to another (Gantenbein, 1992).

Telemonitoring: Remote monitoring of patients' physiological value. This kind of service is used with chronic and/or high-risk patients (Mantas & Hasman, 2002).

Chapter XXIX
Current Telehealth Applications in Telemedicine

Georgios Economopoulos
National and Kapodistrian University of Athens, Greece

ABSTRACT

Rapidly emerging information and communication technologies (ICT) have spurred the recent escalation of various telehealth applications. There is an enormous interest in finding new ways to apply telehealth as much as telemedicine as a special part of telehealth. This chapter has along with providing a better understanding of what telehealth is, investigated the ways in which such an avant-garde, advancing, and newly emerging technology could be used in order to be available in an upper-healthcare level.

INTRODUCTION

Rapidly emerging information and communication technologies (ICTs) have spurred the recent escalation of various telehealth applications (Lehoux, Battista, & Lance, 2000). It is true that there is an enormous interest in finding new ways to apply ICT as much as telemedicine as a special part of telehealth. This chapter, along with providing a better understanding of what telehealth is, investigates the ways in which such an avant-garde, advancing, and newly emerging technology could be used in order to raise the level of healthcare.

First of all, it is necessary to clarify the issue regarding the confusion between the terms telehealth and telemedicine, and even telecare and e-health.

- Telemedicine involves the use of modern information technology, especially two-way interactive audio and video communications, computers, and telemetry, to deliver healthcare to remote patients and to facilitate information exchanges between primary healthcare physicians at some distance from each other (Bashur & Lovett, 1997). It existed long before the Internet. It has been said that telemedicine was present when the term was first established nearly 30 years ago (Willemian et al., as cited in Maheu, Whitten, & Allen, 2001).

- Telecare refers to services that provide care for people away from institutions, typically in their own homes, for example, in the monitoring of elderly people as they lead their normal lives. In other words, it refers to services that provide healthcare no matter where the doctor, the patient, or his or her medical records are (Cornford & Klecun-Dabroeska, 2001).

- E-health is a relatively new term that first appeared in 1999, and it refers to Internet-based healthcare delivery (McClendon, 2000). It includes all forms of healthcare over the Internet (Singh, 2002).

- Telehealth could be considered an umbrella term because the it is seen by authors as being more encompassing of the above terms whereas telemedicine is restricted toward interactive patient-doctor teleconsultations, and e-health refers solely to Internet-based healthcare delivery. It covers a number of different technologies, services, and professions including medicine, health promotion, health administration, social services, and information systems (Cornford & Klecun-Dabroeska, 2001; Singh, 2002).

In order to avoid a misunderstanding, the World Health Organisation (WHO) distinguished the terms telehealth and telemedicine in 1997: "Telehealth is understood to mean the integration of communications systems into the practice of protecting and promoting health, while telemedicine is the incorporation of these terms into curative medicine" (WHO, 1997).

THE HISTORICAL EVOLUTION OF TELEHEALTH

Before an in-depth analysis of current telehealth applications is conducted, it is necessary to examine the historical evolution of telehealth. Nowadays, we consider telehealth as being a matter of high technology, especially associated with the revolution of ICTs such as television, fax, or the Internet. Although we cannot ignore the dependence of telehealth on concurrent developments, it is true that humans have since the early 1900s been communicating information about health long before such new technologies arose (Darkins & Cary, 2000; Singh, 2002).

The first stage of telehealth was in the 1970s when scientists made the first effort to transmit health information in order to provide healthcare to people who were travelling by ships (Maheu et al., 2001). There were also more efforts, especially in the United States, to use telehealth in a productive way, but the efforts were aborted due to high costs and some other reasons, such as insufficient image quality or insufficient acceptance from doctors (Darkins & Cary, 2000; Singh, 2002).

The second stage was in the beginning of the 1990s. Almost 20 years after the first attempt, the conditions were good enough for the telehealth sector to expand. The most important reason for this regeneration of telehealth was the lower cost of technology. Many countries took advantage of that low cost, and a great deal of telehealth applications was adopted. The leading countries were the United States and Norway, but Australia was not far away from developing telehealth applications for its rural areas (Maheu et al., 2001).

The third stage of the telehealth evolution began in the mid-1990s and culminates today. The evolution of technology and communications via the Internet has been really rapid recently, and this seems to have a direct impulse on telehealth (Poulis, 2002).

CURRENT TELEHEALTH APPLICATIONS

There is a great range of telehealth applications. First of all, we should mention that everything that can provide health information in rural areas could be seen as a telehealth application. This means that even the simple and very common household telephone is such an application. We can use the telephone in order to keep in communication with the oldest patients to remind them of simple things like taking their pills or having their examinations (Singh, 2002). Of course, telehealth is applicative in many ways regarding voice and video communication. Videoconference is one of them. In addition, we can use video and voice communication for clinical procedures, particularly for emergency procedures (Matrini, 2003).

In general, doctors have the ability to communicate with their patients, to support them psychologically, and to educate them on how to take care of themselves (Bergman, 1993). Apart from that, videoconferencing can be used for meetings between doctors in a way that reassures the knowledge flow will be constant (Meyer, 1996).

Another issue of increasing interest is telehomecare. There has been an effort in preventing unnecessary hospitalizations, and this can be achieved through telehealth by monitoring patients with chronic conditions or treating sick children at home with the partici-

pation of their parents instead of in hospitals. As we can see, there is a huge space for telehealth's applications regarding telehomecare with multiple benefits: The low cost for institutions, the ability for the patient to remain at home, and the existence of family support are enough to give a boost for telehomecare.

One of the applications of telehealth is to store and forward data and images such as X-rays, CT (computed tomography) scans, and skin images (Matrini, 2003). By storing and forwarding data and images, doctors have the ability to improve diagnoses and to communicate with specialists in order to get a second opinion. This procedure can be done in real time and could prove to be quite vital in case of an emergency.

Telehealth poses a critical role respecting information access, especially in education and training (Matrini, 2003). It is important because through it, everybody can have access to the source of the knowledge no matter if this is a professional doctor, a student, or even a patient or a whole community.

BENEFITS OF TELEHEALTH

The revolution of telehealth is being followed by a number of benefits. Some of them are mentioned as follows:

- Decreased costs for patients because they do not have to travel in order to get to a hospital
- Lower costs for hospitals
- Availability of a wide range of services difficult to access
- Potential constant education
- Prevention of social exclusion, for example, the ability to serve people who live in isolated areas

- Many other parallel benefits such as better feedback for epidemiological research

PROBLEMS WITH TELEHEALTH

Although there are many benefits, the evolution of telehealth faces some problems.

- The situation regarding the reimbursement of telehealth could be prescribed as dim.
- There is no adequate planning for the diffusion of telehealth.
- There are some legal aspects that need to be examined.

THE FUTURE OF TELEMEDICINE

The evolution of telemedicine is without precedent. It has been spread all over the medical practise so that we can talk about telecardiology, teleneurology, teleradiology, teledermatology, telesurgery, and many other specialities as being different fields in medicine (Grigsby & Sanders, 1998). Just a few years before, only a few could imagine that doctors could conduct a surgery while at a distance away. The close relationship between telemedicine and evolution in technology, involving both information and communication, leads us to the thought that the evolution can be even broader. The important thing is to determine the changes that are going to occur. There are many issues that need examination so that we will be able to use telemedicine in the most productive and effective way.

First of all, satellite technology is going to make telemedicine available to even the most isolated areas on the planet. Around 1,700 commercial satellites are scheduled for launch in the next decade worldwide compared to the 150 that are now in orbit (Subba Rao, 2001). Another important issue that is going to affect the future of telemedicine is the relationship between costs and outcomes (Grigsby & Sanders, 1998). For the time being, telemedicine seems to deserve the cost, but we should be careful in order to develop it according to the patients' needs and not to the demand of the industry. Apart from that, telemedicine may result in changes in the relationships between healthcare professionals (Subba Rao). On the one hand, doctors and other scientists will have from now on many ways to communicate and discuss issues about a patient. Additionally, they have at their disposal a great amount of clinical information that can be delivered everywhere in just a few seconds. On the other hand, the role of the teleconsultant seems to draw the attention, so he or she has to depend on high standards. Even more importantly, changes are going to happen in the functioning of the whole healthcare system. It must be mentioned that many changes will involve primary and secondary health are. Using telemedicine, patients can avoid being in a hospital and, thus, administrative change that supports the growth of primary healthcare will be conducted. Another issue that will probably configure the future of telemedicine is that of security. There has been a great discussion about security, and it began right after the discussion about the security of the Internet. The truth is that a great amount of personal data is being transferred via telemedicine through the Internet, and nobody is able to reassure us that it will be safe. The abuse of these personal data could lead to situations like the denial of an insurance company to provide its services. This issue is really crucial and demands very careful consideration.

The future of telemedicine depends on the answer about reimbursement. There are still some unsolved problems about reimbursement and the lack of payment (Greenpope, 2001). The technology of telemedicine and its use generally can be considered avant-garde, so it is understandable that there is still not the right legislation that will provide everybody with the ability to use telemedicine.

CONCLUSION

The use of telehealth and telemedicine seems to have spread like wildfire. It is true that due to the latest technology, many patients who live in rural and isolated areas can have much better healthcare. However, that fast growing must be followed by a number of changes involving administration and reimbursement, which will undoubtedly lead to a better level of services.

REFERENCES

American Nurses Association. (2001). Developing telehealth protocols: A blueprint for success. *Proceedings of the 38ᵗʰ Hawaii International Conference on System Sciences.*

Bashur, R. L., & Lovett, J. (1997). Assessment of telemedicine: Results of initial experience. *Space and Environmental Medicine, 48,* 65-70.

Bergman, R. (1993). Letting telemedicine do the walking: Rural projects use video communications to enhance access to care. *Hospitals & Health Networks.*

Committee on Evaluating Clinical Applications of Telemedicine. (1996). Telemedicine: A guide to assessing telecommunications in health care. *Proceedings of the 38ᵗʰ Hawaii International Conference on System Sciences.*

Cornford, T., & Klecun-Dabrowska, E. (2001). Ethical perspectives in evaluation of telehealth.

Cambridge Quarterly of Healthcare Ethics, 10(2), 161-169.

Darkins, A., & Cary, M. (2000). *Telemedicine and telehealth.* Springer Publishing Company.

Greenpope, D. (2001). *Telemedicine: What it is and how we can use it to achieve better management of health care.*

Grigsby, J., & Sanders, J. (1998). Telemedicine: Where it is and where it's going. *Annals of Internal Medicine,* 129.

Lehoux, P., Battista, R., & Lance, J.-M. (2000). Telehealth: Passing fad or lasting benefits? *Canadian Journal of Public Health, 91,* 277-280.

Maheu, M., Whitten, P., & Allen, A. (2001). *E-health, telehealth and telemedicine.* Jossey Bass Publishers.

Matrini, A. (2003). *Bridging the gap between community participation and policy implementation in health related communication.* Unpublished doctoral dissertation.

McClendon, K. (2000). E-commerce and HIM: Ready or not, here it comes. *Journal of American Health and Information Management, 71,* 22-23.

Meyer, K. (1996). *Can telemedicine deliver what it promises?* American Academy of Family Physicians.

Poulis, S. (2002). *Telemedicine in cardiology.* Unpublished master's thesis.

Singh, H. (2002). *Can telehealth prevent social exclusion and create a fairer health service?* Brunel University, Department of IS and Computing.

Subba Rao, S. (2001). *Integrated health care and telemedicine.* Retrieved from *http://emerald.com*

World Health Organisation (WHO). (1997). *Health care systems in transition.* Copenhagen, Denmark: WHO Regional Office for Europe.

KEY TERMS

Electronic Health Record (EHR): An electronic health record provides an individual in Canada with a secure and private lifetime record of his or her key health history and care within the health system. The record is available electronically to authorized healthcare providers and the individual anywhere, anytime in support of high-quality care.

Information and Communications Technology (ICT): The application of modern electronic and computing capabilities (technology) to the creation and storage of meaningful and useful facts or data (information), and to their transmission to users by various electronic means (communication). The ultimate goal is for ICT to transform data into information, and information into knowledge.

Teleconferencing: Interactive electronic communication between two or more people at two or more sites that makes use of voice, video, and/or data-transmission systems such as audio, audio graphics, and computer and video systems.

Telehealth: The removal of time and distance barriers for the delivery of healthcare services or related healthcare activities (American Nurses Association, 2001).

Telemedicine: The use of electronic information and communications technologies to provide and support healthcare when distance separates the participants (Committee on Evaluating Clinical Applications of Telemedicine, 1996).

Teletriage: A means of providing health information and advice on preferred courses of treatment, usually over the telephone using computerized protocols or algorithms developed by clinical experts.

Chapter XXX
Mobile Telemonitoring Insights

Pantelis Angelidis
Vidavo Ltd., Greece

ABSTRACT

Technology advances create new possibilities for healthcare monitoring, management, and support, focusing on prevention rather than disease management. The provision of personalized healthcare applications is also greatly supported. Developments in the wireless and mobile markets are capitalized by the medical device industry. Services are becoming personalized and location independent to fulfill the increasing patient needs for self-empowerment and quality in the healthcare delivery away from the traditional nursing areas. This overview discusses the new opportunities for the healthcare domain in the mobile times we live.

INTRODUCTION

The healthcare industry is experiencing a substantial shift to care delivery away from the traditional nursing areas due to the convergence of several technology areas. Increasingly capable health-monitoring systems are moving the point of care closer to the patient, while the patient, better informed and aware now, undertakes an active role to self-care and/or -prevention. Emerging ICTs in conjunction with the medical device industry development (intelligent devices, biosensors, novel software, etc.) demonstrate personalized healthcare delivery's potential without geographical limitations.

The concept of prevention prevails now against disease management and treatment plans. As patient-centric processes emerge, the citizens and patients undertake an active role in monitoring their health status. Meanwhile, e-wellness evolves to address the rising expectations of the e-health consumers, who are better informed, more demanding, and empowered. The empowered, worried-well consumers require quality health services on the spot. The drivers are now connectivity, speed, and personalization (McKnight, 2000).

MOBILE HEALTHCARE PROVISION

Waves of technology incorporation and scientific discoveries have driven the sector from reliance on direct communication and physician experience to a higher reliance on technology and community information. This new Web-enabled environment has taken healthcare from local areas, where telemedicine left it, literally into the patient's home and, more recently with m-Internet, to wherever the patient might be and whenever he or she needs it (Simão, 2001).

M-Internet enables information exchange and promotes the availability of services and communication modes to serve working teams with increasing mobility requirements.

Services are becoming personalized and location independent to serve increasing patient needs for self-empowerment and quality in healthcare delivery away from the traditional nursing areas.

Furthering the new approaches in the provision of healthcare services in the frame of e-health, wireless developments create new opportunities for healthcare professionals, individuals and organizations, patients, and health authorities. The scope of mobile health addresses clinical, administrative, and consumer health-information applications and, as it could contribute to the improvement of health outcomes, m-health may be utilized to measure health status and population welfare.

Many healthcare organizations are investing in IT projects that take advantage of new technologies in the mobile healthcare application space. Functionality that augments the capture of evidence-based patient plans of care is essential and must map and bridge the information flow for both inpatient and outpatient work-flow clinical-practice guidelines. As the medical community continues to embrace these new technologies, system integrators must pro-

vide functionality that reduces costs, improves the quality of care, and improves the ease with which caregivers can perform their everyday tasks (Wolf, 2001).

The most significant challenge posed by mobile technology is the seamless integration of multiple hardware and software platforms with reliable, uninterrupted wireless services in a secure manner, which will become mission critical to successful healthcare organizations, payers, and providers (Wolf, 2001).

The current state-of-the-art technology in medical sensors allows for the easy and unobtrusive electronic measurement of several health conditions. The sensors are often stand-alone devices and sometimes comprised of two or more elements connected by a cable or wireless technology. Medical sensors have the capability to measure vital signs such as blood pressure, pulse rate, respiration frequency, and so forth. Based on these medical parameters, the medical professionals can monitor the patient's health condition and act in case of an anomaly.

The application areas of the medical-device wireless telemonitoring capabilities include the following:

1. Assistance in case of accidents and emergencies
2. Increased capacity and lower costs for hospitals
3. Assistance and monitoring in a home-care setting
4. Monitoring of chronically ill patients
5. Patient involvement in setting a diagnosis
6. Medicine dosage adjustment
7. Physical-state monitoring in sports
8. Monitoring of sporadically occurring symptoms
9. Emergency alarms (Fosse & Haug, 2003)
10. Improved health management

As a result, citizens can enjoy quality healthcare provision and an elevated quality of life. As underlined by the European Council objectives set in Lisbon, "effective integration of healthcare and related support services by electronic means, including the widespread use of telecare, could improve the quality of life of citizens by enabling safer independent living and increased social inclusion."

EVOLUTION FORCES AND CHALLENGES

Empowered patients demand advanced wireless health solutions. Similar to most authors, Lerer (2000) suggests that the e-health consumer is being empowered due to an increased ability to obtain health information and to seek health-related offerings via the Internet. A Deloitte Research (2000) study suggests the e-health consumer is a mix of an empowered and an engaged consumer. Recognizing that e-health consumers' empowerment can increase efficiency and reduce health costs, Lerer argues that consumers' education and empowerment should be a key concern for all health players. E-health consumers, he suggests, are not just the ill, but the potentially ill, the worried, and those adjacent to illness, patients, their relatives, and friends. At the first level, e-health services are information-driven activities, which are mostly "event triggered." The Deloitte Research study suggests that the demographic profile of the e-health consumer population reveals a significant population group with economic clout, information sophistication, and technological familiarity, and that is generally wealthy.

An e-health consumer is an individual who is (a) fully involved in the management of health for himself or herself and his or her family, (b) proactively educated about health issues, espe-

cially in the area of prevention, and (c) concerned about the quality of care offered by physicians and institutions, with a willingness to select the highest level of services. In short, an e-health consumer manages health, in all extents possible, as the most important asset of his or her family. The main objective is to maintain the highest level of quality of life (Lerer, 2000)

The rapid proliferation of wireless personal computers, phones, appliances, and other devices will require organizations to look beyond single-platform solutions. System-integration activities have a new level of complexity and cost to support rapidly changing technology (Wolf, 2001). Mobile-health advances generate new capabilities in patient self-care and health-practice administration and reimbursement. Cost-effective solutions minimize effort in monetary and human-input terms, while the creation of new communication modes facilitates both the healthcare professionals and the patients.

When it comes to investing in new technology solutions, affordability is a major milestone to consider. Budget allocation to mobile health applications can be easily influenced both by the technology cost and the user awareness of current and future cost benefits. The complexity and fragmentation of the overall healthcare sector (i.e., centralized vs. decentralized health systems, variations in the public and private funding mix, etc.) often leads to the implementation of fragmented and disposable technological solutions. Interoperability thus is essential for large-scale applications with international scope. Conformance to global (when available) and/or U.S. and European standards enables faster and ubiquitous communications, while also ensuring the compatibility and connectivity of systems and points of care.

According to CEN/TC 251 (2001), the present lack of standardized ICT communication, which prevents appropriate access to health records, may result in important clinical risks for the patients. This is an important safety issue that has not been recognized sufficiently.

Implemented standards are often crucial for any communication, and they are especially important for open, very complex healthcare systems with many different organizations and units, with information systems from different suppliers, providing different parts of the total ICT support.

Furthermore, the wider implementation of mobile solutions requires a robust security plan to reassure the confidentiality of sensitive medical data.

M-HEALTH POTENTIAL

The next few years will witness a rapid deployment of both wireless technologies and mobile Internet-based m-health systems with pervasive computing technologies. The increasing data traffic and demands from different medical applications and roaming applications will be compatible with the data rates of 3G (third-generation) systems in specific mobility conditions. The implementation and penetration of 4G (fourth-generation) systems are expected to help close the gap in medical care. Specifically, in a society penetrated by 4G systems, home medical care and remote diagnosis will become common, checkups by specialists and the prescription of drugs will be enabled at home and in underpopulated areas based on high-resolution image-transmission technologies and remote surgery, and virtual hospitals with no resident doctors will be realized. Preventive medical care will also be emphasized: For individual health management, data will constantly be transmitted to the hospital through a built-in sensor in the individual's watch or another item worn daily, and diagnosis results

will be fed back to the individual (Istepanian et al., 2004)

A fourth-generation m-health solution builds upon the mobile information portal of a 3G solution by adding the multiple devices rendering the capability of the 2G (second-generation) solutions. Now, an end user has the ability to access any application with any device ("Going Mobile," 2001). 4G solutions embrace the distributed and loosely coupled HIS applications throughout a health unit. A 4G solution can allow for the acquisition of data from various sources and for the mobile end user to view, analyze, manipulate, graph, and merge data according to his or her needs right on the mobile device.

In the home of the future, some devices will contribute physiological information about the patient (e.g., heart rate, blood pressure), while other devices in and around the home will contribute information about the patient's environment (e.g., humidity, temperature, carbon-monoxide level). In some cases, groups of devices will have enough collective awareness to function autonomously based on sensor data.

The challenge for healthcare providers and health authorities lies in the comprehension of the end users' needs for the effective integration of new technological capabilities with existing settings in order to leverage their capacities and quality of service.

CONCLUSION

Systematically sensitizing users and providing them with specific information on new mobile and wearable computing technologies will help to discover possible fields of new applications. The initiation of a dialogue between users in healthcare and developers of mobile IT solutions eventually may lead to the identification of new application fields (i.e., medical specialties) and related practices in mobile healthcare provision.

A first step to this end is the identification and definition of mobile-activities profiles, and stakeholder profiles and their level of involvement, as well as mobile application scenarios. Technologies should be designed for people rather than making people adapt to technologies in order to capitalize on the capabilities that wireless technologies create in the healthcare domain.

REFERENCES

CEN/TC 251. (2001). *Report on the Mandate M/255*.

Deloitte Research. (2000). *The emergence of the e-health consumer.*

eHealth in 2010: Meeting the Lisbon objectives with ambient intelligence technologies? (2003). Seville.

Fosse, B., & Haug, B. E. (2003). *A feasibility study and recommendation of technology and solutions for wireless monitoring of biomedical data.* Unpublished master's thesis, Agder University College, Grimstad.

Going mobile: From eHealth to mHealth. A Daou Systems White Paper. (2001).

Istepanian, R., et al. (2004). Non-telephone healthcare: The role of 4G and emerging mobile systems for future m-health systems. In *Medical and Care Compunentics.* IOS Press.

Lerer, L. (2000). *The healthcare 2020 platform: The e-health consumer.* INSEAD.

McKnight, L. (2000). *Internet business models.* Medford, MA: Tufts University.

Simão, C. M. V. Q. (2001). *A study on Internet impact in business designs for the health sector.*

Wolf, J. (2001). *MBA mobile health applications, Version 1.1.*

KEY TERMS

3G and 4G: Third- and fourth-generation wireless Internet devices. The major distinction of 4G over 3G communications is increased data transmission rates. 4G is expected to deliver more advanced versions of the same improvements promised by 3G, such as enhanced multimedia, smooth streaming video, universal access, and portability across all types of devices. 4G enhancements are expected to include worldwide roaming capability and are likely to incorporate global positioning services (GPSs). As was projected for the ultimate 3G system, 4G might actually connect the entire globe and be operable from any location on or above the surface of the earth.

Ambient Intelligence: The concept of ambient intelligence provides a vision of the information society in which the emphasis is on user friendliness, efficient and distributed services support, user empowerment, and support for human interactions. People are surrounded by intelligent, intuitive interfaces that are embedded in all kinds of objects in an environment that is capable of recognizing and responding to the presence of different individuals in a seamless, unobtrusive, and often invisible way.

E-Health Consumer: Self-reliance and empowerment are the core characteristics of the e-health consumer, who actively pursues patient-centric quality services in a frame of information-supported activities.

Empowered Patient: A patient whose self-management is based on informed decisions and who takes into account his or her quality of life, including both physical well-being and psychological state, as well as other dimensions.

E-Wellness: The utilization of Internet capabilities (information, Web-based health services, etc.) in order to maintain a condition of good physical and mental health.

Medical Sensor: A device, such as a photoelectric cell, that receives and responds to a signal or stimulus.

M-Health: Mobile health refers to ambulatory-care provision enabled by third-generation devices that allow for the collection, management, and processing of the patient's vital data. Mobile health services range from the recording of the patient's medical signs and the synchronous or asynchronous communication with health professionals via mobile communication means, to the automatic diagnosis of the data recorded to personal sensors and alarm notices in case of an emergency. Mobile health or m-health is a step beyond electronic healthcare as it enhances ubiquitous health provision regardless of the patient's or physician's geographic location.

Telemonitoring: The science and technology of automatic measurement via medical sensors and the transmission of data by radio or other means from remote sources to receiving stations for recording and analysis. Data transfer can be achieved via wireless communications means and/or via other media, such as a telephone, a computer network, or an optical link.

Vital Signs: The pulse rate, blood pressure, body temperature, and rate of respiration of a person. The vital signs are usually measured to obtain a quick evaluation of the person's general physical condition.

Chapter XXXI
Telepathology
and Digital Pathology

Vincenzo Della Mea
University of Udine, Italy

ABSTRACT

The present chapter deals with state-of-the-art topics related to the application of information and communication technologies to the field of pathology, in particular for what regards telepathology and the so-called digital pathology. A classification of telepathology techniques is provided together with their typical applications. Starting from a definition of virtual or digital slide, digital pathology techniques and issues are then discussed.

INTRODUCTION

In pathology, the sample subject of analysis by the doctor is most often a biological tissue specimen cut in very thin sections, disposed over a glass slide, and coloured with suitable stainings in order to make morphological structures and biochemical components visually apparent. Such a specimen is observed by means of an optical microscope with resolutions up to 0.2 micron.

In the last 40 years, first morphometry (i.e., image analysis applied to the recognition and quantification of biological shapes) and then telepathology have been the two forces driving pathology toward the use of digital images.

In particular, telepathology has been traditionally constituted by the set of techniques for remotely transmitting images acquired from a glass slide through a microscope. The term telepathology was first referred to by R. Weinstein in 1986; he defined it as the "practice of pathology over a long distance," thus encompassing almost every possible application of digital images, including distant diagnosis, expert consultation, distant education, and remote image processing and analysis.

The two usual telemedicine categories of real-time and store-and-forward systems apply to telepathology, too, with the same cost and practical consequences but with peculiar aspects given by the features of the material to be represented by means of digital images.

In the very few last years and thanks to the innovations in the information technology field, a novel acquisition technique has been created that makes it possible to fully digitize a specimen, resulting in billions of pixels. The resulting image is called a virtual slide, virtual microscope, or digital slide, and can be used for most of the usual telepathology applications plus others. This innovation led to the creation of a somewhat new discipline, that is, digital pathology, where the emphasis is no more on the transmission of images, like in telepathology, but more generally on digital-image use.

In the next section, a brief overview of telepathology and digital pathology techniques and applications will be provided.

TELEPATHOLOGY TECHNIQUES: APPLICATIONS AND ISSUES

The approaches to telepathology are classically divided into two categories: store-and-forward and real-time telepathology, respectively based on the asynchronous delivery of images and real-time transmission. Another classification, often used in place of the former but with a slightly different meaning, is such between static and dynamic telepathology, respectively based on still images and live video.

In store-and-forward telepathology (Della Mea, 1999), the sender pathologist is supposed to select some representative image from the specimen to be delivered or simply made available to a remote recipient. Delivery may occur by means of standard e-mail (Della Mea et al., 1996), proprietary systems (Klossa, Cordier,

Flandrin, Got, & Hemet, 1998), or Web-based applications like iPath (Brauchli et al., 2000). Store-and-forward telepathology is the least expensive approach as it can be implemented with very basic technology, and thus it is the most diffused one despite some concerns on the bias inducted by the image selector (Mairinger, Netzer, Schoner, & Gschwendtner, 1998).

In real-time telepathology, a robotized microscope that can be remotely controlled is needed. In this case, the remote user may move the stage, change objectives, and so forth, receiving either still images (Demichelis, Barbareschi, et al., 2001) or live video (Dunn et al., 1997; Nordrum et al., 1991). As live video has lower quality than still images, hybrid approaches have been reported (Della Mea, 2000). Due to the need for quality of service, transmission often occurs through ISDN lines; however, in the past, attempts have been made to use Internet protocols (Wolf, Petersen, Dietel, & Petersen, 1998), which are at present more easily usable.

From the diagnostic point of view, telepathology might be useful in two main areas: second-opinion consultation and intraoperative diagnosis. In the former case, an expert is requested for an opinion regarding a difficult case with loose time constraints. While ordinarily the expert will receive a glass slide by post, with telepathology, he or she may receive a set of selected images (store and forward; Raab et al., 1997) or access to a real-time system (Dunn et al., 1997). In fact, store and forward is mostly used for expert consultation as it overcomes limitations due to different time zones when requesting and consulting pathologists are remotely separated (Della Mea & Beltrami, 1998). In the last years, two official services have been founded for providing consultation through store-and-forward systems: the Armed Forces Institute of Pathology telepathology service and the Union Internationale Centre le Cancer (UICC) consultation service.

Intraoperative diagnosis is made during surgery as quickly as possible to guide the surgeon in his or her work. A rural hospital might not have a pathologist available during operations, so telepathology can be used to deliver the same service from a distance provided that a real-time system is used. For this application, diagnostic performance is comparable to that of the microscope (Dunn et al., 1997; Kayser, Beyer, Blum, & Kayser, 2000; Nordrum et al., 1991); however, concerns are brought up when leaving the macrosampling task to the surgeon or to a technician.

Other applications of telepathology include remote image processing and evaluation, and education. In the former case, selected images can be sent to a remote image-processing service for automatic morphometry or cytometry (Ferrer Roca, Ramos, & Diaz Cardama, 1995; Kunze, Boecking, Haroske, Kayser, Meyer, & Oberholzer, 1998). In the latter, digital imagery may substitute microscope sessions to teach students histology and cytology (Harris, Leaven, Heidger, Kreiter, Duncan, & Dick, 2001).

DIGITAL PATHOLOGY TECHNIQUES: APPLICATIONS AND ISSUES

In a very few years, advances in information technology, including the increase in hard-disk capacity and faster network connections, led to the possibility of digitizing the whole glass slide, thus avoiding the image-selection bias reported for traditional store-and-forward telepathology. The digitized slide is then viewed by means of suitable software that emulates the features of a real microscope and is often able to connect to remote cases through the Internet.

The basic equipment for doing this is similar to those needed for real-time telepathology, that is, a robotized microscope driven by software able to scan the whole glass-slide surface and acquire all fields. More sophisticated devices have been developed in the form of either slide scanners or array microscopes (Weinstein et al., 2004).

The practice of digitizing large parts of a glass slide has been known since its beginnings as virtual microscopy (Ferreira et al., 1997), and the digitized slide has thus been called a virtual slide or digital slide; sometimes the viewing software is referred to as a virtual microscope.

Typical applications of the digital slide include education (Ferreira et al., 1997), quality control (Demichelis, 2002; Taylor, Gagnon, Lange, Lee, Draut, & Kujawski, 1999), and image processing and analysis (on tissue microarray slides; Dell'Anna, Demichelis, Barbareschi, & Sboner, 2005); informal reports have been made on their use for telediagnosis and long-term storage, too.

The main problems with digital slides are related to their size. A full slide (e.g., a Pap test) is made of up to 30GB of data when uncompressed, which when compressed may become just 1GB. This is an issue of storage; for remote viewing this is not a great problem as often a slide is only partially viewed to render a diagnosis (Tsuchihashi et al., 1999).

The size influences acquisition time, too, which when using tools based on robotized microscopes is measured in hours, although new developments like the array microscope (Weinstein et al., 2004) strongly reduce it. A secondary yet important problem is given by the fact that, although rarely, there is not a single focus plane. So, at least in some visual fields, it is necessary to acquire more than one image to capture all information.

DISCUSSION

Telepathology and digital pathology provide for three telemedicine techniques still in use due to their different features and issues.

In fact, while real-time telepathology and digital slides may provide the same amount of information to the distant user, the former is needed in urgency while the latter needs time for acquisition. On the other hand, digital slides automatically provide for long-term storage, while classical real-time pathology cannot in an easy way.

In addition, store-and-forward telepathology based on selected images still represents the most used technique due to its low cost and ease of use, which makes it suitable, for example, for supporting developing countries; good examples are the UICC telepathology centre and the consultation communities born around the free iPath software (Brauchli et al., 2000).

REFERENCES

Barbareschi, M., Demichelis, F., Forti, S., & Dalla Palma, P. (2000). Digital pathology: Science fiction? *International Journal of Surgical Pathology, 8,* 261-263.

Brauchli, K., Christen, H., Meyer, P., Haroske, G., Meyer, W., Kunze, K. D., et al. (2000). Telepathology: Design of a modular system. *Analytical Cellular Pathology, 21*(3-4), 193-199.

Costello, S. S., Johnston, D. J., Dervan, P. A., & O'Shea, D. G. (2003). Development and evaluation of the virtual pathology slide: A new tool in telepathology. *Journal of Medical Internet Research, 5*(2), e11.

Dell'anna, R., Demichelis, F., Barbareschi, M., & Sboner, A. (2005). An automated procedure to properly handle digital images in large scale tissue microarray experiments. *Computer Methods and Programs in Biomedicine, 79*(3), 197-208.

Della Mea, V. (1999). Store-and-forward telepathology. In B. Hernandez & R. Wootton (Eds.), *European telemedicine 1998/99.* London: EHTO, RSM Press, & Kensington Publications.

Della Mea, V., & Beltrami, C. A. (1998). Telepathology applications of the Internet multimedia electronic mail. *Medical Informatics, 23,* 237-244.

Della Mea, V., Forti, S., Puglisi, F., Bellutta, P., Finato, N., Dalla Palma, P., et al. (1996). Telepathology using Internet multimedia electronic mail: Remote consultation on gastrointestinal pathology. *Journal of Telemedicine and Telecare, 2,* 28-34.

Demichelis, F., Barbareschi, M., Boi, S., Clemente, C., Dalla Palma, P., Eccher, C., et al. (2001). Robotic telepathology for intraoperative remote diagnosis using a still-imaging-based system. *American Journal of Clinical Pathology, 116*(5), 744-752.

Demichelis, F., Barbareschi, M., Dalla Palma, P., & Forti, S. (2002). A new method to completely digitise cytological and histological slides. *Virchows Archive, 441*(2), 159-164.

Demichelis, F., Della Mea, V., Forti, S., Dalla Palma, P., & Beltrami, C. A. (2002). Digital storage of glass slides for quality assurance in histopathology and cytopathology. *Journal of Telemedicine and Telecare, 8*(3), 138-142.

Dunn, B. E., Almagro, U. A., Choi, H., Sheth, N. K., Arnold, J. S., Recla, D. L., et al. (1997). Dynamic-robotic telepathology: Department of Veterans Affairs feasibility study. *Human Pathology, 28,* 8-12.

Ferreira, R., Moon, B., Humphries, J., Sussman, A., Saltz, J., Miller, R., et al. (1997). The virtual microscope. *Proceedings of AMIA Annual Fall Symposium* (pp. 449-453).

Ferrer Roca, O., Ramos, A., & Diaz Cardama, A. (1995). Immunohistochemical correlation of steroid receptors and disease-free interval in 206 consecutive cases of breast cancer: Validation of telequantification based on global scene segmentation. *Analytical Cellular Pathology, 9*, 151-163.

Foran, D. J., Meer, P. P., Papathomas, T., & Marsic, I. (1997). Compression guidelines for diagnostic telepathology. *IEEE Transactions on Information Technology in Biomedicine, 1*, 55-60.

Harris, T., Leaven, T., Heidger, P., Kreiter, C., Duncan, J., & Dick, F. (2001). Comparison of a virtual microscope laboratory to a regular microscope laboratory for teaching histology. *The Anatomical record, 265*(1), 10-14.

Kayser, K., Beyer, M., Blum, S., & Kayser, G. (2000). Recent developments and present status of telepathology. *Analytical Cellular Pathology, 21*, 101-106.

Klossa, J., Cordier, J. C., Flandrin, G., Got, C., & Hemet, J. (1998). A European de facto standard for image folders applied to telepathology and teaching. *International Journal of Medical Informatics, 48*, 207-216.

Kunze, K. D., Boecking, A., Haroske, G., Kayser, K., Meyer, W., & Oberholzer, M. (1998). Remote quantitation in the framework of telepathology. *Advances in Clinical Pathology, 2*(2), 141-143.

Mairinger, T., Netzer, T. T., Schoner, W., & Gschwendtner, A. (1998). Pathologists' attitudes to implementing telepathology. *Journal of Telemedicine and Telecare, 4*, 41-46.

Nordrum, I., Engum, B., Rinde, E., Finseth, A., Ericsson, H., Kearney, M., et al. (1991). Remote frozen section service: A telepathology project in northern Norway. *Human Pathology, 22*(6), 514-518.

Raab, S., Robinson, R. A., Snider, T. E., McDaniel, H. L., Sigman, J. D., Leigh, C. J., et al. (1997). Telepathologic review: Utility, diagnostic accuracy, and interobserver variability on a difficult case consultation service. *Modern Pathology, 10*, 630-635.

Taylor, R. N., Gagnon, M., Lange, J., Lee, T., Draut, R., & Kujawski, E. (1999). CytoView: A prototype computer image-based Papanicolaou smear proficiency test. *Acta Cytologica, 43*(6), 1045-1051.

Tsuchihashi, Y., Mazaki, T., Nakasato, K., Morishima, M., Nagata, H., Tofukuji, I., et al. (1999). The basic diagnostic approaches used in robotic still-image telepathology. *Journal of Telemedicine and Telecare, 5*(Suppl. 1), S115-S117.

Weinstein, R. S. (1986). Prospects for telepathology. *Human Pathology, 17*(5), 433-434.

Weinstein, R. S., Descour, M. R., Liang, C., Barker, G., Scott, K. M., Richter, L., et al. (2004). An array microscope for ultrarapid virtual slide processing and telepathology: Design, fabrication, and validation study. *Human Pathology, 35*(11), 1303-1314.

Wolf, G., Petersen, D., Dietel, D., & Petersen, I. (1998). Telemicroscopy via the Internet. *Nature, 391*, 613-614.

KEY TERMS

Digital Pathology: The set of image acquisition, storage, transmission, and processing techniques based on the digital slide.

Real-Time Telepathology: Synchronous form of telepathology in which the distant operator is able to drive a remote robotized microscope by using software simulating the behaviour of a microscope.

Store-and-Forward Telepathology: Asynchronous form of telepathology based on the exchange of still images selected from a glass slide, often used for second-opinion consultation.

Telepathology: Practice of pathology over a long distance. It includes telediagnosis.

Virtual Microscope: The system constituted by one or more virtual slides and the viewer software needed for their examination. The term is also used to identify the viewer alone.

Virtual Slide (Digital Slide): A digital copy of a complete glass slide or of a substantially large part of it.

Chapter XXXII
Collaborative Environments for the Health Monitoring of Chronically Ill Children

G. Ganiatsas
University of Ioannina, Greece

K. Starida
University of Ioannina, Greece

Dimitrios I. Fotiadis
University of Ioannina, Greece
Biomedical Research Institute—FORTH, Greece
Michaelideion Cardiology Center, Greece

ABSTRACT

A revolution is taking place in the healthcare field with information technology (IT) playing an increasingly important role in its delivery. Healthcare providers are exploring IT opportunities in reducing the overall costs of healthcare delivery while improving the quality of its provision to citizens. Healthcare services have accumulated great benefits from the application of information technologies, telecommunications and management tools. Internet, wireless, and handheld technologies have the capability to affect healthcare by improving quality, efficiency, and cost-effectiveness of work. Healthcare information systems include a wide range of applications ranging from diagnostic tools to health management applications and from inpatient to outpatient monitoring services. Home-care systems address patients and their families and provide the means to manage their health status related to a specific health problem. Home-care systems include a wide variety of offered services such as: (a) directory services (hospital location, doctor specialties), (b) computer patient records (CPR) along with interfaces for interoperability, (c) certified medical information provision, (d) interfacing to specialized medical monitoring devices, and (e) synchronous and asynchronous collaboration services. All these services are offered, most of the time, through secure and seamless networks.

INTRODUCTION

A revolution is taking place in the healthcare field with information technology playing an increasingly important role in its delivery. Further exponential growth is expected as the healthcare industry implements electronic medical records, upgrades hospital information systems, sets up intranets for sharing information among related participants, and uses public networks to distribute health-related information and provide remote diagnostics via telemedicine (Directorate-General Information Society & Immarsat Ltd, 1999). Today's healthcare providers, faced with an unprecedented era of competition, are exploring IT opportunities in reducing the overall costs of healthcare delivery while improving the quality of its provision to citizens.

Healthcare services have accumulated great benefits from the application of information technologies, telecommunications, and management tools. The Internet and wireless and handheld technologies have the capability to affect health care by improving the quality, efficiency, and cost effectiveness of work (Eder & Darter, 1998). By integrating data from disparate sources—various medical departments, billing systems, insurers, and other medical information resources—into a single point of reference and making them available at anytime and anyplace via the Internet and wireless technology on a handheld computer, health-care professionals are able to provide the most effective patient care at the point of care.

Healthcare information systems include a wide range of applications ranging from diagnostic tools to health-management applications, and from inpatient to outpatient monitoring services. During the last few years, advances in telecommunications, Internet technologies, and specialized lightweight medical devices have advanced development in healthcare, enabling the deployment of healthcare systems for children who are chronically ill and need continuous monitoring of their health conditions (Southall et al., 2000). Asthma, diabetes, and chronic heart problems are among those that raised the demand for continuous monitoring systems, and several services and products became available powered by different technologies.

Asthma is defined as a chronic inflammatory disease of the airways; this inflammation is responsible for the appearance of symptoms associated with reversible airway obstruction, both spontaneous as well as following treatment, and is a determining factor of concomitant airway hyperresponsiveness. The clinical situation of acute asthma may be classified as mild, moderate, or severe. Moderate asthma is accompanied by tachypnoea, the use of accessory muscles for respiration, and the inhibition of physical activity. In severe asthma, wheezing may no longer be audible, cyanosis and shortness of breath are present with the contraction of the thoracic muscles, and the patient is compelled to stay in bed; the heart rate exceeds 120 beats per minute, and PEF and FEV1 are lower than 50% (Lung Association, n.d.).

Diabetes mellitus is a condition in which the amount of glucose (sugar) in the blood is too high because the body cannot use it properly. Glucose comes from the digestion of starchy foods such as bread, rice, potatoes, chapatis, yams, and plantain, from the digestion of sugar and other sweet foods; and from the liver, which makes glucose. There are two main types of diabetes. Type 1 diabetes, also known as insulin-dependent diabetes, develops if the body is unable to produce any insulin. This type of diabetes usually appears before the age of 40. Type 2 diabetes, also known as non-insulin-dependent diabetes, develops when the body can still make some insulin, but not enough, or when the insulin that is produced does not work properly (known as insulin resistance). This type of diabetes usually appears in people over 40 years old, though in South Asian and African-Caribbean people, it often appears in those over 25 years old (American Diabetes association, n.d.).

BACKGROUND

Home-care systems address patients and their families and provide the means to manage their health status related to a specific health problem (Tatman, Woodroffe, Kelly, & Harris, 2001). Home-care systems include a wide variety of offered services such as (a) directory services (hospital location, doctor specialties), (b) computer patient records (CPRs) along with interfaces for interoperability, (c) certified medical information provision, (d) interfacing to specialized medical monitoring devices, and (e) synchronous and asynchronous collaboration services. All these services are offered, most of the time, through secure and seamless networks. The following section provides an insight on the most commonly used home-care services and applications.

Directory Services

A directory provides a consistent way to name, describe, locate, access, manage, and secure information. A directory is used to store information that must be shared between applications in a network environment. Information is organized as a hierarchy of objects with their associated attributes. A directory service makes this information available as named objects that can be found using familiar white-page-style lookups or yellow-page-style searches. There is currently a huge amount of interest, comment, and speculation within the industry about

directory services (Howes, Smith, & Good, 1998).

Computer Patient Records and Interoperability Mechanisms

A computer-based patient-record system adds information-management tools to provide the maintenance of records, clinical reminders and alerts, linkages with knowledge sources for health-care decision support, analyzes of aggregate data, and so forth. An important issue when designing and implementing computer patient records lies in the interoperability with existing legacy systems.

The most common method used for interoperability is the Health Level 7 (HL7) protocol. HL7 is a messaging protocol for electronic data exchange in health-care environments. It defines transactions for transmitting data about patient registration, insurance, billing, orders and results for laboratory tests, physiology, image studies, observations, diet orders, pharmacy orders, and supply orders. The HL7 standard is message based and uses an event-trigger model that causes the sending system to transmit a specified message to the receiving unit, with a subsequent response by the latter (Heath Level 7, n.d.). HL7 handles transactions for exchanging information about patient administration (admission, discharge, transfer, outpatient registration), patient accounting (billing), appointment scheduling, problem lists, clinical-trial enrollments, patient permissions, voice dictations, advanced directives, and physiologic signals.

Another method for interchanging medical information relies on the Digital Imaging and Communications in Medicine (DICOM) standard (American College of Radiology/National Electronic Manufacturers Association, 1983; *Digital Imaging and Communications in Medicine*, n.d.). This is a specification that describes the formatting and exchanging of medical images and associated information. It relies on standard communication protocols and addresses the communication of images from digital modalities such as CT, MR, ultrasound, nuclear medicine, digital cardiology, and angiography and RF equipment, as well as radiation-therapy devices. It also allows the exchange of patient demographics, exam status, and scheduling information.

Certified Medical Content

A widely used home-care service is found in the provision of certified medical content through the delivery of personalized medical information or educational material for the patients and their family. These services range from simple Web pages to more advanced, personalized Web applications. They usually provide healthcare tips and instructions on how to manage various situations related to the patient's status. The increasing availability of large bodies of medical literature online (journal articles, encyclopedias, patient records) fuels the development of applications based on some kind of knowledge processing. Examples of such applications include concept-based indexing and retrieval, question answering, and, more generally, text understanding, as well as medical corpus or database mining. A sound representation of the medical domain, or ontology, is needed by all of these applications (Medical Ontology Research, n.d.).

Interfacing to Specialized Medical Monitoring Devices

These services include the monitoring of chronic diseases through the use of appropriate equipment, for instance, portable devices for peak expiratory flow or blood-glucose monitoring in order to deal with asthma or diabetes, respec-

tively. Patients use specialized medical devices to acquire measurements related to their specific diseases, and they communicate the results to medical professionals using either device software or communication-link applications by inserting the acquired values to specific fields (Philips Medical Systems, n.d.). Existing home-care services often provide communication with healthcare experts through various means, although this is not mandatory.

Synchronous and Asynchronous Collaboration Services

Online collaboration among health specialists can be based on advanced telemedicine and teleconference tools of high cost with which healthcare centers and organizations are equipped. Collaboration falls into two main categories: synchronous collaboration, in which users communicate with each other at the same time, and asynchronous collaboration, in which the communication of the users is achieved at different times (Microsoft, n.d.). Based on these categories, collaboration tools and services are further classified into the following functional categories.

Synchronous Collaboration

- Electronic meeting systems.
- Real-time conferencing systems (local and remote) as well as collaborative presentation systems (*Data Protocols for Multimedia Conferencing*, 1996).
- Desktop video and real-time data conferencing focusing on real time rather than BBS or Notes. All products in this category store documents, and/or allow others to see and work on documents simultaneously or on each other's screen or a whiteboard.

- Group document handling, including group editing, shared-screen editing work, group document and image management, and document databases.

Asynchronous Collaboration

- Electronic mail and messaging, including messaging infrastructures and e-mail systems.
- Group calendaring and scheduling, including products for meeting and resource coordination.
- Non-real-time data conferencing. Asynchronous conferencing is similar to a bulletin board, in which the user carries on a conversation over time by leaving and answering messages. These messages can be public, as in a BBS, or private, as in a Notes discussion database.
- Work-flow-process diagramming and analysis tools, work-flow enactment engines, electronic forms that route products.

Security and Privacy

Security mechanisms include all technological and operational measures to safeguard the confidentiality and privacy of personal data, as well as to protect the services and the operators from liability exposure and possible legal sanctions.

The usual security and privacy practices of most of the existing home-care systems involve a number of steps.

- **Protection of Resources:** To protect both data and services from a number of external threats, firewalls are incorporated into the system (Stallings, 1999).
- **User Authentication:** The identities of legitimate users are verified by means of digital certificates.

- **User Authorization:** Whenever access to the services, the data repositories, or the shared resources of the system is required, an access-control mechanism is invoked, involving access-control lists and security filters. A hierarchy of authorization levels is built in order to model the different privileges of the system users.
- **Privacy of Transmission:** The secure exchange of health records, personal information, and management plans over the Web is achieved by employing a PKI scheme by means of secure network protocols like S-HTTP and SSL (Data Protection Working Party, n.d.).
- **Security Policies:** Administrative procedures and physical safeguards secure data integrity, confidentiality, and availability.

MAIN THRUST

The existing home-care systems are either Web-based or stand-alone applications that act as health-management tools for child patients suffering from chronic diseases. The following section presents the main characteristics, technical features, and services of the major home-care systems available.

LifeChart

LifeChart has created a system to collect and store personal health information from individuals with chronic diseases. Individuals monitor their health using personal electronic monitors and transmit their results to LifeChart through the public telephone network. The information resides in a robust relational database that allows sophisticated query and analysis. Information collected from the remote monitor is formatted into reports available for transmission by automated fax to the healthcare professional's fax number listed on the patient's enrollment in the LifeChart information service. The collected information can be made available to health-care professionals to assist clinicians in treating their patients' diseases; it is also available for cross-sectional analysis to assist in disease management.

Transtelephonic Home-Care Services

Transtelephonic monitoring (TTM) is a technology that allows patients to report symptoms and/or transmit data from a medical device (usually a pacemaker or implanted cardioverter defibrillator) over the phone for medical evaluation by their physician. TTM may be used to allow patients to have their pacemaker or ICD checks done over the phone, or to transmit data from an electrocardiograph (EKG) machine over the phone for evaluation. Signals from the devices are converted into sound waves, sent over the phone, received by the monitoring station at the other end of the phone, and reconverted back into the original signals (Mednet Healthcare Technologies, n.d.).

MyHealthyLife Network

Protocol Driven HealthCare Inc. (PDHI) has developed 10 channels in major disease areas that can be configured, privately labeled, and integrated with a customer Web strategy. Access to any of these sites requires registration and is password protected. Nonetheless, the service is free of charge. PDHI health channels allow users to do the following:

- Input data about their condition, symptoms, and lifestyle
- Receive immediate feedback in the form of graphs, scores, and reminders, rein-

forcing successes and highlighting areas that need further work

- Communicate with nurses and other healthcare professionals via a secure messaging system for support, advice, and education
- Allow their physician to review their personal charts and diaries
- Share their experiences and receive peer group support through bulletin boards

CHILDCARE

The CHILDCARE system supports the out-of-hospital, continuous health-care management of chronically ill children. CHILDCARE is a complete home-care system designed to promote collaboration between health professionals. Enhancing this collaboration with intelligent features can improve the prevention, early detection, prognosis, and treatment of children's diseases while at the same time facilitating access to best medical practice regardless of the child's location (*CHILDCARE Project*, n.d.).

Special focus is placed on the utilization of the latest technology accomplishments toward the incorporation of teleconference sessions, collaborative spaces, and intelligent add-ons over a common secure platform. This combination allows for (a) remote communication between health experts and the child's family, (b) efficient collaboration between the responsible doctor and healthcare professionals, (c) the interfacing of legacy hospital information systems to obtain health records, (d) the setup, execution, and monitoring of health-management plans, (e) ubiquitous access from multiple devices, (f) role-based management of the actors with respect to their actual involvement in the healthcare process, and (g) confidentiality and security at all levels.

CHILDCARE services are built reflecting the most urgent needs of real users: electronic medical records, communication between the patient and the doctor, ability for remote examination and online consultation, automated tracking of the health condition based on monitored indicators, collaboration between the responsible doctor and specialized health professionals, delivery of personalized information about the illnesses, provision of yellow-pages information on healthcare resources, and unification and flexibility in accessing the services. Privacy and Web-based-service security mechanisms are integrated in the CHILDCARE platform, thus safeguarding both the CHILDCARE data and its services. All these end up creating a system that advances quality in pediatric home care.

CHILDCARE is based on a modular and flexible design that focuses on the unified integration of technologies, the utilization of well-established experience, the adopting of powerful standards in the exchange of healthcare records, and the representation of medical information, while at the same time advancing current information-processing technologies. CHILDCARE encourages the initiative and effort of all the involved actors. This is achieved through ubiquitous and secure services at all levels that can be accessed through a vast variety of fixed and wireless network interfaces.

The CHILDCARE framework addresses the management of chronic conditions—currently asthma and diabetes—but it can easily be customized to other chronic diseases. The mentioned diseases have been most favored by pediatricians (89% and 93%, respectively) as far as monitoring through the use of telemedicine services is concerned. The criteria for selecting diabetes and asthma among other diseases are that they are serious, common, amenable to improved outcomes through better manage-

ment, and have clearly defined parameters of well-being. CHILDCARE also incorporates the management of the normal development of neonates, despite the fact that neonatal development is far from a chronic condition. This target group provides added value to the system since neonates are most common and have a great impact on the public.

CONCLUSION

It is easily understood why chronically ill children and adults feel more comfortable receiving care at home rather than having to visit a healthcare facility. Usually, they are frightened and under stress, not only due to their medical condition, which might be a chronic disease, but also because they are in a place completely foreign to them. Yet, providing these people with a telemedicine tool is not an adequate solution since ongoing health care involves more than just the patient and the doctor. The medical professional needs to work in close cooperation with a variety of health specialists and the patient's family for delivering the best care. For this reason, a great variety of home-care systems and services has been developed. The most common services provided through these systems include (a) electronic medical records, (b) streamlined communication between patient and doctor, (c) cooperation among health professionals over a virtual collaborative space, (d) the exchange of medical data, (e) the interfacing of medical equipment that measure medical indicators, and (f) alerts and reminders that relate to the obtained measurement. The related legal and ethical implications or constraints that concern home-care systems and medical procedures are taken into account so as to ensure that all the appropriate technological and operational measures are delivered.

REFERENCES

American Diabetes Association. (n.d.). Retrieved January 15, 2005, from http://www.diabetes.org.uk/

CHILDCARE project. (n.d.). Retrieved January 10, 2005, from http://www.childcare-eu.com

Data Protection Working Party. (n.d.). *Privacy on the Internet: An integrated EU approach to on-line data protection* (5063/OO/EN/FINAL, Article 29). Retrieved February 8, 2005, from http://europa.eu.int/comm/internal_market/en/dataprot/wpdocs/wp37en.pdf

Data protocols for multimedia conferencing (Recommendation T.120). (1996). Retrieved February 5, 2005, from http://www.itu.int/rec/recommendation.asp

Digital imaging and communications in medicine (DICOM). (n.d.). Retrieved from http://medical.nema.org

Directorate-General Information Society & Immarsat Ltd. (1999). Telemedicine in the 21st century: Opportunities for citizens, society and industry. An international space university workspace. In *Proceedings of Telemedicine in the 21st century.* Strasbourg, France.

Eder, L. B., & Darter, M. E. (1998). Physicians in cyberspace. *Communications of the ACM, 41*(3), 52-54.

Health Level 7. (n.d.). Retrieved January 26, 2005, from http://www.hl7.org

Howes, T., Smith, M., & Good, G. (1998). *Understanding and deploying LDAP directory services.* London: MacMillan Technical Publications.

Lung Association. (n.d.). Retrieved February 16, 2006, from http://www.lung.ca/asthma

Medical Ontology Research. (n.d.). Retrieved from February 7, 2006, http://lhnbc.nlm.nih.gov

Mednet Healthcare Technologies. (n.d.). Retrieved February 8, 2005, from http://www.mednethealth.net

Microsoft. (n.d.). Retrieved February 20, 2005, from http://www.microsoft.com/ms.htm

Philips Medical Systems. (n.d.). Retrieved March 5, 2005, from http://www3.medical.philips.com/

Southall, D., Burr, S., Smith, R. D., Bull, D. N., Randford, A., Williams, A., et al. (2000). The child-friendly healthcare initiative (CFHI): Healthcare provision in accordance with the UN Convention on the Rights of the Child. *Pediatrics, 106*(5), 1054-1064.

Stallings, W. (1999). *Cryptography and network security: Principles and practice* (2nd ed.). Upper Saddle River, NJ: Prentice Hall.

Tatman, M. A., Woodroffe, C., Kelly, P. J., & Harris, R. J. (2001). Paediatric home care in tower hamlets: A working partnership with parents. *Quality in Health Care, 1*, 98-103.

KEY TERMS

Chronic Diseases: Diseases that have one or more of the following characteristics: They are permanent, leave residual disability, are caused by nonreversible pathological alteration, require special training by the patient for rehabilitation, and/or may be expected to require a long period of supervision, observation, or care.

Computer Patient Record (CPR): A repository of electronically maintained information about an individual's lifetime health status and health care, stored in such a way so as to be able to serve the multiple legitimate users of the record.

CPR Interoperability: The ability of two or more computer patient-record systems or their components to exchange medical information and to use medical information that has been exchanged.

Home-Care Products: Medical devices that enable patients to monitor their health status (e.g., by providing the ability to measure certain vital indicators), but that can also be integrated with other applications that are developed for this purpose.

Home-Care Services: Complete applications that provide the means to allow medical professionals to monitor and manage their patients' health status.

Medical Ontology: The terminology used to refer to the shared understanding of some domain of interest, which may be used as a unifying framework to solve the problem of dispersed medical information.

Real-Time Conferencing Systems: Composed of software and services that provide a real-time venue for the exchange, creation, and viewing of information by users in real time.

Chapter XXXIII
Electronic Submission of New Drugs in Europe

A. Susanne Esslinger
Friedrich-Alexander-University, Germany

Daniela Marschall
Friedrich-Alexander-University, Germany

ABSTRACT

All over the world, drugs and drug applications have to be submitted to and approved by an admission office before they may be sold on the market. All procedures are extensive, time-consuming, and costly. To simplify the process, it could be organised electronically. In an economic perspective, there are many benefits by using the electronic form for the pharmaceutical industry: managing knowledge, cost advantages, and time savings. All, pharmaceutical industry and institutions have undertaken lots of efforts to enforce the electronic solutions. They focus on international standards in order to harmonise structures and processes. It would be necessary to reduce paper and copies, especially if the electronic solution takes place. This method will simplify the way to deal with data and documents and reduce process time and costs.

INTRODUCTION

The pharmaceutical industry is characterised by high expenditures on research and development. In 2003 in Germany, over 3.56 billion euros were spent for the development of new drugs and new drug applications (Bundesverband der Pharmazeutischen Industrie e.V., 2004a). In the year 2004, almost 9,000 drugs were listed in the *Rote Liste*, a compendium of all medication patients may get (Bundesverband der Pharmazeutischen Industrie e.V., 2004b). The developing process for a new product lasts on average between 8 and 11 years and costs about 800 million euros (Bundesverband der Pharmazeutischen Industrie e.V., 2004a). The duration of a patent for a new drug or new drug application lasts 20 years. Usually, in the product-development process, the application for a letters patent takes place early. Therefore, the patent time for the producer, the time in which they can promote the drug on the market and amortise the costs of research and development, is reduced to about 10 years (Bundesverband der Pharmazeutischen Industrie e.V., 2004a). Thus, time to market is a critical issue for firms in order to economically succeed in a long-term perspective. The duration for research and development of a drug usually is fixed. But the time for the submission of a new medicine, which takes about 2 years, may be reduced. If firms do so, they may gain profit.

Electronic solutions are more and more common in the healthcare sector (e.g., electronic prescription), and it may be useful to submit pharmaceutical products electronically. This article will give a closer look on the opportunities of electronic submission concerning processes, time, and costs.

SUBMISSION OF DRUGS

All over the world, drugs and drug applications have to be submitted to and approved by an admission office before they may be sold on the market (Jordan, 2002). Usually, for the submission, the producer has to get in contact with the local admission office (for example, in Germany, it is the Bundesinstitut für Arzneimittel und Medizinprodukte, BfArM, 2004) and with the European Medicines Evaluation Agency (EMEA; Europäische Arzneimittel-Agentur, 2003). The firm has to send a submission dossier to the office. It contains information about the harmlessness, effectiveness, and quality of the drug. For some medicines, registration is sufficient for the firms: No clinical evaluations or pharmacological-toxicological tests have to be conducted by the producer. Within Europe, several regulations, directives, legal decisions, and guidelines have to be considered (Bundesverband der Arzneimittel-Hersteller, n.d.). They are especially concerned with technical aspects and harmonisation, form, and content. The detailed Common Technical Document (CTD) has existed since 2003. It is a guideline for the technical documentation of any drug in Europe, the United States, or Japan and was established in the International Conference on Harmonisation (ICH; BfArM, 2003). Formal aspects of the dossier are shown in the European standardised *Notice to Applicants* (NTA; Wagner, 2000). The content specifications are described in EU (European Union) guidelines or country-specific rules. In Germany, for instance, firms must fulfill diverse criteria set by the Arzneimittelgesetz (AMG), the AMG-Einreichungsverordnung, the Verwaltungsverfahrensgesetz, and the Arzneimittelzulassungsgesetz. Products released in just one country might be accredited just for this region. But drugs that are placed on the European market have to fulfill European standards. Depending on the requested licensing, the submission dossier for a new drug or drug application will be made up of about 1,000 folders and more than 500,000 pages (Mitteleuropäische Gesellschaft für Regulatory Affairs, n.d.).

As one can imagine, all procedures are extensive, time consuming, and costly. To simplify the process, it could be organised electronically. Doing so, in 1985, the United States founded the Computer Assistance in New Drug Applications (CANDA) project. In 1994, the SMART (Submission Management and Tracking System) project displaced the labor-intensive CANDA project. This system is based on the guideline "Providing Regulatory Submissions in Electronic Format: General Considerations." It is a data-oriented approach with a general and a specific section. Thus, the evaluation is based on data and supported by statements of experts and textual documentation.

The legal framework of SMART is the Electronic Records and Electronic Signatures Regulation (21 CFR Part 11; U.S. Department of Health and Human Services, Food and Drug Administration [FDA], CDER, & CBER, 1999). Today in the United States, over 80% of all submissions, including new-drug applications, are conducted electronically, and the process time has been reduced by more than half a year in each of the cases (Food and Drug Administration, 2004).

The DAMOS Initiative

In Europe in the year 1989, the DAMOS (Drug Application Methodology with Optical Storage) project was the first to submit drugs electronically (Franken, 2003a). In 1993, the admission office started the pilot. Two years later, in 1995, a software developer offered the first electronic dossiers on the market. At the same time, the firm started to invent a review tool for the admission office. In 1998, DAMOS was officially accepted as a possible way to hand in the electronic dossier for the submission of a new drug. Documents from experts are evaluated in the first step, and data in the second step (top-down process). Therefore, the focus in electronic documents is on text besides data, which is different from the SMART solution. DAMOS is structured in two parts. One part only illustrates the structure of the complete dossier, and the other part is content (Franken, 2003a).

In Europe, submission processes are still country specific. However, lots of efforts are undertaken concerning worldwide harmonisation (ICH). Thus, as an example, the German BfArM would accept the format of the DAMOS but prefers the electronic CTD (eCTD) format. This format has assumed the basic structure and specification of DAMOS and will displace it completely in the close future. It can be observed that in Germany, nobody hands in DAMOS-based dossiers. In fact, the CTD format has been obligatory in Europe since July 2003.

The Electronic Common Technical Document

According to eCTD (2005):

The eCTD is defined as an interface for industry to agency transfer of regulatory information while at the same time taking into consideration the facilitation of the creation, review, lifecycle management and archival of the electronic submission. The eCTD specification lists the criteria that will make an electronic submission technically valid. The focus of the specification is to provide the ability to transfer the registration application electronically from industry to a regulatory authority.

Besides the transfer:

the eCTD and related standards will help pharmaceutical companies to control global submissions, product life cycle, time to market and supply chain cost-effectiveness (eCTD, 2005).

The guidelines are based, as mentioned above, on the CTD. In order to send data via Web browsers, the format of the data is XML (Extensible Markup Language; Franken, 2003b).

"The consequence of this approach is that in order to receive, validate and review eCTD compliant applications, regulatory authorities need to have a system in place." In this context, the most critical initial user requirement of such a system is actually the European Union Review System (EURS, 2002). Besides the eCTD, firms need an information-management system (IMS). According to PIM (2005):

PIM is a system to be introduced by the EMEA in the first instance in November 2005. It has been conceived as a means of: a) increasing the efficiency of the management and exchange of product information (summary of product characteristics, package leaflet and labelling) by all parties involved in the evaluation process through the structuring of the information and its exchange by electronic means; and b) improving the quality and consistency of the published product information.

Within Europe, experts still have problems with complete electronic submission because of security concerns. In the EU Directive 1999/93/EG, the common frames for electronic signatures are set already. The directive may differ in the various European countries (Hock & Jostes, 2003). If a pharmaceutical producer decides to hand in the complete documents in an electronic form, he or she still has to hand in a textual version. The latter is still the only one legally accepted (Europäische Arzneimittel-Agentur, 2004), and it is still necessary to sign some of the needed documents in most European countries. Besides this, the pharmaceutical firms may send their electronic versions. In order to do so, they have to consider, as it was said earlier, a wide range of regulations.

ECONOMICAL ASPECTS

Benefits

From an economic perspective, there are many benefits by using the electronic form for the pharmaceutical industry: managing knowledge, cost advantages, and time savings.

First of all, it is of high importance to reveal implicit knowledge and make it transparent. This is an essential success factor for pharmaceutical firms as their success is mainly based on research and development. Economies of scope may be gained easily (Erhard, 2003), and organisational learning in a long-term perspective is possible. Also, the quality of the documents will be improved (Vis-à-Vis, 2002) because of well-informed employees. It might also be possible to standardise processes due to routines.

Second, cost advantages may be realised: Costs of paper, copies, mailing, and storage may be saved. Firms using electronic submission do not need plenty of bookshelves to store the documents. Above all, they do not need the laborious transportation of documents from their offices to the archive or from expert to expert. In consequence, logistical overhead will be reduced.

Third, time savings are possible. The electronic submission of new drugs allows the admission office to access the complete documentation with one click. Thus, searching for one specific aspect one might need for the submission will proceed more quickly.

All these benefits allow the firms to speed up the submission process significantly. Time to market for a new drug or a new-drug application is improved (Vis-à-Vis, 2002). The pharmaceutical producer will be able to profit from this pioneering. Being the first in the market, the company skims the payers' high willingness to pay for a new innovative drug. The medicine is known as a brand. Thus, the firm gains market shares. On the basis of pioneer experiences of the drug, they may further improve the quality of other drugs and create bonding of the patient and doctors on the firm's brands.

Actually, the measurement of the benefits in firms and institutions is still difficult. There are some explorative data. It was measured that the time of the submission process was reduced by over 75% (Höniger, 2003) through electronic submission. Also, costs for the process were reduced by over 60% (Witzel, Yamaguchi, & Lorenz, 1998). Have a product on the market one day earlier creates an added daily average turnaround of more than 1 million euro (Baldowski, 2000; Kainz & Harmsen, 2003; Schmitt, 2003).

Costs

The electronic submission of drugs does not only create cost advantages. Some investments have to be made. For realising electronic submission, the pharmaceutical firms have to implement management information systems. For this reason, they have to invest in hardware and software. These costs (e.g., for the search and selection of adequate software) are of high importance especially for the pharmaceutical industry because information techniques do not necessarily belong to their core competencies. The configuration and maintenance of the system may even require employing specialists. Training is necessary in order to achieve the organisational learning of the employees mentioned above. Additionally, a professional support system for the users has to be assured. The firms also have to install firewalls in order to protect their data.

Depending on the implemented system, experts estimate that the investment at least takes 250,000 euro, and the amortisation of the investment takes at least 12 months (Zimmer, 2003).

Cost calculation concerned with reorganisation and process optimisation is a difficult task. Also, costs related to amortisation, the maintenance of software, network administration, and support for users are difficult to measure. Nevertheless, it is very important to compare the realisable benefits with the calculated costs.

CONCLUSION

The electronic submission of drugs today is reality. All pharmaceutical industry and software firms as well as institutions have undertaken lots of efforts to enforce electronic solutions. They focus on international standards in order to harmonise structures and processes. The problem is still the electronic signature. It will be necessary to reduce paper and copies, especially if the electronic solution takes place. Still, there are some pharmaceutical firms that have no need to change to the electronic system. But if they think it over, this method will simplify the way they deal with data and documents, and reduce process time and costs.

REFERENCES

Baldowski, N. (2000). Elektronische arzneimittelzulassung verkürzt die behandlung der anträge. *Computerwoche, 20*, 75-77.

Bundesinstitut für Arzneimittel und Medizinprodukte (BfArM) (Ed.). (2003). *Hinweise zum einreichen von zulassungsanträgen im CTD: Format beim bundesinstitut für arzneimittel und medizinprodukte.* Retrieved November 10, 2004, from http://www.bfarm.de/de/Arzneimittel/zul/CTD.pdf

Bundesinstitut für Arzneimittel und Medizinprodukte (BfArM) (Ed.). (2004). *Erläuterungen zum vollzug der verordnung über die einreichung von unterlagen in verfahren für die zulassung und verlängerung der zulassung von arzneimitteln (AMG-Einreichungsverordnung: AMG-EV), Version 4.09.* Retrieved November 10, 2004, from http://www.bfarm.de/de/Arzneimittel/amg_ev/Erl-V4-9.pdf

Bundesverband der Arzneimittel-Hersteller e.V. (Ed.). (n.d.). *ICH: International conference on harmonisation of technical requirements for registration of pharmaceuticals for human use.* Retrieved November 10, 2004, from http://www.bah-bonn.de/arzneimittel/europa/ich.htm

Bundesverband der Pharmazeutischen Industrie e.V. (Ed.). (2004a). Pharmadaten 2004. 34.

Bundesverband der Pharmazeutischen Industrie e.V. (Ed.). (2004b). *Pharmadaten 2004 kompakt.* Retrieved November 10, 2004, from http://www.bpi.de/internet/download/pharmadaten_2004_kompakt.pdf

Electronic common technical document (eCTD). (2005). Retrieved July 22, 2005, from http://www.ectd.com/about.htm

Erhard, D. (2003). Erfolgskriterien für die einrichtung eines elektronischen dokumentenmanagament-systems zur unterstützung der erstellung von zulassungsdossiers. *Pharmind: Die Pharmazeutische Industrie, 65*(5a), 498-502.

Europäische Arzneimittel-Agentur. (Ed.). (2003). Explanatory note on fees payable to the EMEA.

Europäische Arzneimittel-Agentur. (Ed.). (2004). *Practical guidance for electronic submission of regulatory information in support of a marketing authorisation applica-tion using the electronic common technical document ("eCTD") following the centralised procedure.* Retrieved from November 10, 2004, from http://esubmission.eudra.org/EMEA%20eCTD%20Guidance%200.4-Draft.doc

European Union Review System (EURS). (2002). Requirements document for EURS version 1: Telematics Implementation Group on Electronic Submissions (TIGes).

Food and Drug Administration. (Ed.). (2004). *Electronic common technical document (eCTD).* Retrieved November 26, 2004, from http://www.fda.gov/cder/regulatory/ersr/ectd.htm

Franken, A. (2003a). eSubmission management im regulatorischen umfeld von arzneimittelzulassungen. *Pharmind: Die Pharmazeutische Industrie, 65*(5a), 463-472.

Franken, A. (2003b). Zukunft des regulatorischen e-managements bei der arzneimittelzulassung. *Pharmind: Die Pharmazeutische Industrie, 65*(5a), 491-497.

Hock, S., & Jostes, T. (2003). Gesetzliche regelungen zu elektronischen unterschroften bei der einreichung von zulassungsunterlagen für arzneimittel. *Pharmind: Die Pharmazeutische Industrie, 65*(5a), 476-484.

Höniger, L. (2003). Einführung und nutzung von elektronischen verfahren bei der arzneimittelzulassung: Dargestellt am beispiel von regierungsaktivitäten in den länern mittel- und osteuropas. *Pharmind: Die Pharmazeutische Industrie, 65*(5a), 520-524.

Jordan, H. (2002). Regulatory affairs. In O. Schöffski, F. U. Fricke, W. Guminski, & W. Hartmann (Eds.), *Pharmabetriebslehre* (pp. 177-193).

Kainz, A., & Harmsen, S. (2003). Einsatz eines dossier-management-systems in der arzneimittelindustrie: Auswahl, einführung und praktische erfahrungen. *Pharmind: Die Pharmazeutische Industrie, 65*(5a), 511-519.

Mitteleuropäische Gesellschaft für Regulatory Affairs e.V. (Ed.). (n.d.). *Die aufgaben einer zulassungsabteilung & arzneimittel und regulatory affairs.* Retrieved November 10, 2004, from http://www.megra.org/html/affairs.htm

PIM (Ed.). (2005). *EU-telematics.* Retrieved July 22, 2005, from http://pim.emea.eu.int/

Schmitt, A. (2003). Umgang mit anforderungen der elektronischen einreichung von arzneimitteln beim pharmazeutischen unternehmner: Dargestellt am beispiel von änderungsanzeigen. *Pharmind: Die Pharmazeutische Industrie, 65*(5a), 525-530.

U.S. Department of Health and Human Services, Food and Drug Administration (FDA), CDER, & CBER (Eds.). (1999). *Guidance for industry. Providing regulatory submission in electronic format: General considerations.* Retrieved November 10, 2004, from http://www.fda.gov/cder/guidance/2867fnl.pdf

Vis-à-Vis (Ed.). (2002). *COI-PharmaSuite: Zulassung leicht gemacht!* Retrieved August 18, 2004, from http://www.visavis.de/modules.php?name=News&file=article%sid=254

Wagner, S. A. (2000). Europäisches zulassungssystem für arzneimittel und parallelhandel unter besonderer berücksichtigung des deutschen arzneimittelrechts.

Witzel, W., Yamaguchi, A., & Lorenz, R. (1998). Damos experience report.

Zimmer, G. (2003). Dokumenten-management-systeme als basis für die einreichung von arzneimittel-zulassungsdossiers. *Pharmind: Die Pharmazeutische Industrie, 65*(5a), 537-545.

KEY TERMS

Benefits: The positive implications, both direct and indirect, resulting from some action. They include both financial and nonfinancial information.

Costs: The total spent for goods or services including money, time, and labor.

Drug: A substance that is used as a medicine or narcotic.

Economical Aspects: Factors relating to an economy. Practically, it is using the minimum time or resources necessary for effectiveness.

Electronic Signature: A paperless way to sign a document using an electronic symbol or process attached or associated with the document.

Electronic Submission: Submission made via a modem or computer disk. Very few editors accept electronic submissions of unsolicited manuscripts.

Guideline: A detailed plan or explanation to guide one in setting standards or determining a course of action.

Time to Market: The period between product development and launch on the market.

Chapter XXXIV
Semantic Web Services for Healthcare

Christina Catley
Carleton University, Canada

Monique Frize
Carleton University, Canada
University of Ottawa, Canada

Dorina Petriu
Carleton University, Canada

ABSTRACT

This chapter explores the ongoing efforts to integrate Web services and the Semantic Web for the purposes of sharing knowledge, enabling access to services, and application integration in distributed clinical environments. Combining the Semantic Web and Web services in relation to the healthcare domain, results in Semantic Web services for healthcare, which will enable intelligent interpretation of healthcare data by services such as clinical decision support systems. Critical issues in ontology standardization and security are discussed. The multidisciplinary problem of service composition is presented with emphasis on the role healthcare experts play in identifying value-added medical services.

NEXT-GENERATION INTERNET: THE SEMANTIC WEB AND WEB SERVICES

The Semantic Web and Web services are two complementary and evolving technologies that will change the face of healthcare delivery. Healthcare IT experts predict that in the future, healthcare services will be offered as inter-changeable Semantic Web services used in distributed but related medical domains. According to Hoffman (2003, p. 54), "Entire eco-systems of electronic services will be built around specific industries, providing specific processes to solve specific problems for specific types of customers, through specific transaction chains."

Web services constitute an important emerging technology for which potential applications are unlimited. Stafford (2003, p. 27) explains that "if a provider can imagine a way of delivering something of value to a customer to provide some usefulness ... they have a viable Web service." Web services are based on a service-oriented system architecture, in which providers assess which applications they can offer as services to different groups of potential users. There are three main roles in a service-oriented architecture: a provider, a consumer, and a directory. In the case of a Web-services system, the provider publishes descriptions of its Web services in a directory, which is accessible by the consumer. Once the consumer selects a service, the consumer and the service are dynamically bound, for example, at run time. The publish-find-bind model of interaction enables the loose coupling of providers and consumers and, thus, increases the agility, flexibility, and adaptability of distributed systems (Tosic, 2004).

Web services facilitate integration and interoperability because the underlying implementation and deployment platform are not relevant to the application invoking the service. There are three key components of Web-service systems with three major corresponding XML- (extended markup language) based standardization initiatives proposed by the World Wide Web Consortium (W3C) to support the interactions among Web services.

- **Delivery:** Comprises all technologies required to transport a service request from the client to the server, including XML for message encoding, and SOAP (previously known as the simple object access protocol, now considered a misnomer) for handling the transmission of XML-formatted data.

- **Description:** A Web-service interface provides a collection of operations accessible through standardized XML messaging. This interface is described using the Web services description language (WSDL), which specifies the operations provided by a Web service (Graham, 2003).
- **Discovery:** The service requestor discovers the Web service via discovery agencies, such as universal description discovery and integration (UDDI), which allows service descriptions to be published and discovered.

Adding semantics to the Web is a necessary component toward realizing Web services' goal of application-to-application integration. To this end, the next-generation Internet will be the Semantic Web. The vision of the Semantic Web is to associate meaning to all Web resources such that they can be discovered and consumed autonomously by applications (Berners-Lee, Hendler, & Lasilla, 2001), making the Semantic Web a meaningful indexed repository of documents and services (Lee, Patel, Chun, & Geller, 2004). Currently, the interpretation of Web-based information requires human knowledge and intuition; both humans and machines could interpret the Semantic Web.

Schweiger, Brumhard, Hoelzer, and Dudeck (2005, p. 274) claim that because the Web and healthcare systems are both "little organized systems of distributed data," innovations in Web technology are particularly relevant to the healthcare industry. As such, the development of the Semantic Web will impact healthcare in numerous ways, such as in retrieving information from multiple disparate databases so that patient mobility will not affect the continuity of individual care and the transfer of patient information (Sun, 2004), and in enabling machines to capture and provide clinicians with the information stored in clinical guidelines and scientific publications.

SEMANTIC WEB SERVICES FOR HEALTHCARE

The healthcare domain is defined by a plethora of distributed data and knowledge from which complex and timely high-value decisions must be made in a low-tolerance environment (Turner, Rigby, et al., 2004). Wreder and Deng (1999, p. 250) elaborate: "How to migrate from stovepipe systems to the next generation of open healthcare information systems that are interoperable, extensible and maintainable is increasingly a pressing problem for the healthcare industry." Semantic Web services are being advocated as a logical means of achieving open healthcare systems. Current applications span a range of healthcare domains (Catley, Frize, Petriu, Walker, & Yang, 2004; Chatterjee, 2003; Lee et al., 2004; Turner, Rigby, et al.) and encompass services with diverse goals, from knowledge management, to application integration, to clinical decision support.

With the ability to offer sophisticated applications to consumers via Semantic Web services, a new dimension emerges: applying the service-oriented concept to data and software. Turner, Budgen, and Brereton (2003) have coined the terms software as a service (SaaS) and data as a service (DaaS). The vision is to eliminate many of the problems that occur with developing, updating, and evolving software systems (Turner, Rigby, et al., 2004) and, indirectly, the data accessed by these systems. The implications for healthcare mean offering the potential to easily share distributed heterogeneous medical data between researchers and allied healthcare professionals, and facilitating data processing by medical software.

Although there is a need for clinical decision-support systems (CDSSs) to aid physicians in making optimum diagnoses and reducing medical errors (Committee on Quality of Health Care in America, Institute of Medicine, 2000; Wilson, Runciman, & Gibberd, 1995), from a technical perspective, the advancement of CDSSs has been severely hampered by two key factors. First, clinical data are intended for use by humans; even in the case of electronic patient records (EPRs), the data have no attached Semantic meaning and are primarily intended for human viewing. Second, the clinical data needed to make decisions are constantly increasing, heterogeneous, fragmented, and distributed geographically, making it difficult to both train and deploy CDSSs. This problem is compounded by the implicitly private nature of healthcare data and the resulting restrictions from an ethical viewpoint.

Kwon (2003) reports that as decision-support-system environments are rapidly changing from centralized and closed to distributed and open, scalability and interoperability features are becoming more crucial to CDSS development. Combining the Semantic Web and Web services offers a solution, providing physicians with instant access to knowledge, not just data, in real-time decision-making environments.

A sophisticated healthcare example involves using Semantic Web services to reduce the waiting times for noncritical surgery (Motta, Domingue, Cabral, & Gaspari, 2003) by providing five interacting Semantic Web services: (a) a diagnostic service to diagnose conditions based on a set of symptoms, (b) a yellow-page service indicating which hospitals in Europe provide specific medical services, (c) a cost-query service to provide the cost of medical services on a per-hospital basis, (d) an ambulance service to determine the cost of transporting patients between hospitals, and (e) an exchange-rate service for converting between European currencies. Semantic Web services are also being applied to artificial-intelligence-based CDSSs. Other work describes a Web-services infrastructure for linking obstetrical, perinatal, and NICU (neonatal intensive care unit) data with CDSSs for the purposes of predicting preterm birth, exploring indicators of cesarean birth (Catley, Frize, Petriu, et al., 2004), and predicting critical outcomes in the NICU, such as mortality, length of stay, and duration of ventilation (Frize, Ennett, Stevenson, & Trigg, 2001; Tong, Frize, & Walker, 2002). The CDSSs offered as Web services in the infrastructure include (a) trained artificial neural networks for outcome prediction (Ennett & Frize, 2003), (b) case-based reasoners for matching an individual patient's condition to the most similar past cases (Frize & Walker, 2000), (c) alert generation for notifying physicians of potential complications via mobile devices (Catley, Frize, Walker, & St-Germain, 2003), and (d) an ethical decision-support tool for parents of very sick infants to help them make difficult decisions, such as withholding or terminating critical care (Frize, Yang, Walker, & O'Connor, in press).

CRITICAL ISSUES

While some large healthcare systems use a common data model to integrate information from multiple facilities, the majority of existing clinical information is stored in heterogeneous databases using different names and different data models (Sun, 2004). Although the Semantic Web provides a means to attach meaning to data, there is no guarantee that everyone agrees with this meaning; in order to deal with numerous and heterogeneous data formats, ontolo-

gies are needed to define healthcare standards and the mapping between them. In simplest terms, ontologies define the common words and concepts used to describe and represent an area of knowledge (Daconta, Obrst, & Smith, 2003). Standard ontologies, schemas, and vocabularies are a prerequisite for the Semantic Web (Schweiger et al., 2005). In describing their experience in creating a healthcare information broker, Turner, Rigby, et al. (2004) state that future work will require an ontology service comprising multiple ontologies as this is considered the only viable option for providing a global view of an information space. While efforts such as Health Level 7 (HL7) and Digital Imaging and Communications in Medicine are providing a common ground for describing healthcare information, they are not currently at a level to resolve all relevant interoperability issues (Lee et al., 2004).

While Web services offer benefits and opportunities, they also present many challenges in healthcare environments, such as the need to comply with health-insurance regulations, and increased requirements for reliability, security, and monitoring (Chatterjee, 2003). Currently, one of the biggest obstacles in deploying Semantic Web services is security (Daconta et al., 2003); this is of particular concern in healthcare when maintaining the privacy of sensitive patient data is paramount. Authentication, authorization, confidentiality, data integrity, and nonrepudiation are all security concerns that relate to Web services and must be addressed before such services can be exposed externally. The Web-services industry is working to overcome security concerns with initiatives such as XML signatures for validating message integrity and nonrepudiation, XML encryption for data confidentiality, the security assertion markup language (SAML), an OASIS (Organization for the Advancement of Structured Information Standards) standard that provides assertions of trust between parties, and WS-Security, which combines XML signatures and XML encryption with standard SOAP messaging. Given that Web-service security is still evolving, the majority of applications described in the literature are based on the deployment of Web services on intranets, which nevertheless provides great potential for the integration of data and services across large healthcare organizations.

FUTURE TRENDS

Automatic Web service composition has recently taken center stage as an emerging research area (Medjahed, Bouguettaya, & Elmagarmid, 2003). As more Web services become available, it is possible to offer consumers more complex services by combining simple ones. Candidate Web services can be categorized as being either core or composite services. A *core Web service* offers basic functionality that will potentially be required by multiple higher level applications. *Composite Web services* represent these higher level applications, which combine two or more core services to offer a complete system application as seen from the user's perspective; the complete application is referred to as a *composition scenario*.

While Web-service delivery, description, and discovery are largely technical problems under the domain of IT experts, service composition represents a complex multidisciplinary problem. Healthcare experts are needed to identify value-added medical services and to determine appropriate service composition scenarios, including contextual knowledge that indicates when and why certain services should be combined. Due to the more complex nature of interdisciplinary work, service composition in healthcare is currently an evolving research area.

A notable composition initiative is the work by Lee et al. (2004) on Semantic medical services. Their team is determining how heterogeneous medical Web services interoperate in a medical service flow for the cardiovascular domain using three kinds of knowledge: syntactic, Semantic, and contextual. First the syntactic constraints must be met; an example would be obtaining a valid patient identifier before allowing the invocation of a service. The Semantic knowledge constrains the order in which services are invoked and requires input from domain experts, such as those with knowledge of healthcare policies, health insurance, and drug regulations. Contextual knowledge identifies the situations in which a service should be used; for example, if a service for choosing a blood lab returns multiple options, the system could select the lab closest to the patient. Contextual constraints are sophisticated and involve detailed knowledge of the patient's preferences.

Efforts are also under way to deploy mobile applications based on loosely coupled Web services. Chatterjee (2003) claims that the combination of lightweight and almost ubiquitous Web services together with around-the-clock access to mobile devices represents a powerful platform for the development and delivery of pervasive and cost-effective healthcare applications and systems.

CONCLUSION

Based on the acceptance of Web services predicted by IT experts (Daconta et al., 2003; Kreger, 2003; Lea & Vinoski, 2003), many healthcare providers are starting to leverage Web services as a solution to data and application integration (Chatterjee, 2003). The Semantic Web provides a mechanism for adding meaning to data, essential in healthcare when the same clinical information can have many different representations. Combining the Semantic Web and Web services in relation to the healthcare domain results in semantic Web services for healthcare, which will ultimately enable the automated interpretation of clinical data. Semantic Web services for healthcare open new possibilities in knowledge management, clinical decision support, and application integration. Semantic Web services have the potential to support an advanced healthcare environment, offering new applications and services to health networks. Primary issues of concern are data security and confidentiality.

REFERENCES

Berners-Lee, T., Hendler, J., & Lasilla, O. (2001). The Semantic Web. *Scientific American, 284*(5), 34-43.

Catley, C., Frize, M., Petriu, D. C., Walker, C. R.., & Yang, L. (2004). Towards a Web services *infrastructure for perinatal, obstetrical, and neonatal clinical decision support.* Proceedings of the 26ᵗʰ Annual International Conference of the IEEE Engineering in Medicine and Biology Society, San Francisco.

Catley, C., Frize, M., Walker, C. R., & St-Germain, L. (2003). Integrating clinical alerts into an XML-based healthcare framework for the neonatal intensive care unit. *Proceedings of the 25ᵗʰ Annual International Conference of the IEEE Engineering in Medicine and Biology Society* (pp. 1276-1279).

Chatterjee, S. (2003). Developing enterprise Web services and applications: Opportunities and best practices for the healthcare industry. *Fifth International Workshop on Enterprise Networking and Computing in Healthcare Industry* (p. 159).

Committee on Quality of Health Care in America, Institute of Medicine. (2000). *To err is human: Building a safer health system.* Washington, DC: National Academy Press.

Daconta, M. C., Obrst, L. J., & Smith, K. T. (2003). *The Semantic Web: A guide to the future of XML, Web services, and knowledge management.* Indianapolis, IN: Wiley Publishing, Inc.

Ennett, C. M., & Frize, M. (2003). Weight-elimination neural networks applied to coronary surgery mortality prediction. *IEEE Transactions of Information Technologies in Biomedicine, 7*(2), 86-92.

Frize, M., Ennett, C. M., Stevenson, M., & Trigg , H. C. E. (2001). Clinical decision-support systems for intensive care units using artificial neural networks. *Medical Engineering & Physics, 23*, 217-225.

Frize, M., & Walker, C. R. (2000). Clinical decision-support systems for intensive care units using case-based reasoning. *Medical Engineering and Physics, 22*(9), 671-677.

Frize, M., Yang, L., Walker, R. C., & O'Connor, A. (in press). Conceptual framework of knowledge management for ethical decision-making support in neonatal intensive care. *Transactions of Information Technology in Biomedicine.*

Graham, S. (2003). *Building Web services with Java: Making sense of XML, SOAP, WSDL, and UDDI.* Indianapolis, IN: SAMS Publishing.

Hoffman, D. (2003). Marketing + MIS = e-service. *Communications of the ACM, 46*(6), 29-34.

Kreger, H. (2003). Fulfilling the Web services promise. *Communications of the ACM, 46*(6), 29-34.

Kwon, O. B. (2003). Meta Web service: Building Web-based open decision support system based on Web services. *Expert Systems with Applications, 24*(4), 375-389.

Lea, D., & Vinoski, S. (2003). Middleware for Web services. *IEEE Internet Computing, 7*(1), 28-29.

Lee, Y., Patel, C., Chun, S. A., & Geller, J. (2004). Compositional knowledge management for medical services on Semantic Web. *Proceedings of the 13ᵗʰ International World Wide Web Conference on Alternate Track Papers & Posters* (pp. 498-499).

McIlraith, S. A., & Martin, D. L. (2003). Bringing semantics to Web services. *IEEE Intelligent Systems, 18*(1), 90-93.

Medjahed, B., Benatallah, B., Bouguettaya, A., Ngu, A. H. H., & Elmagarmid, A. K. (2003). Business-to-business interactions: Issues and enabling technologies. *The International Journal on Very Large Data Bases, 12*(1), 59-85.

Medjahed, B., Bouguettaya, A., & Elmagarmid, A. K. (2003). Composing Web services on the Semantic Web. *The International Journal on Very Large Data Bases, 12*(4), 333-351.

Motta, E., Domingue, J., Cabral, L., & Gaspari, M. (2003). IRS-II: A framework and infrastructure for Semantic Web services. *International Semantic Web Conference 2003* (pp. 306-318).

Schweiger, R., Brumhard, M., Hoelzer, S., & Dudeck, J. (2005). Implementing health care systems using XML standards. *International Journal of Medical Informatics, 74*(2-4), 267-277.

Stafford, T. (2003). E-services. *Communications of the ACM, 46*(6), 26-28

Sun, Y. (2004). Methods for automated concept mapping between medical databases. *Journal of Biomedical Informatics, 37*(3), 162-178.

Tong, Y., Frize, M., & Walker, R. (2002). Extending successful predictions of ventilation needs using artificial neural networks from adult to neonatal ICU patients. *IEEE Transactions on Information Technology in Biomedicine, 6*(2), 188-191.

Tosic, V. (2004). *Service offerings for XML Web services and their management applications.* Unpublished doctoral dissertation, Carleton University, Tosic, Ottawa, Canada.

Turner, M., Budgen, D., & Brereton, P. (2003). Turning software into a service. *IEEE Computer, 36*(10), 38-44.

Turner, M., Rigby, M., Zhu, F., Kotsiopoulus, I., Russell, M., Budgen, D., et al. (2004). Using Web service technologies to create an information broker: An experience report. *Proceedings of the 26ᵗʰ International Conference on Software Engineering* (pp. 552-561).

Wilson, R. M., Runciman, W. B., & Gibberd, R. W. (1995). The quality in Australian health care study. *Medical Journal of Australia, 163*, 458-471.

Wreder, K., & Deng, Y. (1999). Architecture-centered enterprise system development and integration based on distributed object technology standard. *Proceedings of the 23ʳᵈ Annual International Computer Software and Applications Conference* (pp. 250-258).

KEY TERMS

Clinical Decision-Support System: A computer program designed to aid physicians and others (parents, patients, clinicians) in the decision-making process. Applications include generating alerts, diagnostic assistance, and therapy planning.

Integration: Implies both semantic and technical interoperability, as well as a logical integration flow between interoperable modules.

Interoperability: The ability of two or more systems or components to exchange information and to use the information that has been exchanged.

Ontology: An explicit, formal specification representing the knowledge entities in a domain, such as objects and concepts, and the relationships between them.

Semantic Web: The next-generation Internet in which semantic meaning will be associated with all Web resources, both data and services, such that they can be discovered and consumed autonomously by applications.

Semantic Web Service: Using Semantic Web technology to describe a Web service's capabilities and content in an unambiguous, computer-interpretable language (McIlraith & Martin, 2003).

Web Service: Software applications that can be discovered, described, and accessed based on XML and standard Web protocols over intranets, extranets, and the Internet (Daconta et al., 2003).

World Wide Web Consortium (W3C): A forum for information, commerce, communication, and collective understanding that develops open Web standards and guidelines with the goal of achieving Web interoperability.

XML: A standard from the World Wide Web Consortium that provides the tagging of information content within documents. XML offers a means for representing content in a format that is both human and machine readable.

Section IX
Image Processing and Archiving Systems

The rapid progress in imaging technologies during the last decades has stimulated many developments and applications in medicine, biology, industry, aerospace, remote sensing, meteorology, oceanography, and the environment. New developments are continually making the technology faster, more powerful, less invasive, and less expensive. Imaging technology was primarily used in medical diagnosis initially, but it is being increasingly used in pure neuroscience, psychological research, and in many other fields. The quantitative nature of data will be relevant for the effective diagnostic as well as therapeutic management of patients, whichever diseases they have. In this section, various imaging technologies and their applications in biomedicine are clearly presented.

Chapter XXXV
Imaging Technologies and their Applications in Biomedicine and Bioengineering

Nikolaos Giannakakis
National and Kapodistrian University of Athens, Greece

Efstratios Poravas
National and Kapodistrian University of Athens, Greece

ABSTRACT

New developments are making the technology faster, more powerful, less invasive, and less expensive. While the technology evolves, new devices are developed, in purpose to be used in the hospitals. Many new imaging methods are used in biomedical applications today and can predict the growth of a tumor or detect a disease. The advantages are numerous, but the problems, during the acquisition and use by the staff, are also remarkable.

INTRODUCTION

We have come from the family doctor's signature black bag in the first half of the 20th century to the powerful scanning equipment of the modern medical center, from tens of thousands dying in influenza epidemics to hundreds of thousands of seniors receiving their annual flu shots, and from an average life expectancy of about 50 years to our present expectancy of 75 years. The biomedical community is taking advantage of the power of computing and technology so as to manage and analyse data. Imaging technologies save day to day more and more people.

X-rays, endoscopes, CT (computed tomography) scans, MRI (magnetic resonance imaging), digital mammography—these imaging technologies make it possible for medical scientists to peer into the body without cutting through the skin. With video monitors and robotic equipment, surgery becomes less invasive and less traumatic to the body (Sawchuck, 2000). Noninvasive means of looking into the human body are now being used to diagnose a wide variety of diseases, including cancer, Alzheimer's disease, stroke, heart failure, and vascular disease (President's Committee of Advisors on Science and Technology, 2000). The first imaging technologies, the X-ray (discovered by W. K. Roentgen) and EEG (electroencephalogram), were primitive by today's standards, but both have been considerably improved and provided the conceptual base of the other amazing imaging technologies that have recently emerged.

The most common, CAT (computer-assisted tomography) scans, combine X-rays with computer technology to create cross-sectional images of the patient's body, which are then assembled into a three-dimensional picture that displays organs, bones, and tissues in great detail. MRI scanners use magnets and radio waves instead of X-rays to generate images that provide an even better view of soft tissues, such as the brain or spinal cord (President's Committee of Advisors on Science and Technology, 2000).

Much of today's imaging technology relies on microprocessors and software. In addition, the great advances in noninvasive sensing, tomography, and imaging technologies now allow repeated studies with minimal stress and damage (National Research Council, & Institute for Laboratory Animal Research, 2002).

Medical imaging is often thought of as a way of viewing anatomical structures of the body. Indeed, X-ray computed tomography and magnetic resonance imaging yield exquisitely detailed images of such structures. It is often useful, however, to acquire images of physiologic function rather than of anatomy. Such images can be acquired by imaging the decay of radioisotopes bound to molecules with known biological properties. This class of imaging

techniques is known as nuclear medicine imaging.

Although the mathematical sciences were used in a general way for image processing, they were of little importance in biomedical work until the development in the 1970s of computed tomography for the imaging of X-rays (leading to the CAT scan) and isotope-emission tomography (leading to positron-emission tomography [PET] scans and single-photon-emission computed tomography [SPECT] scans). In the 1980s, MRI eclipsed the other modalities in many ways as the most informative medical imaging methodology (Webb, 1988).

Table 1 summarises some of the imaging methods used in biomedical applications.

Technologies such as those in Table 1 are all being investigated in small-animal models. The goal is to marry fundamental advances in molecular and cell biology with those in biomedical imaging to advance the field of molecular imaging (TA-Datenbank-Nachrichten, 2001). The two basic starting points in evaluating the overall utility of a medical technology are efficacy and safety. If a technology is not efficacious, it should not be used. In addition, efficacy and safety data are needed to evaluate the cost

Table 1. Imaging methods used in biomedical applications

X-ray projection imaging (discovered in 1895)
X-ray CT (1972)
MRI (1980)
Magnetic resonance spectroscopy (MRS)
SPECT
PET (1974)
Gamma camera (1958)
Nuclear magnetic resonance (NMR, 1946)
Ultrasonics
Electrical source imaging (ESI)
Electrical impedance tomography (EIT)
Magnetic source imaging (MSI)
Medical optical imaging
Micro computerised axial tomography (MicroCAT)
Optical and thermal diagnostic imaging (OCT, DOT)

effectiveness of a technology (Banta, Clyde, & Williams, 1981).

Biomedical imaging devices have been used to obtain anatomical images and to provide localised biochemical and physiological analysis of tissues and organs. The ability of these devices to provide anatomical images and physiological information has provided unparalleled opportunities for biomedical and clinical research, and has the potential for important improvements in the diagnosis and treatment of a wide range of diseases (National Institute of Biomedical Imaging and Bioengineering [NIBIB], 2002).

Technological devices visualise and enlarge somatic space, rendering images of our most infinitesimal cells, molecules, and genetic structures, which allows for a more precise manipulation of our muscles, tissues, and bones (Sawchuck, 2000). Imaging tests now provide much clearer and more detailed pictures of organs and tissues. New imaging technology allows us to do more than simply view anatomical structures such as bones, organs, and tumours. Functional imaging—the visualisation of physiological, cellular, or molecular processes in living tissues—enables us to observe activity such as blood flow, oxygen consumption, or glucose metabolism in real time.

Imaging technology already has had lifesaving effects on our ability to detect cancer early and more accurately diagnose the disease (especially the PET device). Generally, the

purpose of the biomedical imaging techniques is the early detection, clinical diagnosis, and staging of a disease, and therapeutic applications (*Biomedical Imaging Symposium: Visualizing the Future of Biology and Medicine*, 1999). Imaging technologies have many applications in biomedicine. Oncology, cardiology, and ophthalmology are only some of its sections that use these technologies, which everyday are developed more and more.

PROBLEMS AND DISADVANTAGES OF IMAGING TECHNOLOGIES

Despite all the promises, the use of imaging technologies in biomedicine and bioengineering evoke many problems. All biomedical imaging devices suffer from various limitations that can restrict their general applicability. Some major limitations are sensitivity, spatial resolution, temporal resolution, and the ease of the interpretation of data. One way to circumvent these limitations is to develop technological and methodological approaches that improve and extend the sensitivity and the information content of individual imaging techniques. Another way is to combine two or more complementary biomedical imaging techniques (like MRI and PET, MRI and MEG, and optical MRI).

Table 2 summarises some problems of the imaging technologies.

Table 2. Problems and disadvantages of imaging technologies

The high cost of equipment and their maintenance, which aggravates the national economy for medicine
Wasteful expenditures because of bad usage by users and technical staff (20 to 40%)
The technology changes rapidly and devices may become out of date
Users need education to learn how to break the new technologies in
Physicians and the nursing staff must continuously be acquainted through articles related to the new technologies and equipment
New technologies cause disruption and disappointment for staff
They are venturous for patients because the levels of radiation they are exposed to may be too high

There is no crystal ball to predict the future of medical imaging technologies. New applications continue to be explored for both diagnosis and treatment (Canadian Institute for Health Information, http://www.cihi.ca). Biomedical imaging has seen truly exciting advances in recent years. New imaging methods can now reflect internal anatomy and dynamic body functions heretofore only derived from textbook pictures, and applications to a wide range of diagnostic and therapeutic procedures can be envisioned. Not only can technological advances create new and better ways to extract information about our bodies, but they also offer the promise of making some existing imaging tools more convenient and economical.

Advances based on medical research promise new and more effective treatments for a wide variety of diseases. New noninvasive imaging techniques for the earlier detection and diagnosis of disease are essential to take full advantage of new treatments and to promote improvements in healthcare. The development of advanced genetic and molecular imaging techniques is necessary to continue the rapid pace of discovery in molecular biology. Several breakthrough imaging technologies, including MRI and CT, have been developed primarily abroad (American Institute for Medical and Biological Engineering, http://www.aimbe.org).

Key paradigms of emerging imaging technologies from different technological areas will be presented, and the engineering principles and research findings leading to the design of efficient bioimaging technologies will be introduced and analysed. Specifically, imaging technologies from space or aerospace research have been identified and successfully applied toward the development of novel high-resolution, multisensor medical imaging systems, with potential applications in digital radiography and CT. Similarly, experimental research findings for defence applications have been applied toward the development of multifusion optical sensing imaging systems and techniques for efficient disease detection (Giakos, 2003).

Today, as for all products and services in all sectors, there exists the DICOM (Digital Imaging and Communications in Medicine) Standards Committee. Its purpose is to create and maintain international standards that help the allocation of medical pictures (like radial tomographies, magnetic tomographies, etc.), and the communication of biomedical diagnostic and therapeutic information in disciplines that use digital images and associated data (DICOM, 2004). DICOM is used or will be used by every medical profession that utilises images within the healthcare industry.

CONCLUSION

The rapid progress in imaging technologies during the last decades has stimulated many developments and applications in medicine, biology, industry, aerospace, remote sensing, meteorology, oceanography, and the environment.

New developments are continually making the technology faster, more powerful, less invasive, and less expensive. Imaging technology was primarily used in medical diagnosis initially, but it is being increasingly used in pure neuroscience, psychological research, and many other fields. The quantitative nature of data will be relevant for the effective diagnosis as well as therapeutic management of patients, whichever disease they have ("Nuclear Medicine Sextet," 1999).

REFERENCES

Banta, H. D, Clyde, J. B., & Williams, J. S. (1981). *Toward rational technology in medi-*

cine: Considerations for health policy. New York: Springer Verlag.

Biomedical Imaging Symposium: Visualizing the Future of Biology and Medicine. (1999, June 25-26). Natcher Conference Center, National Institutes of Health, Bethesda, MD. Sponsored by the NIH Bioengineering Consortium (BECON), the American Institute for Medical and Biological Engineering (AIMBE), and the Radiological Society of North America (RSNA). Retrieved from http://www.becon.nih.gov/report_19990625.pdf

Digital Imaging and Communications in Medicine (DICOM). (2004). *Scope of DICOM: Strategic document, Version 4.0*. VA: National Electrical Manufacturers Association.

Giakos, G. (2003). *Emerging imaging technologies: Technology identification transfer and utilization for bioengineering applications*. McMaster University. Retrieved October 28, 2003, from http://www.ece.mcmaster.ca/news/seminars/giakos_sem.htm

National Institute of Biomedical Imaging and Bioengineering (NIBIB). (2002). *Improvements in imaging methods and technologies*. Retrieved from http://www.nibib1.nih.gov

National Research Council (U.S.), & Institute for Laboratory Animal Research (U.S.) (2002, April 17-19). *International perspectives: The future of non-human primate resources. Proceedings of the Workshop*. Retrieved from http://www.nap.edu/catalog/10774.html

Nuclear medicine sextet. (1999, August 21). *The Lancet*, 665.

President's Committee of Advisors on Science and Technology (2000, Spring). *Chapter 3. Biomedical technologies*. In *Wellspring of prosperity: Science and technology in the U.S. economy*. Washington, DC: Office of

Science and Technology Policy. Retrieved from http://www.ostp.gov

Sawchuck, K. (2000). *Digibodies online exhibition and Synapse online forum*. Retrieved from http://www.digibodies.org/synapse/intro.html

TA-Datenbank-Nachrichten. (2001). *Nr. 1/10. Jahrgang: März, S. 13-22*. Retrieved from http://www.itas.fzk.de

Webb, S. (1988). The physics of medical imaging. *Magnetic Resonance Imaging and Biophysics and Medical Imaging*. Retrieved from http://newton.ex.ac.uk/teaching/modules/PHYM433.html

KEY TERMS

Assessment of Imaging Technology: Research on and development of methods for the evaluation and comparison of new and existing imaging technologies to establish their effectiveness, robustness, and range of applicability.

Bioengineering: The application of engineering principles to the fields of biology and medicine, as in the development of aids or replacements for defective or missing body organs. It is also called biomedical engineering.

Biomedicine: A branch of medical science concerned especially with the capacity of human beings to survive and function in abnormally stressful environments and with the protective modification of such environments. Broadly, it is medicine based on the application of the principles of the natural sciences, especially biology and biochemistry.

Development of Imaging Devices: Research and development of generic biomedical imaging technologies before specific applications are demonstrated.

Diagnostic Imaging: A study section reviews applications dealing with the development and evaluation of new technology for imaging, including instrumentation and software for producing, evaluating, storing, and transmitting images for anatomical, physiological, metabolic, diagnostic, and therapeutic information.

Image Exploitation: Development, design, and implementation of algorithms for image processing and information analysis, including advanced methods for the acquisition, storage, and display of images; research and development on image-guided procedures; and techniques for using multidimensional images to understand physiology and normal and abnormal function.

Medical Device: Any instrument, apparatus, appliance, material, or other article, whether used alone or in combination, including the software necessary for its proper application, intended for the purpose of the diagnosis, prevention, monitoring, treatment, alleviation, or investigation of a disease, injury, or handicap.

Medical Imaging: Term describing the various technologies that produce pictures or images of the body and its structures. Imaging technologies include X-ray, CT scanning, PET scanning, and ultrasound. This term also includes technology such as digital cameras, which produce digital images.

Medical Imaging Technologies: A study section reviews all modalities of medical imaging, including gamma ray; MRI; functional MRI; PET; SPECT; X-ray; CT; visible, infrared, and ultraviolet photons; and optical, photo-acoustic, microwave-acoustic, and exotic imaging methods.

Minimally Invasive Technologies: Basic research involving the use of robotics technologies for actuation, sensing, control, programming, and the human-machine interface, and the design of mechanisms to determine research end points such as diagnosis and the automated or remote treatment of disease.

Chapter XXXVI
Medical Image Compression Using Integer Wavelet Transforms

B. Ramakrishnan
M.I.T. Manipal, India

N. Sriraam
Multimedia University, Malaysia

ABSTRACT

In this chapter, we have focused on compression of medical images using integer wavelet transforms. Lifting transforms such as S, TS, S+P(B), S+P(C), 5/3, 2+@, 2, 9/7-M and 9/7-F transforms are used to evaluate the performances of lossless and lossy compression. Four medical images, namely, MRI, CT, ultrasound, and angiograms are used as test data sets. It is found from the experiments that, among the different transforms, the 9/7-M wavelet transform is identified as the optimal method for lossless and lossy compression of medical images.

INTRODUCTION

Compression of medical images is an area of discussion among the medical community due to the fact that compressing an image could lead to vital diagnostic information being lost. On the other hand, images obtained from imaging modalities such as computed tomography (CT), magnetic resonance imaging (MRI), ultrasound (US), and other modalities require large amounts of space for storage and also pose a problem during transmission. Hence, there is a need to achieve high compression and at the same time preserve the image quality. In telemedicine applications, the compression of medical images plays a paramount role in reducing the image file size, thereby reducing the bandwidth for transmission over a network.

There has been a tremendous increase in the use of wavelets as image-compression tools due to their ability to achieve high compression while sustaining image quality (Antonini,

Barlaud, Mathieu, & Daubechies, 1992; Averbuch, Lazar, & Israeli, 1996). One of the advantages of wavelet-based compression is that it supports progressive lossy to lossless reconstruction (Adams & Kossentini, 2000; Said & Pearlman, 1996a, 1996b; Sheng, Bilgin, Sementilli, & Marcellin, 1998). The Joint Photographic Experts Group (JPEG2000) compression standard is based on wavelets. Wavelet-based entropy coders have been developed to enhance compression that exploits the spatial similarities among the wavelet coefficients. These coders, called zero-tree coders, include embedded zero-tree wavelet (EZW; Shapiro, 1993), set partitioning in hierarchical trees (SPIHT; Said & Pearlman, 1996a, 1996b), an advancement of EZW, and embedded block coding with optimized truncation (EBCOT; Taubman, 2000). With the development of integer wavelets, lossless compression could be realized (Calderbank, Daubechies, Sweldens, & Yeo, 1997, 1998). Integer wavelets generate integer coefficients, whereas the conventional wavelets generate floating-point coefficients. Lossless compression could not be achieved with the conventional wavelets due to having to round off these floating-point values. Integer wavelets are possible with the construction of wavelets based on the lifting scheme (Sweldens, 1998). The lifting scheme provides fast, efficient, and in-place calculation of the wavelet transform.

The main objective of this work is to evaluate different integer wavelets on the basis of their lossy and lossless compression performance for various medical images. The core idea behind compression is that in an image, there exists some correlation among the neighborhood pixels. The task is to decorrelate the image data so as to eliminate the redundancy and reduce the entropy of the image. The general architecture for a lifting-based wavelet compression scheme is depicted in Figure 1.

The image is first transformed from a spatial domain to a wavelet domain using two-dimensional lifting wavelet transform (2D-LWT). The resulting wavelet coefficients are entropy coded to obtain a compressed image. In this chapter, SPIHT is used for entropy coding as it is fast and easy to implement and provides superior compression among the wavelet-based coders. To reconstruct the image, the process is reversed. The compressed image is first entropy decoded and then two-dimensional inverse lifting wavelet transform (2D-ILWT) is applied to obtain the original image.

The chapter is arranged as follows. In the next section, a brief description of the lifting wavelet transform will be presented, followed by the description of the SPIHT coder. A number of integer wavelets for various medical images are then analyzed based on their lossless and progressive lossy compression performance.

LIFTING WAVELET TRANSFORM

The lifting approach of constructing wavelets was proposed by Sweldens (1998). It allows fast, efficient, and in-place calculation of the wavelet transform. Besides this, it is feasible to construct integer wavelets based on this scheme.

Consider an image I of size N x N with N being an integer power n of 2. and each row and column consisting of 2^n pixels. The two-dimensional wavelet transform is performed by first applying one-dimensional wavelet transform along the columns and then applying one-dimensional wavelet transform along the rows or vice-versa. Therefore, we can treat the image as N x N one-dimensional vectors with each vector consisting of 2^n pixels. Hereafter, we refer to the one-dimensional vector as a signal x_n. Applying wavelet transform to x_n divides it into coarse s_{n-1} values and detail d_{n-1} values,

Figure 1. *Compression scheme*

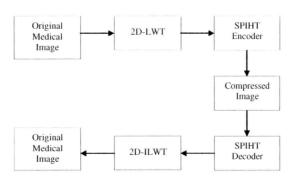

Figure 2. *Different levels of dyadic (pyramid) decomposition*

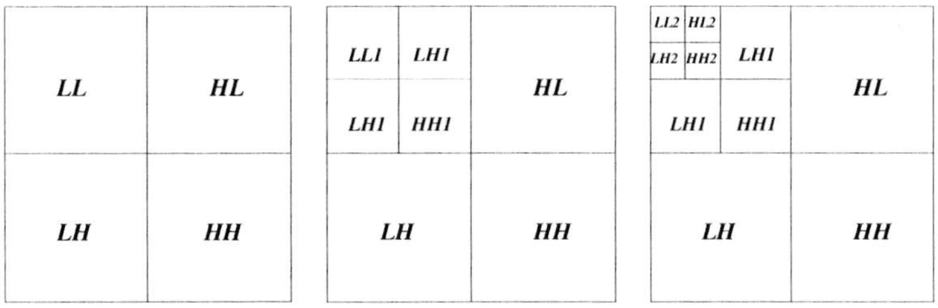

both consisting of 2^{n-1} pixels. This step is performed for each column and the result is used as input for row transformation. After one sequence, the image will be divided into four bands, LL, LH, HL, and HH, with each column and row in a band consisting of 2^{n-1} pixels. The wavelet transformation is then performed on the LL sub-band, resulting in the division of the band into four sub-bands. This procedure can be repeated until the LL sub-bands consist of only one pixel. This decomposition is referred to as dyadic or pyramid decomposition (Figure 2) and provides a multiresolution representation of the image.

The lifting approach of wavelet transform consists of the following operations:

- **Split:** In this operation, the signal x_n is split according to even x_{2j} and odd x_{2j+1} elements ($0 \le j \le 2^{n-1}$). The even elements represent the coarse s_n values while the odd elements represent the detail d_n values. This step is also referred to as lazy wavelet transform.

- **Predict:** In the prediction or dual lifting step, the odd elements are predicted from the even elements. Then the detail d_{n-1} is the difference between its prediction and the odd element. The odd element is replaced by its detail. The procedure is described by the equation

$$d_{n-1} = d_n - P(s_n) \qquad (1)$$

where P is the prediction operator.

Figure 3. Forward lifting wavelet transform

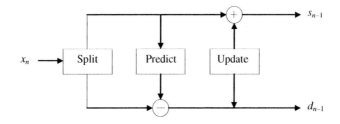

Figure 4. Inverse lifting wavelet transform

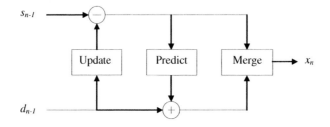

- **Update:** In the update or primal lifting step, the even elements are replaced by an average. The coarse s_{n-1} is calculated as follows:

$$s_{n-1} = s_n + U(d_{n-1}) \qquad (2)$$

where U is the update operator.

The preceeding process is illustrated in Figure 3.

The inverse lifting wavelet transform is performed by the following operations:

- **Undo Update:** Given s_{n-1} and d_{n-1}, the even elements are recovered as described in the equation

$$s_n = s_{n-1} - U(d_{n-1}). \qquad (3)$$

- **Undo Predict:** Once the even elements are recovered, the odd elements are found as follows:

$$d_n = d_{n-1} + P(s_n). \qquad (4)$$

- **Merge:** With both even and odd elements recovered, the original signal x_n is obtained by combining the even and odd elements.

The preceeding process is depicted in Figure 4.

Figures 3 and 4 represent a one-pair predict and update process. This process is repeated for L pairs until the even elements become the coarse values (low-pass coefficients) and the odd elements become the detail values (high-pass coefficients). The predictor and update operators can be thought of as filters with their values constructed depending on the choice of the wavelet. In general:

$$d_{i,j} = d_{i-1,j} - \sum_k p_{i,k} s_{i-1,j-k} \qquad (5)$$

and

$$s_{i,j} = s_{i-1,j} - \sum_k u_{i,k} d_{i,j-k} \,, \qquad (6)$$

where the following applies:

- k: filter coefficient
- i: level of decomposition or reconstruction, $1 \leq i \leq n$
- j: element in the vector, $1 \leq j \leq 2^n$

The integer version of the lifting process can be built by truncating the filter output to the nearest integer in both the predict and update operations. Equations 5 and 6 then becomes

$$d_{i,j} = d_{i-1,j} - \left\lfloor \sum_k p_{i,k} s_{i-1,j-k} + 1/2 \right\rfloor \qquad (7)$$

and

$$s_{i,j} = s_{i-1,j} - \left\lfloor \sum_k u_{i,k} d_{i,j-k} + 1/2 \right\rfloor. \qquad (8)$$

The wavelet transforms are either represented by their vanishing moments $(W, \hat{W})$, where W is the number of vanishing moments of the analyzing high-pass filter and $\hat{W}$ is the number of vanishing moments of the synthesizing low-pass filter, or by their filter lengths f/r, where f represents the low-pass filter length and r represents the high-pass filter length. For example, $(2, 2)$ transform is also referred to as 5/3 transform. Table 1 lists the wavelet transforms used for evaluation along with their forward lifting equations (Calderbank et al., 1998).

Table 1. Transforms and their forward lifting equations

Transform	Forward Lifting Equation
(1,1) or S	$d_j = x_{2j+1} - x_{2j}$ $s_j = x_{2j} + \lfloor d_j / 2 \rfloor$
(3,1) or TS	$d_{1,j} = x_{2j+1} - x_{2j}$ $s_j = x_{2j} + \lfloor d_{1,j} / 2 \rfloor$ $d_j = d_{1,j} + \lfloor 1/4(s_{j-1} - s_{j+1}) + 1/2 \rfloor$
(2,1) or S+P(B)	$d_{1,j} = x_{2j+1} - x_{2j}$ $s_j = x_{2j} + \lfloor d_{1,j} / 2 \rfloor$ $d_j = d_{1,j} + \lfloor 1/8(2s_{j-1} + s_j - 3s_{j+1} + 2d_{j+1}) + 1/2 \rfloor$
(2,1) or S+P(C)	$d_{1,j} = x_{2j+1} - x_{2j}$ $s_j = x_{2j} + \lfloor d_{1,j} / 2 \rfloor$ $d_j = d_{1,j} + \lfloor 1/16(-s_{j-2} + 5s_{j-1} - 4s_j - 8s_{j+1} + 6d_{j+1}) + 1/2 \rfloor$
(2,2) or 5/3	$d_j = x_{2j+1} - \lfloor 1/2(x_{2j} + x_{2j+2}) + 1/2 \rfloor$ $s_j = x_{2j} + \lfloor 1/4(d_{j-1} + d_j) + 1/2 \rfloor$
(4,2) or 2+2,2	$d_{1,j} = x_{2j+1} - \lfloor 1/2(x_{2j+2} + x_{2j}) \rfloor$ $s_j = x_{2j} + \lfloor 1/4(d_{1,j-1} + d_{1,j}) + 1/2 \rfloor$ $d_j = d_{1,j} - \lfloor 1/16(-s_{j-1} + s_j + s_{j+1} - s_{j+2}) + 1/2 \rfloor$
(4,2) or 9/7-M	$d_j = x_{2j+1} - \lfloor 9/16(x_{2j} + x_{2j+2}) - 1/16(x_{2j-2} + x_{2j+4}) + 1/2 \rfloor$ $s_j = x_{2j} + \lfloor 1/4(d_{j-1} + d_j) + 1/2 \rfloor$
(4,4) or 9/7-F	$d_{1,j} = x_{2j+1} + \lfloor 203/128(-x_{2j+2} - x_{2j}) + 1/2 \rfloor$ $s_{1,j} = x_{2j} + \lfloor 217/4096(-d_{1,j-1} - d_{1,j}) + 1/2 \rfloor$ $d_j = d_{1,j} + \lfloor 113/128(s_{1,j} + s_{1,j+1}) + 1/2 \rfloor$ $s_j = s_{1,j} + \lfloor 1817/4096(d_{j-1} + d_j) + 1/2 \rfloor$

SET PARTITIONING IN HIERARCHICAL TREES

The final step in compression is the entropy coding of the decorrelated image data. The entropy coder should take advantage of this decorrelation. SPIHT is a progressive transmission coder and produces embedded bit streams. It works on the principle that there exists a spatial relationship among the wavelet coefficients at different levels and frequency sub-bands in the pyramid structure. A wavelet coefficient at location (i,j) in the pyramid representation has four direct descendants (offspring) at locations:

$$O(i,j) = \{(2i,2j), (2i,2j+1), (2i+1,2j), (2i+1,2j+1)\}, \quad (9)$$

and each of them recursively maintains a spatial similarity to its corresponding four offspring. This pyramid structure is commonly known as the spatial orientation tree. For example, Figure 5 shows the similarity among sub-bands within levels in the wavelet space. If a given coefficient at location (i,j) is significant in magnitude, then some of its descendants will also probably be significant in magnitude. The SPIHT algorithm takes advantage of the spatial similarity present in the wavelet space to optimally find the location of the wavelet coefficients that are significant by means of a binary search algorithm.

The SPIHT algorithm sends the top coefficients in the pyramid structure using a progressive transmission scheme. This scheme is a method that allows the obtaining of a high-quality version of the original image from the minimal amount of transmitted data. The pyramid wavelet coefficients are ordered by magnitude and then the most significant bits are transmitted first, followed by the next bit plane and so on until the lowest bit plane is reached. This reduces the mean square error (MSE) for every bit plane sent.

To take advantage of the spatial relationship among the coefficients at different levels and frequency bands, the SPIHT coder algorithm partitions all the coefficients $C_{i,j}$ according to a number of sets T_k and performs the significance test:

$$\max_{i,j \in T_k} |C_{i,j}| \geq 2^n \quad (10)$$

on each set T_k, with n being the bit plane. If the result of the significance test is *yes*, then, using the same rule, T_k is partitioned into subsets, and the same significance test is performed on all the subsets. This partitioning is continued until all the significance tests are reduced to size 1. The significance test performed on a set T can be summarized by:

$$S_n(T) = \begin{cases} 1, & \max_{i,j \in T_k} |C_{i,j}| \geq 2^n \\ 0, & otherwise \end{cases}. \quad (11)$$

Wavelets coefficients that are not significant at the nth bit-plane level may be significant

Figure 5. Offspring dependencies in the pyramid structure

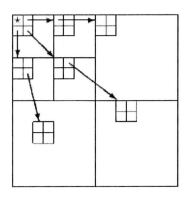

Figure 6. Test images of (a) MRI brain, (b) CT abdomen, (c) ultrasound, and (d) angiogram

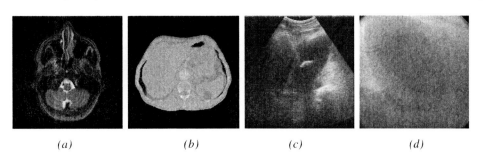

(a)   (b)   (c)   (d)

at the (*n*-1)th bit plane or lower. This information is arranged, according to its significance, in three separate lists: the list of insignificant sets (LIS), the list of insignificant pixels (LIP), and the list of significant pixels (LSP). In the decoder, the SPIHT algorithm replicates the same number of lists.

EXPERIMENTAL RESULTS

The analysis was performed on MRI brain, CT abdomen, ultrasound, and angiogram images (Figure 6). All images are of size 512x512 with 8-bit resolution.

Lossless Compression

The test images were evaluated for lossless compression using the transforms listed in Table 1. The performance results are defined in terms of their bit rates (Equation 12) and tabulated in Table 2.

$$\text{Bit Rate} = \frac{\text{no. of bits in the original image} \times \text{resolution of the image}}{\text{no. of bits in the compressed image}}$$

$$(12)$$

We can infer from Table 2 that no single transform performs best for all medical images. In the case of the MRI image, the S+P(C) transform yields the best compression due to the fact that MRI images have high contrast but give poor results for other images. For CT and angiogram images with low contrast, the 9/7-M transform performs the best. For the ultrasound image, the 2+2,2 transform works better than other transforms. The 9/7-M transform performs consistently well for all images, and the 9/7-F, S, and TS transforms perform the worst.

Lossy Compression

The test images were evaluated for progressive lossy compression by varying the bit rates. The results are tabulated in Table 3. Unlike in the conventional transform where the magni-

Table 2. Lossless compression results

Image	Bit rate (bpp)							
	S	TS	S+P(B)	S+P(C)	5/3	2+2,2	9/7-M	9/7-F
br	3.931	3.671	3.539	**3.443**	3.569	3.474	3.476	3.546
abd	1.799	1.658	1.589	1.591	1.583	1.588	**1.568**	1.733
us	3.631	3.178	3.111	3.129	3.064	**3.019**	3.040	3.315
angio	4.473	4.364	4.292	4.315	4.241	4.210	**4.189**	4.296

Table 3. Lossy compression results

MRI

Bit Rate (bpp)	PSNR (dB)							
	S	TS	S+P(B)	S+P(C)	5/3	2+2,2	9/7-M	9/7-F
0.1	29.45	30.74	31.15	30.94	**31.81**	31.74	31.21	**31.81**
0.5	34.19	35.09	34.80	34.26	36.26	36.26	35.96	**36.43**
1.0	36.61	37.58	37.17	36.76	38.98	**39.06**	38.73	38.87
2.0	39.49	40.41	40.19	39.95	**42.70**	42.65	42.26	41.55

CT

Bit Rate (bpp)	PSNR (dB)							
	S	TS	S+P(B)	S+P(C)	5/3	2+2,2	9/7-M	9/7-F
0.1	32.79	35.68	35.56	34.52	36.34	36.09	**36.97**	36.89
0.5	38.23	41.94	40.97	39.54	**45.05**	44.53	43.81	43.68
0.7	41.02	44.32	43.81	42.82	**47.38**	46.88	46.28	45.25
1.0	44.53	47.29	46.72	45.97	**50.04**	49.59	49.14	46.11

US

Bit Rate (bpp)	PSNR (dB)							
	S	TS	S+P(B)	S+P(C)	5/3	2+2,2	9/7-M	9/7-F
0.1	29.76	30.58	30.52	29.74	31.22	30.93	30.46	**31.25**
0.5	34.25	35.06	36.59	36.58	**37.86**	37.70	37.13	37.84
1.0	37.74	38.27	38.58	38.25	41.07	41.38	**41.41**	40.11
2.0	40.19	41.51	41.88	41.32	**46.87**	46.47	46.01	43.17

ANGIO

Bit Rate (bpp)	PSNR (dB)							
	S	TS	S+P(B)	S+P(C)	5/3	2+2,2	9/7-M	9/7-F
0.1	32.92	30.25	32.62	32.21	33.16	32.11	32.65	**33.26**
0.5	34.24	32.33	34.75	34.08	35.08	34.61	34.71	**35.10**
1.0	36.61	35.92	37.14	36.79	**40.78**	38.40	38.98	38.47
2.0	38.68	38.06	39.41	38.91	**44.11**	43.51	43.75	40.04

tudes of coefficients are unitary, the lifting approach produces coefficients that are not unitary. SPIHT works on unitary transformation, wherein the larger magnitudes at the higher sub-bands are transmitted first, thereby reducing MSE. The lifting wavelet transform is thus adapted for SPIHT by scaling the wavelet coefficients in each sub-band of each level accordingly. The scaling is done intrinsically in the SPIHT coder, as reported by Said and Pearlman (1996a).

The lossy compression performance is evaluated in terms of the peak signal-to-noise ratio (PSNR) described by Equation 13.

$$PSNR(dB) = 20\log_{10}\frac{[\max(I)]^2}{MSE}, \qquad (13)$$

where $\max(I)$ is the maximum pixel value of the original image I. The MSE is given by:

$$MSE = \frac{\sum[I-I']^2}{N^2}, \qquad (14)$$

where I' is the reconstructed image and N^2 is the total number of pixels in the image.

From Table 3, the results indicate that at lower compression ratios, the 5/3 transform performs better than other transforms, whereas at higher compression ratios, the 9/7-F transform gives the best result. The 9/7-F, 9/7-M, 2+2,2, and 5/3 transforms have the best performance, whereas the S+P(B), S+P(C), TS, and S transforms have the worst performance.

CONCLUSION

A number of integer wavelets were evaluated for various medical images based on their lossless and progressive lossy performance. No one transform has superior lossless or lossy compression performance. In general, the 9/7-M transform gives consistent results for both lossless and lossy compression and could therefore be accepted as the optimum wavelet for medical image compression.

REFERENCES

Adams, M. D., & Kossentini, F. (2000). Reversible integer-to-integer wavelet transforms for image compression: Performance evaluation and analysis. *IEEE Transactions on Image Processing, 9*(6), 1010-1024.

Antonini, M., Barlaud, M., Mathieu, P., & Daubechies, I. (1992). Image coding using wavelet transform. *IEEE Transactions on Image Processing, 1*(2), 205-220.

Averbuch, A., Lazar, D., & Israeli, M. (1996). Image compression using wavelet transform and multiresolution decomposition. *IEEE Transactions on Image Processing, 5*(1), 4-15.

Calderbank, A. R., Daubechies, I., Sweldens, W., & Yeo, B.-L. (1997). Lossless image compression using integer to integer wavelet transforms. *Proceedings of IEEE International Conference on Image Processing* (Vol. 1, pp. 596-599).

Calderbank, A. R., Daubechies, I., Sweldens, W., & Yeo, B.-L. (1998). Wavelet transforms that map integers to integers. *Applied and Computational Harmonic Analysis, 5*(3), 332-369.

Said, A., & Pearlman, W. A. (1996a). An image multiresolution representation for lossless and lossy compression. *IEEE Transactions on Image Processing, 5*(9), 1303-1310.

Said, A., & Pearlman, W. A. (1996b). A new fast and efficient image codec based on set partitioning in hierarchical trees. *IEEE Transactions on Circuits and Systems for Video Technology, 6*(3), 243-249.

Shapiro, J. M. (1993). Embedded image coding using zerotrees of wavelet coefficients. *IEEE Transactions on Signal Processing, 41*(12), 3445-3462.

Sheng, F., Bilgin, A., Sementilli, P. J., & Marcellin, M. W. (1998). Lossy and lossless image compression using reversible integer wavelet transforms. *Proceedings of IEEE International Conference on Image Processing* (Vol. 3, pp. 876-880).

Sweldens, W. (1998). The lifting scheme: A construction of second generation wavelets. *SIAM Journal on Mathematical Analysis, 29*(2), 511-546.

Taubman, D. (2000). High performance scalable image compression with EBCOT. *IEEE Transactions on Image Processing, 9*(7), 1151-1170.

KEY TERMS

Bandwidth: The amount of data that can be transferred in a given time period.

Decoder: Algorithm that does the reverse of an encoder, undoing the encoding so that the original information can be retrieved. The same method used to encode is usually just reversed in order to decode.

Encoder: Algorithm used to encode a bit stream into a form that is acceptable for transmission or storage.

Entropy: Minimum channel capacity required to reliably transmit the source as encoded binary digits.

Multiresolution Analysis: The study of signals at various resolutions and scales. A signal, when wavelet transformed, provides this representation.

Progressive Transmission: Type of transmission in which the image is displayed from a low-quality scale to a high-quality scale.

Rate-Distortion Theory: Branch of information theory addressing the problem of determining the minimal amount of entropy that should be communicated over a channel such that the source (input signal) can be reconstructed at the receiver with given distortion.

Source Coding: Process of encoding information using fewer bits.

Telemedicine: The use of modern telecommunication and information technologies for the provision of clinical care to individuals located at a distance and for the transmission of information to provide that care.

Wavelet Transform: Transformation to basis functions that are localized in scale and in time as well.

Chapter XXXVII
Three Dimensional Medical Images

Efstratios Poravas
National and Kapodistrian University of Athens, Greece

Nikolaos Giannakakis
National and Kapodistrian University of Athens, Greece

Dimitra Petroudi
National and Kapodistrian University of Athens, Greece

ABSTRACT

The revolution of technology has lead to a change; from the analogic to the digital function of medical devices. Some of them were produced in the last years to improve the quality of images. Although the procedure of acquiring and using the devices has been very complicated, the analysis of the images is so dependable that a big amount of the annual budget is spent for their acquisition.

INTRODUCTION

The rapid development of science and the continuous manufacture of pioneer medical technological products, together with the modern requirements for high-quality medical services, led to the growth and introduction of modern technologies in the health sector. This development has been really impressive and rapid.

At the beginning of the 20th century, the progress of applied sciences, such as chemistry, physics, microbiology, physiology, pharmacology, and so forth enforced medical research, which resulted in the continuous discoveries in medical technology. In 1895, W. K. Roentgen discovered X-rays, which was a turning point for medical imaging and diagnostics in general. In the 1950s, there was the development of computerized systems, while in the 1960s, there were applications such as the transport of biological signals from equipped space missions and teletransfers of information.

Figure 1. Three dimensional imaging

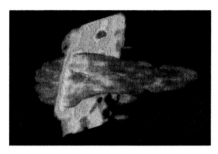

To be more specific, the dynamic entry and the enforced intervention of sciences such as informatics gave an enormous impulse to the medical field and created new data for treatment and diagnosis. Thus, we now have the interaction and participation of many different scientific sectors, which aim at the best medical care. One of these sectors is the imaging and treatment of medical pictures, whose development and use are a crucial point in modern therapeutics.

Medical imaging is related to issues such as the descriptive principles of medical images and their elaboration, together with whatever they include. Therefore, it is easy for someone to understand the importance and the role of imaging in diagnosis, treatment, and recovery in general.

This chapter will discuss the basic concepts, such as the analysis of medical images, their elaboration, various uses and applications, as well as an analysis of the functional requirements of such applications in order for them to be fulfilled.

DIGITAL ELABORATION OF IMAGES

The digital elaboration of images is actually a new sector of informatics and has been applied

for only 15 years. Its development is revolutionary in the health field and constitutes a major contribution for the promotion of health.

The vast amount of optical information and the need for elaborating them led scientists and technicians to the discovery of storage means for the images and their elaboration by using computers combined with the development and improvement of biomedical equipment.

Digital elaboration, as the title itself declares, deals with the digital registration of images and their elaboration by computers. The objective of elaboration can be the quality improvement of images, the straining of recording or transmission noises, the compression of the amount of information, the storage of images, and their digital transmission and depiction.

In the picture below, we schematically represent all the necessary equipment that is needed to fulfill a digital registration of images to be elaborated by the appropriate personnel in order to give all the necessary information and conclusions.

Thus, everyone can understand that for the elaboration of three-dimensional medical images, a device for the admission of images is required, and this can be an axial tomographer, a magnetic tomographer, an ultrasound device, or even more developed depiction systems. A computer is also required, with all the necessary equipment in order to elaborate the images, analyse them, and store and transmit them, and finally all the appropriate exit devices that will project the images will be needed, which can be terminal stations, special films, and printers. Finally, it is very important that the whole system will support network communications so that all information can be available to the scientific community fast and safely with both quality and reliability. Before we introduce some of the depiction devices of three-dimensional medical images that are widely used by the scientific community nowadays, it is important to study some necessary notions for the comprehension of the way this elaboration of three-dimensional images occurs.

An image is a two-dimensional signal. Thus, for the analysis and elaboration of this signal, all the techniques and mathematic relations of digital signal elaboration can be used. Specifically, in the health field, we introduce the notion of modality, which is a biomedical signal that represents one view or one function of the organization. Therefore, the depiction devices receive modalities and with the appropriate processes turn them into images. The dimension of a signal depends on the number of independent variables it has. Consequently, the two-dimensional signals have as independent variables the two dimensions of the surface.

Therefore, the elements that should be included in a digital system for the elaboration of images are the following:

- **Image Elaborator:** This is the hardcore of the system that receives the image, temporarily stores and elaborates it on a low level, and finally demonstrates it on a primary level.
- **Digitizer:** It arithmetically represents the image in order for it to be received by a computer.
- **Digital Computer:** It performs an extensive elaboration.
- **Storage Devices**
- **Screens and Recording Devices**

We will now proceed to analyse the above elements in order to realize their participation in the elaboration of images, and at the same time we will present all the processes that occur at each level.

Image Elaborator

The evolution of technology, as mentioned above, was the vaulting bar for the development and

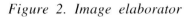

Figure 2. Image elaborator

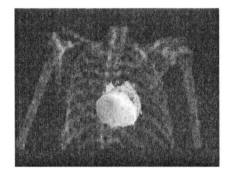

evolution of medical depiction devices and machines, something that proved to be beneficial for health services. Today, there is a large number of medical apparatuses that fills any kind of diagnostic demands. More specifically, in the three-dimensional depiction area, there are now many options that suit every demand. The categories of medical images are as follows.

- Digital abstraction angiography
- Ultrasound system
- Computed tomography (CT)
- Magnetic resonance imaging (MRI)
- Gamma camera
- Computed tomographies of nuclear medicine (single-photon-emission computed tomography [SPECT] and positron-emission tomography [PET])

Digital Abstraction Angiography

It is a medical diagnostic examination that depicts the condition of the vessels. It is extremely useful in the sector of cardiology and helps to with the prevention of many diseases of the cardiac system. Its characteristic is that it produces a vast number of data, especially as we move from one-dimensional systems to two-dimensional ones and from a still image to a moving one (video).

Figure 3. Digital angiography

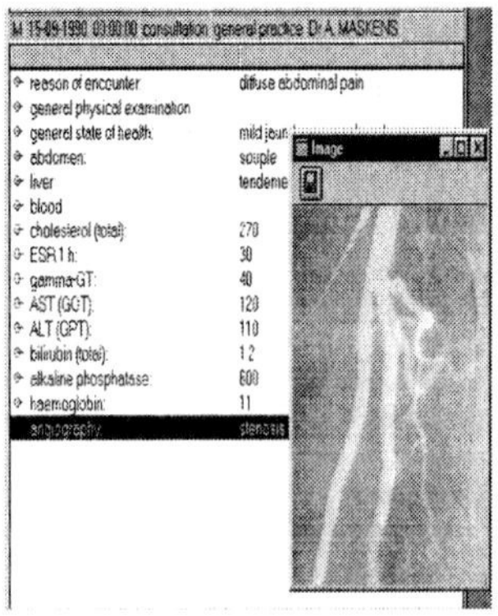

Figure 4. MRI depiction

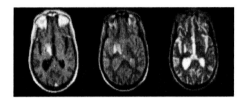

Ultrasound System

It depicts the resonance of high-frequency sound waves, which depend on the auditory properties of tissues that are produced by different organs and are examined as brightness in the image. One application of the ultrasound system is the ultrasound of the heart and vessels (Doppler), which is developed in real time and depicts the flux speed of the blood.

Computed Tomography

It uses X-rays for the creation of images, which means that the patient is exposed to radiation during the examination. The part of the body that needs to be examined receives X-rays through different transmission angles. With the use of mathematic transformations and calculations on the counted prices from these different angles, we receive images that are cross and plane sections. Each ray penetrating the body is recording densities of tissues.

Magnetic Tomography

It is a nonpenetration diagnostic method that produces a series of images that represent biological differences among tissues. Further-

more, the patient does not have to be exposed to harmful radiation. It is based on the application system of a magnetic field in order to obtain magnetic tomographies.

By applying a magnetic field, the cells orient to the rotation frequency and thus we have the production of resonance through the pulse of radiofrequency. Afterward, we have a rest so that the cells can reorient to their initial positions. The produced signal depends on the density and type of cells and, thus, magnetic tomographies show a high contrast on the soft tissues.

Gamma Camera

It is a diagnostic method that belongs to the field of nuclear medicine. It is based on the calculation of the position and concentration of a radioactive isotope that is provided to the patient before the examination. It gathers clinical information about the normal function while its discernibility is very low.

Computed Tomographies of Nuclear Medicine (PET and SPECT)

This section is about diagnostic examinations that are related to the physiology of the organization and are the most modern in technological terms in the field of diagnostics. SPECT involves the computed tomography of photon transmission, something that shows that the

Figure 5. Depiction in SPECT

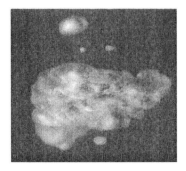

signal-production process is based on photon transmission. PET involves tomography with positron transmission.

The diagnostic devices mentioned are the means of acquiring medical images in analogous or digital forms. The device used may have the ability to store digitally; otherwise, the digitalization occurs with the use of a digitizer before storage. Next we have the process of compressing images.

Digital Image Compression

The term compression is mentioned in a number of technicalities and algorithms aiming to reduce the required memory for the representation and storage of digital images. The storage of a digitalized image leads to a squandering of the memory of the computing system. Thus, in the medical field, where the amount of image information is enormous, a major problem rises because of the amount of memory required for image storage. For this reason, faster compression and decompression algorithms for images have been searched for. Besides sparing memory, compression provides a reduction in the time and the width needed for transmission.

The techniques for the compression of digital images can be divided into two categories.

In medicine, where even the smallest detail in depiction can be of vital importance, we choose lossless techniques.

Compression is based on redundant information that is included in the images. The more redundancy there is, the more is the achieved compression. The whole process is called source coding, and it is based on a system that includes the following:

- **Transformer:** It transforms the initial image into a more appropriate one for compression.
- **Quanter:** It quants the transformed image either with graduation or with vector.
- **Coder:** A sequence of bits corresponds with each quant level. The code can be of a specific or variable length.

Compression with no losses does not use a quanter system because a quant always shows a loss of information.

The used patterns of image compression are as follows:

- G3, G4, GBIG—binary images
- JPEG—firm images
- H.261 MPEG1, MPEG2, MPEG4, MPEG7—movable images

After the compression process, we have the process of storage to the PACS system and recuperation from RIS.

Storage of Medical Images and Their Recuperation

Medical images, according to the diagnostic device used, have large sizes due to the need for high-quality analysis and clearness, thus demanding a large storage space. The recuperation time differs according to the kind of examination and the demanded number of images in each examination.

When the image reaches the final stage of elaboration, the goals are then the improvement of the quality of the given information with the use of the appropriate graphic-elaboration software (e.g., clearness, brightness, contrast), and also the exploitation of specific information with the use of special operations and transformations like division and recombining.

Quality Improvement of Images

The quality improvement of images is achieved with the use of software that helps to reach the desired levels of analysis aiming to exploit and evaluate the information given from an image. During the process of recording images, certain deformities appear. These are:

- Dimness,
- Noise of recording, and
- Geometrical deformities.

All these deformities should be corrected in order to eliminate all kinds of alterations. The elimination of dimness is done with the process of restoration. The process of restoration is extremely important in the elaboration of moving images because movement creates dimness. In most cases, a filtering of the image is also required in order to remove sound. This can be achieved with various linear or nonlinear filters. Usually, nonlinear filters are preferred because they preserve the contrast of outlines, which are an important factor for human vision. Moreover, the general contrast of the image can be improved with special nonlinear techniques.

One other important procedure for image analysis is the recognition of outlines. Usually, the areas of an image are coloured with false colours.

Finally, we achieve improvement of quality by adjusting the proper clearness, brightness, and contrast with the use of appropriate technical equipment that allows us to exploit all

these tools provided by the graphic software for quality improvement.

Image Division

By dividing a medical image, we are able to divide the image in different sections that show some cognitive interest according to the speciality under examination. Thus, according to the reason why the diagnostic examination occurs, the scientist can focus on a specific part of the image to process suitably and find the needed information without the redundancy of information to trouble him or her.

Furthermore, with the appropriate software, we can store to the computed system only those parts of the image that interest us, thus sparing storage space and making it more easy to recuperate the images from the used medical databases.

Medical Image Recombination

With medical image recombination, we can have a combination of different views from various depiction examinations (e.g., ultrasound+CT, MRI+PET, MRI+SPECT), giving us a three-dimensional representation of composition.

Indeed, medical image recombination is extremely important in medical depiction. Each diagnostic examination allows the scientist to

Figure 6. Division of image received by an MRI

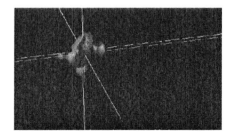

Figure 7. Image recombination MRI + PET + CT

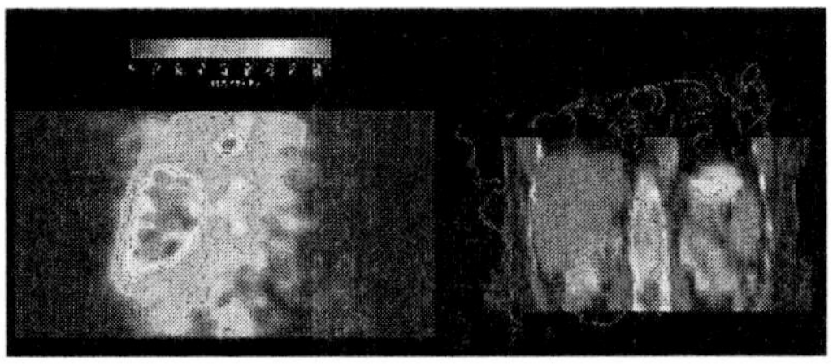

Figure 8. Image recombination SPECT + CT

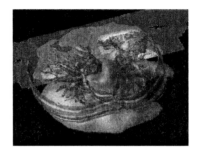

extract specific information through it. With this recombination method, the scientist can have the elements and information provided by different diagnostic examinations in only one image, can elaborate them and analyse them in any way he or she desires, and, finally, can reproduce them in a three-dimensional environment. The whole undertaking occurs through complex graphic software, which should have certain characteristics in order to be an actual diagnostic tool in the hands of the scientist vs. an obstacle in his or her effort to do the job.

The characteristics of the elaboration software include the following:

- Friendly user interface
- Large number of choices that are easy to overcome
- Support of the established models of compression and image management
- Support of future applications

- Safe use
- Is easy to learn

CONCLUSION AND PERSPECTIVES

Three-dimensional image elaboration is a very strong tool in medical diagnostics. Many of the diseases of tissue and microscopic interest are able to be diagnosed early and therefore can be cured. Especially benefited are the fields of research in medicine, pharmacology, and genetics, where the elaboration and depiction of three-dimensional models is extremely crucial for their development. The appearance of more and more evolved depiction devices and the growth of more powerful and more complete software for digital graphic elaboration will predispose even bigger steps of evolvement in the near future.

Chapter XXXVIII
Imaging the Human Brain with Magnetoencephalography

Dimitrios Pantazis
University of Southern California, USA

Richard M. Leahy
University of Southern California, USA

ABSTRACT

Magnetoencephalography is a relatively new medical imaging modality for the monitoring and imaging of human brain function. Extracranial magnetic fields produced by the working human brain are measured by extremely sensitive superconducting sensors, called SQUIDs, enclosed in a liquid helium-filled dewar. Mathematical modeling allows the formation of images or maps of cortical neuronal currents that reveal neural electrical activity, identify cortical communication networks, and facilitate the treatment of neuronal disorders, such as epilepsy.

INTRODUCTION

Magnetoencephalography (MEG) is a noninvasive technique for measuring neuronal activity in the human brain. Electrical currents flowing through neurons generate weak magnetic fields recorded using magnetic sensors surrounding the head. The MEG method is part of a broad area of research referred to as biomagnetism, which involves studies of magnetic fields emanating from several organs of the human body, notably the brain and heart.

The temporal resolution of MEG is in the millisecond (ms) range, the timescale at which neurons communicate. Therefore, we can follow the rapid cortical activity reflecting ongoing signaling between different brain areas. This is a great advantage compared to other medical imaging modalities such as functional magnetic resonance imaging (fMRI) and positron emission tomography (PET), where temporal resolution is on the order of seconds. Furthermore, unlike other methodologies that measure brain metabolism or the relatively slow hemodynamic response, MEG directly measures electrical brain activity. Electroencephalography (EEG) is a complimentary method to MEG, measuring electrical scalp potentials rather than magnetic fields. It offers similar temporal resolution to MEG, but the spatial resolution is less accurate because electrical potentials measured on the scalp are heavily influenced by strongly inhomogeneous conductivity of the head, whereas magnetic fields are mainly produced by currents that flow in the relatively homogeneous intracranial space.

NEURAL BASIS OF ELECTROMAGNETIC SIGNALS

A neuron consists of the cell body (or soma), which contains the nucleus; branching dendrites, which receive signals from other neurons; and a projection called an axon, which conducts the nerve signal. When a pulse arrives at an axon of a presynaptic cell, neurotransmitter molecules are released from the synaptic vesicles into the synaptic cleft. These molecules bind to receptors located on target cells, opening ion channels (mostly Na^+, K^+, and Cl^-) through the membrane. The resulting flow of charge causes an electrical current along the interior of the postsynaptic cell, changing the postsynaptic potential (PSP). When an excitatory PSP reaches the firing threshold at the axon hillock, it initiates an action potential that travels along the axon with undiminished amplitude.

The conservation of electric charge dictates that intracellular currents, commonly called primary currents, give rise to extracellular currents flowing through the volume conductor. Both primary and volume currents contribute to magnetic fields outside the head; however, only locally structured arrangements of cells can achieve sufficient coherent superposition of

Figure 1. Cerebral frontal cortex drawn by Ramón y Cajal using a Golgi staining technique. Pyramidal (A, B, C, D, E) and nonpyramidal (F, K) cells are clearly depicted. Currents flowing in the dendritic trunks of pyramidal cells are believed to be the primary generators of magnetic signals outside the head.

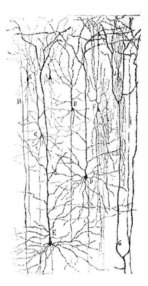

currents as to produce measurable external fields. Clusters of thousands of synchronously activated pyramidal cortical neurons are believed to be the main generators of MEG signals (Figure 1). In particular, the currents associated with large dendritic trunks, which are locally oriented in parallel and perpendicular to the cortical surface, are believed to be the primary source of the neuromagnetic fields outside the head. In contrast, the temporal summation of currents for action potentials, which have duration of only 1 ms, is not as effective as for dendritic currents flowing in neighboring fibers, so action potentials are believed to contribute little to MEG measurements.

INSTRUMENTATION

Empirical observations indicate that we observe sources on the order of 10 nA-m, and consequently, the neuromagnetic signals are typically 50 to 500 fT, that is, 10^9 or 10^8 times smaller that the geomagnetic field of the earth (Hämäläinen, Hari, Ilmoniemi, Knuutila, & Lounasmaa, 1993). The only detector that offers sufficient sensitivity to measure such fields is the superconducting quantum interference device (SQUID) introduced in the late 1960s by James Zimmerman (Zimmerman, Thiene, & Harding, 1970). The first measurement of brain magnetic fields using a SQUID magnetometer was carried out by David Cohen (1972) at the Massachusetts Institute of Technology, and it consisted of the spontaneous alpha activity of a healthy participant and abnormal brain activity in an epileptic patient.

The SQUID is a superconducting ring interrupted by thin insulating layers to form one or two Josephson junctions (Barone & Paterno, 1982). One important property associated with Josephson junctions is that magnetic flux is quantized in units of $\Phi_0 = 2.0678x10^{-15}$ tesla·m^2. If a constant biasing current is maintained in the SQUID device, the measured voltage oscillates as the magnetic flux increases; one period of voltage variation corresponds to an increase of one flux quantum. Counting the oscillations allows one to evaluate the flux change that has occurred, and therefore detect magnetic fields on the order of a few fT. The sensitivity of the SQUID can be increased to 1 fT by attaching a coil of superconducting wire or flux transformer. The latter is placed as close to the human head as possible, and depending on its shape, it can be configured as a first-order planar or axial gradiometer, a second-order axial gradiometer, or a simple magnetometer (Hämäläinen et al., 1993). The gradiometer configurations produce measurements proportional to the spatial gradient of the magnetic field, thus offering robustness to interference from distant magnetic field sources.

Modern MEG systems consist of a few hundred SQUID sensors placed in a liquid-helium-filled dewar, with the flux-transformer pickup coils surrounding a helmet structure (Figure 2). Worldwide, three companies build the majority of whole-head MEG systems: 4-D Neuroimaging (formerly Biomagnetic Technologies Bti), Elekta Neuromag Oy, and VSM MedTech Ltd. (manufacturers of the CTF Systems). In recent years, all three vendors have introduced dense arrays comprising over 200 SQUID channels.

Brain magnetic signals are very weak compared to ambient noise. Outside disturbances include fluctuations of the earth's geomagnetic field, power-line fields, electronic devices, elevators, and radio-frequency waves. Nearby artifacts are caused by instrumentation noise and body interference, such as heart, skeletal muscle, and spontaneous or incoherent background brain activity. Shielded rooms made of successive layers of mu-metal, copper, and aluminum effectively attenuate high-frequency

Figure 2. Whole-head CTF Omega MEG system with 275 axial gradiometers (left), and MEG sensors using low-temperature electronics cooled by liquid helium (right)

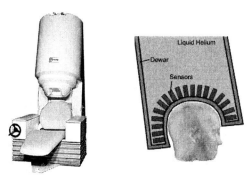

disturbances. Furthermore, gradiometer flux transformers cancel distant noise sources that produce magnetic fields with small spatial gradients.

MODELING

To estimate the neural sources of magnetic fields, one must first solve the associated forward problem, that is, the forward model that maps sources of known location, strength, and orientation to the MEG sensors. The most common source model is the current dipole (Baillet, Mosher, & Leahy, 2001), used to approximate the flow of an electrical current in a small area of the brain. The typical strength of a current dipole, generated by the synchronous firing of thousands of neurons, is 10 nA-m. Alternatively, to avoid the identifiability problem that arises when too many small regions and their dipoles are required to represent a single large region of coherent activation, we can use multipolar models, consisting of dipoles, quadrupoles, octupoles, and so on (Mosher, Leahy, Shattuck, & Baillet, 1999).

Since the useful frequency spectrum for electrophysiological signals is largely below 100 Hz, the physics of MEG can be described with the quasistatic approximation of Maxwell's equations. The propagation of electromagnetic fields inside the head is estimated based on the conductivities of the scalp, skull, gray and white matter, cerebrospinal fluid, and other tissue types. Head models that consist of a set of nested concentric spheres with isotropic and homogeneous conductivities have closed-form solutions. Even though spherical head models work surprisingly well, more accurate solutions use realistic head models based on anatomical information from high-resolution magnetic resonance (MR) or x-ray computed tomography (CT) volumetric images. To estimate the parameters of these models, numerical solutions using boundary-element methods (BEMs), finite-element methods (FEMs), or finite-difference methods (FDMs) are necessary (Darvas, Pantazis, Kucukaltun-Yildirim, & Leahy, 2004).

To make inferences about the brain activity that gives rise to a set of MEG data, we must solve the inverse problem, that is, find a neuronal current-source configuration that explains the MEG measurements. Inverse methods for MEG can be roughly categorized into two classes: imaging methods and dipole-fitting or-scanning methods. The imaging approaches are based on the assumption that the primary sources are intracellular currents in the dendritic trunks of cortical pyramidal neurons that are aligned normally to the cortical surface. Consequently, a tessellated representation of the cerebral cortex is extracted from a

Figure 3. MEG model depicting: (a) Sensor arrangement of a 275-channel CTF MEG system, (b) topography of sensor measurements, and (c) minimum-norm inverse solution on a tessellated cortical surface

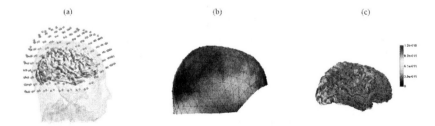

coregistered MR image, and the inverse problem is solved for a current dipole located at each vertex of the surface. In this case, since the position and orientation of the dipoles are fixed, image reconstruction is a linear problem and can be solved using standard techniques. The dipole-fitting or -scanning methods assume that the sources consist of only a few activated regions, each of which can be represented by an equivalent current dipole of unknown location and orientation. The standard approach to localization is to perform a least-squares fit of the dipole model to the data (Lu & Kaufman, 2003). More recently, scanning methods have been developed that are also based on the dipole model, but involve scanning a source volume or surface and detecting sources at those positions at which the scan metric produces a local peak (Baillet et al., 2001). Examples of these methods include the MUSIC (multiple signal classification) algorithm (Mosher, Leahy, & Lewis, 1992) and the LCMV (linearly constrained minimum variance) beamformer (VanVeen, van Drongelen, Yuchtman, & Suzuki, 1997).

Due to intrinsic spatial ambiguities of the electromagnetic principles that underlie MEG, the spatial resolution is lower than that of PET and fMRI. These ambiguities force a choice between low-resolution linear cortical imaging methods, or potentially higher resolution methods based on parametric models, or Bayesian or other nonlinear imaging methods incorporating physiological priors that reflect the expected characteristics of neural activation. A consensus is developing in the research community that no single method suits all MEG applications; each method has strengths and weaknesses, reflecting the ill pose of the inverse problem. The characteristics of expected neural activation, as well as model-fitting techniques, can facilitate the proper choice of inverse methodology.

STATISTICAL ANALYSIS

Given the large number of localization methodologies, it is important to perform validation and statistical analysis under different experimental settings, such as the number, location, and time series of neuronal sources. Furthermore, several methods require the fine-tuning of parameters, such as the subspace correlation threshold for the MUSIC algorithm. The receiver operating characteristic (ROC) curve is a standard tool to evaluate the trade-off between sensitivity and specificity, and to compare different inverse methods. By varying a threshold applied to localization maps, we can estimate two performance measures: the sensitivity or true positive fraction (TPF), and 1-specificity or false positive fraction (FPF). The ROC curve is a plot of the TPF vs. FPF as a detection threshold is varied. When comparing two detection methods, the one whose ROC curve gives higher sensitivity at matched specificity, and vice versa, for all points on the curve is the better detector. A simple metric to compare methods is the area under the ROC curve (AUC), where the method with the largest AUC is superior. The use of free-response ROC, an ROC variant that can handle the presentation and detection of multiple targets per image, is demonstrated in Yildirim, Pantazis, and Leahy (in press) for the evaluation of minimum-norm and scanning-inverse methods.

In addition to evaluating the relative performance of different methods, it is important to establish some degree of confidence in the results of real data analysis. Dipole-scanning methods often produce unstable solutions, and the reproducibility of the reconstructed dipoles is not guaranteed. A number of different approaches have been investigated for assessing dipole-localization accuracy, including Cramer Rao lower bounds, perturbation analysis, and Monte Carlo simulation. To avoid strict distributional assumptions, a resampling alternative based on bootstrap theory was proposed in Darvas, Rautiainen, et al. (2005). The principle underlying the bootstrap theory is that although the distribution of the data is unknown, it can be approximated by the empirical distribution of a set of independent trials. By sampling with replacement over independent trials collected during an event-related MEG study, the position, variance, and time series of current dipoles can be estimated reliably.

In contrast to dipole-scanning methods, imaging methods are hugely underdetermined, resulting in low-resolution localization maps; interpretation is further confounded by the presence of additive noise exhibiting a highly nonuniform spatial correlation. In this case, we need a mechanism to decide which features in the data are indicative of true activation vs. those that are noise artifacts. To determine a suitable threshold for detecting statistically significant activation, the familywise error rate (FWER), that is, the chance of any false positives under the null hypothesis of no activation (Type 1 error), is typically controlled. Parametric random-field methods and nonparametric permutation methods are used to estimate familywise-corrected thresholds in Pantazis, Nichols, Baillet, and Leahy (2005). Alternatively, the control of the false discovery rate (FDR), that is, the proportion of false positives among those tests for which the null hypothesis is rejected, can produce more sensitive thresholds.

Recent literature in MEG statistical analysis has been mostly limited to pairwise comparisons at each cortical surface element for event-related averages. However, extensions of this methodology to the investigation of multiple effects using analysis of variance (ANOVA) and analysis of covariance (ANCOVA) in individuals and groups is possible, as, for example, in Brookes et al. (2004).

APPLICATIONS

Applications in MEG include both basic and clinical research. One of the most important clinical applications is the detection, classification, and localization of abnormal neuronal activity in epilepsy patients. MEG has been successfully used to localize three different spontaneous interrictal signal components: epileptic spikes, slow-wave activity, and fast-wave activity (Lu & Kaufman, 2003). The neurosurgical planning of medically intractable epilepsy often includes the identification of epileptogenic lesions with MEG (Ossadtchi, Baillet, Mosher, Thyerlei, Sutherling, & Leahy, 2004; Stefan et al., 2003). Furthermore, recent literature investigates the possibility of seizure prediction based on a drop in the complexity of neural activity immediately before seizures (Maiwald, Winterhalder, Aschenbrenner-Scheibe, Voss, Schulze-Bonhage, & Timmer, 2004).

In addition to the diagnosis of epilepsy, MEG is currently used for functional brain mapping. Evoked response fields have been used to identify somatosensory-, motor-, and vision-related activity (Lu & Kaufman, 2003). Several MEG studies (Pantazis, Merrifield, Darvas, Sutherling, & Leahy, 2005) have localized language-specific cortical activity using either equivalent current dipoles or distributed cortical imaging, with promising results for clinical application in neurosurgery. Time-frequency analysis of MEG oscillatory-evoked responses (Pantazis, Weber, Dale, Nichols, Simpson, & Leahy, 2005) has detected networks of cortical interactions and determined the functional specificity of several frequency bands. A wide range of signal-processing techniques including image modeling and reconstruction, blind source separation, phase synchrony estimation, nonlinear analysis, and chaos theory are under investigation to reveal complex cognitive processes such as attention and working memory.

Recent literature investigates how evoked response fields relate to neuronal disorders, such as Alzheimer's disease, autism, dyslexia, brain tumors, and Parkinson's disease. Furthermore, MEG has been used in conjunction with transaxial magnetic stimulation to ameliorate abnormal brain activity (Anninos, Tsagas, Sandyk, & Derpapas, 1991).

CONCLUSION

Magnetoencephalography is a relatively new medical imaging modality for the monitoring and imaging of human brain function. While spatial resolution is significantly lower than that of PET and fMRI, the ability to monitor neuronal activation at the millisecond time scale makes this modality, together with EEG, a unique window on the human brain. Recent developments in instrumentation have lead to the manufacture of whole-head MEG arrays with an excess of 300 magnetometers. Coupled with new data-analysis tools for mapping brain function from MEG data, these systems will lead to important new insights into the workings of the human brain with applications in both clinical and cognitive neuroscience.

REFERENCES

Anninos, P. A., Tsagas, N., Sandyk, R., & Derpapas, K. (1991). Magnetic stimulation in the treatment of partial seizures. *International Journal of Neuroscience, 60*, 141-171.

Baillet, S., Mosher, J. C., & Leahy, R. M. (2001). Electromagnetic brain mapping. *IEEE Signal Processing Magazine, 18*(6), 14-30.

Barone, A., & Paterno, G. (1982). *Physics and applications of the Josephson effect.* Wiley.

Brookes, M. J., Gibson, A. M., Hall, S. D., Furlong, P. L, Barnes, G. R., Hillebrand, A., et al. (2004). A general linear model for MEG beamformer imaging. *Neuroimage, 23*, 936-946.

Cohen, D. (1972). Magnetoencephalography: Detection of the brain's electrical activity with a superconducting magnetometer. *Science, 175*, 664-666.

Darvas, F., Pantazis, D., Kucukaltun-Yildirim, E., & Leahy, R. M. (2004). Mapping human brain function with MEG and EEG: Methods and validation. *Neuroimage, 23*(Suppl. 1), S289-S299.

Darvas, F., Rautiainen, M., Pantazis, D., Baillet, S., Benali, H., Mosher, J. C., et al. (2005). Investigations of dipole localization accuracy in MEG using the bootstrap. *Neuroimage, 25*(2), 355-368.

Hämäläinen, M., Hari, R., Ilmoniemi, R. J., Knuutila, J., & Lounasmaa, O. V. (1993). Magnetoencephalography: Theory, instrumentation, and applications to noninvasive studies of the working human brain. *Reviews of Modern Physics, 65*(2), 413.

Lu, Z.-L., & Kaufman, L. (Eds.). (2003). *Magnetic source imaging of the human brain.* Mahwah, NJ: Lawrence Erlbaum Associates, Inc.

Maiwald, T., Winterhalder, M., Aschenbrenner-Scheibe, R., Voss, H. U., Schulze-Bonhage, A., Timmer, J. (2004). Comparison of three nonlinear seizure prediction methods by means of the seizure prediction characteristic. *Physica D, 194*, 357-368.

Mosher, J., Leahy, R., & Lewis, P. (1992). Multiple dipole modeling and localization from spatiotemporal meg data. *IEEE Transactions on Biomedical Engineering, 39,* 541-557.

Mosher, J. C., Leahy, R. M, Shattuck, D. W., & Baillet, S. (1999). MEG source imaging using multipolar expansions. *Proceedings of the 16th Conference on Information Processing in Medical Imaging, IPMI'99* (pp. 15-28).

Ossadtchi, A., Baillet, S., Mosher, J. C., Thyerlei, D., Sutherling, W., & Leahy, R. M. (2004). Automated interrictal spike detection and source localization in magnetoencephalography using independent components analysis and spatio-temporal clustering. *Clinical Neurophysiology, 115*(3), 508-522.

Pantazis, D., Merrifield, W., Darvas, F., Sutherling, W., & Leahy, R. M. (2005). Hemispheric language dominance using MEG cortical imaging and non-parametric statistical analysis. *WSEAS Transactions on Biology and Biomedicine, 2*(3), 318-325.

Pantazis, D., Nichols, T. E., Baillet, S., & Leahy, R. M. (2005). A comparison of random field theory and permutation methods for the statistical analysis of MEG data. *Neuroimage, 25*(2), 383-394.

Pantazis, D., Weber, D. L., Dale, C. C., Nichols, T. E., Simpson, G. V., & Leahy, R. M. (2005). Imaging of oscillatory behavior in event-related MEG studies. In C. A. Bouman & E. L. Miller (Eds.), *Proceedings of SPIE, Computational Imaging III, 5674* (pp. 55-63).

Stefan, H., Hummel, C., Scheler, G., Genow, A., Druschky, K., Tilz, C., et al. (2003). Magnetic brain source imaging of focal epileptic activity: A synopsis of 455 cases. *Brain, 126*(11), 2396-2405.

VanVeen, B., van Drongelen, W., Yuchtman, M., & Suzuki, A. (1997). Localization of brain electrical activity via linearly constrained minimum variance spatial filtering. *IEEE Transactions on Biomedical Engineering, 44*(9), 867-880.

Yildirim, E. K., Pantazis, D., & Leahy, R. M. (in press). Task-based comparison of inverse methods in MEG. *IEEE Transactions on Biomedical Engineering.*

Zimmerman, J. E., Thiene, P., & Harding, J. T. (1970). Design and operation of stable rf-based superconducting poinst-contact quantum devices and a note on the properties of perfectly clean metal contacts. *Journal of Applied Physics, 41*, 1572-1580.

KEY TERMS

ANOVA and ANCOVA: Analysis of variance or covariance is a collection of statistical models and their associated procedures that compare means by splitting the overall observed variance into different parts.

Current Dipole: Popular source model in MEG, representing a point's current source. It is a convenient representation for the coherent activation of a large number of pyramidal cells, possibly extending over a few square centimeters of gray matter.

EEG: Electroencephalography measures neuronal activity by recording electrical potentials with electrodes attached on the human scalp. The resulting waveforms are used to localize brain activity and assess brain damage, epilepsy, or even in some cases brain death.

fMRI: Functional magnetic resonance imaging uses powerful magnets to create a field that resonates the nuclei of atoms in the body. The oscillating atoms emit radio signals that are converted by a computer into 3-D images of the human body and cerebral blood flow.

LCMV Beamformer: Linearly constrained minimum-variance beamformer applies spatial filtering to sensor array data to discriminate between signals from a location of interest and those originating elsewhere. In the application to MEG, the goal is to find a spatial filter that minimizes the output power of the beamformer subject to a unity gain constraint at the desired location on the brain.

MUSIC: Multiple signal classification is a localization algorithm that uses the subspace correlation between the data and model sub-space to identify the origin of signals. It is often used in MEG to estimate the location, orientation, and strength of current dipoles.

PET: Positron emission tomography is a noninvasive imaging modality that measures the distribution of radioactive-labeled molecules inside a biological system. By using molecular probes that have different rates of uptake depending on the type of tissue involved, PET can localize lesions, and detect regional blood flow and gene expression among others.

Chapter XXXIX
Region of Interest Coding in Medical Images

Sharath T. Chandrashekar
Sarayu Softech Pvt Ltd., India

Gomata L. Varanasi
Samskruti, India

ABSTRACT

To provide efficient compression of medical images, identifying and extracting the region of interest from the entire image and coding the specific region to accuracy is important. This chapter introduces the basics of region of interest coding, an overview of the coding methods available and their main features for the benefit of learners and researchers. The special focus is on JPEG-2000-based algorithms.

INTRODUCTION

One of the main aims in medical image processing is to extract important features from radiological image data, called the region of interest (ROI), for accurate diagnostic analysis, interpretation, and better patient treatment. Coding the region of interest is significant for easy, rapid transmission, and also for efficient storage. This is useful in the application areas of teleradiology, picture archiving and communication systems (PACSs), and hospital information systems (HISs; http://www.dclunie.com).

What is the Region of Interest?

ROI is the region of image that is of clinical or diagnostic interest to the doctor, radiologist, or image analyst. Its shape may be regular, as shown in Figure 1, or arbitrary and irregular, as in Figure 2.

Multiple ROIs

There could be more than one region of interest within a given image, leading to multiple ROIs as shown in Figure 3.

Figure 1. UltraSound image ROI is fetus zone—regular shape

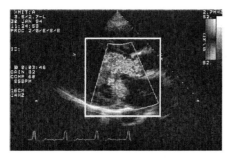

Figure 2. CT image—ROI is heart—arbitrary shape

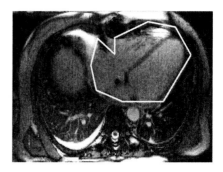

Identifying and Extracting

Identifying and extracting the region of interest is required before compressing and coding the image that includes the region of interest. Identifying a region is done by manual and/or automatic segmentation methods. The segmentation procedure used is based on the input image data, the nature of the information sought by the end user from the segmented image, and the application (Grimes, 2004).

ROI Compression and Coding

With the growing interest in the areas of telemedicine and health informatics, compressing and coding ROI is a necessity. The following are some of the compression schemes employed in this area of image coding.

Image compression usually can be lossy or lossless. Lossless compression methods are preferred for high-value content, such as medical imagery or image scans made for archival purposes. Lossy methods are especially suitable for natural images in applications where minor (sometimes imperceptible) loss of fidelity is acceptable to achieve a substantial reduction in bit rate.

Lossy Compression Schemes

Totally lossy schemes result in image alteration, which might entail a loss of diagnostic or scientific utility. Sometimes lossy compression may deliver exquisite quality and yet can introduce medically unacceptable artifacts into the image. These are less popular in medical situations.

Lossless Compression Schemes

The following are categorized as lossless compression schemes in different contexts based on the end user or observer:

- **Visually Lossless:** Nonclinical human observer

Figure 3. Lesions are the ROIs in brain MRI slice

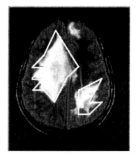

Figure 3a. ROI, the cube representing the wavelet coefficients of Figure 5. Surface of the cube represents the most significant bit, MSB of the coefficients. Each of the coding method scales this height for ROI.

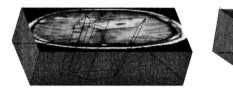
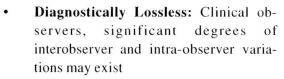

- **Diagnostically Lossless:** Clinical observers, significant degrees of interobserver and intra-observer variations may exist
- **Quantifiably Lossless:** Mostly nonhuman observers, computer-assisted detection

Lossless schemes cannot offer high compression ratios, yet they are preferred in certain situations where the data is needed without much loss (Clunie, n.d.).

Regionally Lossless Compression Schemes

These are a special case of lossless coding schemes based on a certain region of interest (Christopoulos, Askelöf, & Larsson, 2000). A chosen ROI is encoded with higher quality than the background (BG). The ROI can either be static or dynamic. Static ROIs are defined at coding time. The user defines dynamic ROIs interactively while they are progressively transmitted and decoded.

After segmenting an image into regions (either automatically or manually), it is possible for a compression algorithm to deliver different levels of reconstruction quality in different spatial regions of the image. One could accurately preserve the features needed for medical diagnosis or for scientific measurement while achieving high compression overall by allowing the degradation of data in unimportant regions.

Uses of Compression

In radiology, compression can be done in many ways and has the following uses:

- Compression before primary diagnosis (for rapid transmission)
- Compression after primary diagnosis (for long-term archiving in a PACS)
- Compression for database browsing (where progression in quality and resolution would be useful)

Region of Interest Coding

ROI coding is a process performed mostly at the encoder end. The encoder decides which ROI is to be coded with better quality than the background. If the encoder does not know the ROIs in advance, there is still a possibility for the decoder to receive only the data that is requested using some end-user specification. This case is also explained in one of the coding algorithms mentioned in later sections.

Coding Methods: Encoding End

The JPEG2000 standard (Christopoulos, Skodras, & Ebrahimi, 2000; Clunie, n.d.; Marcellin, Gormish, Bilgin, & Boliek, 2000) is a wavelet-based still-image compression standard. This compression standard is adopted in DICOM format (Digital Imaging and Communications in Medicine; http://www.dclunie.com; http://www.rsna.org), commonly used for medical images. Two of the ROI coding methods defined in JPEG2000 are the following:

- Generic scaling-based method
- Maximum shift (Maxshift) method

Other than these, the following are also being used and have different advantages based on the application:

- Most significant bit-plane shift (MSBShift) method
- Bit-plane-by-bit-plane shift (BbBShift) method

Coding algorithms used in any of these methods are derived based on the standard image-compression schemes (Bhaskaran & Konstantinides, 1997). Along with the color transform, discrete wavelet transform, quantization, image coding, rate control, and entropy coding, these methods include additional processing related to ROI compression (Figure 5 and Figure 6). The information provided in this article is only at an overview level, and it is highly suggested that the readers consult the references for all the details.

Generic Scaling Method

The following is the overview of this method and its features (Christopoulos, Askelöf, et al., 2000):

- Part 2 of the JPEG2000 standard (Christopoulos, Skodras, et al., 2000) supports the general scaling method.
- **ROI in Higher Bit Planes:** The bits of BG coefficients are downshifted toward

the least significant bit plane (LSB) so that the ROI-associated bits are placed in the higher bit planes. This can also be viewed as ROI mask coefficients shifted up (Figure 4). This relative scaling value between ROI and BG is recorded.

- **Multiple ROIs:** The generic scaling method allows for multiple ROIs; each ROI is upshifted by a different value. The upshift value is recorded in the codestream header for each ROI.
- **Multiple Overlapped ROIs:** If the different ROIs overlap, the overlapped region is coded as belonging to the highest quality ROI. Because this method does not result in an easily identifiable ROI mask, it must be made available to the decoder.
- **Fine Control:** As any scaling value is supported, the generic scaling-based method allows fine control on the relative importance between ROI and BG.
- **Shape Coding Needed:** The ROI shape information has to be coded, and this significantly increases the complexity and reduces the coding efficiency.
- **Restricted Shapes:** Regular ROI shapes (rectangle and ellipse) are supported in this method. This restriction may limit the real application of ROI coding and the compression efficiencies that can be achieved.

Coding Algorithm

The general scaling-based method is implemented as follows, and it is very familiar amongst image-compression communities.

Encoding ROI:

1. The color transform is performed on the entire image, and the discrete wavelet transform is calculated as in JPEG2000 (Bhaskaran & Konstantinides, 1997).

Figure 4. Generic scaling method. ROI-1-star: coefficients are raised to higher scale—2 and ROI-2—the elliptical brain slice. Different ROIs can be raised to different scales.

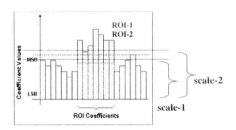
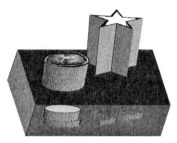

2. If the ROI is identified, then an ROI mask is derived extracting the region, indicating the set of coefficients that are required for lossless ROI reconstruction.

3. The wavelet coefficients are quantized. These coefficients are stored in a sign magnitude representation. Magnitude bits comprise the most significant part of the implementation precision used.

4. The coefficients that are out of the ROI are scaled up or down by a specific scaling value. If there are more than one ROI, these can be multiple coded with different scaling values.

5. The resulting coefficients are progressively entropy encoded (with the most significant bit planes first). As overhead information, the scaling value assigned to the ROI and the coordinates of the ROI are added to the bit stream. The decoder performs also the ROI mask generation, but scales up the background coefficients in order to recreate the original coefficients.

Decoding ROI: The decoder reverses the steps of encoding to reconstruct the image as in Figure 6 (Bhaskaran & Konstantinides, 1997). At the decoder, the bit planes are first reconstructed from the most significant bit plane to the least significant bit plane. Then, according

to the shape information of the ROI included in the code stream, the BG coefficients are located and scaled up to their original places before the inverse wavelet transform is applied to reconstruct the image.

Maxshift Method

The following is the overview of this method and its features:

•   Maxshift scaling is supported in Part 1 of the JPEG2000 standard.

•   **Special Case of General Scaling:** This can be viewed as a particular case of the generic scaling-based method when the scaling value is so large that there is no overlap between BG and ROI bit planes, as seen in Figure 7. After scaling, all bits of the ROI coefficients will be in higher bit planes than all the bits associated with the BG.

•   **Larger Scaling and Less Compression:** Compared with the generic scaling-based method, the Maxshift method uses larger scaling values and reduces the compression efficiency by introducing more bit planes.

•   **Multiple ROIs:** A single scale value is used for all the ROIs. When multiple ROIs with different priorities may be in-

Figure 5. Encoding algorithm

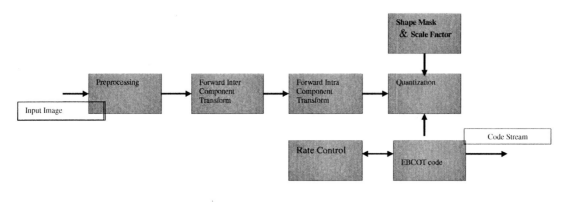

Figure 6. Decoding algorithm

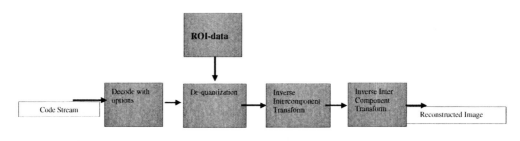

volved, the Maxshift method cannot support the concept like the generic scale-based method.

- **Arbitrary-Shape Coding Support:** Arbitrary shapes are supported. The shape of the ROI is encoded and sent. It is available implicitly for the decoder.
- **No Fine Control:** Unlike the generic scaling-based method, the Maxshift method cannot control the relative importance between ROIs and the BG. No BG information can be received until all ROI coefficients are decoded fully.
- **No ROI Mask Generation in Decoder:** The ROI mask is easy to find because of the scaling value mentioned along with the location and shape of the ROI. This means also that the decoder does not have to

perform ROI mask generation, either (this might still be needed at the encoder).

Coding Algorithm
Encoding ROI: The coding algorithm is almost the same as the generic scaling method. It differs after the first two steps as follows:

- The wavelet coefficients are quantized. The encoder scans the quantized coefficients and chooses a scaling value S such that the minimum coefficient belonging to the ROI is larger than the maximum coefficient of the background (non-ROI area).
- It shifts the ROI mask coefficients up such that their LSBs are higher than the most significant non-zero bit of all background coefficients.

Figure 7. MaxShift method. ROI-1 and ROI-2 both are scaled up to the MSB level. Green cylinder and star show the location. But no ROI coefficients are there below MSB level.

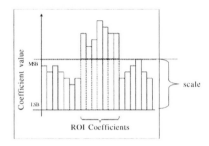 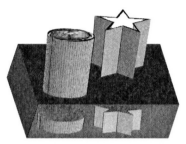

Decoding ROI: At decoding, the BG and ROI coefficients can be identified easily according to the bit-plane positions. Every coefficient that is smaller than the scale belongs to the background and is therefore scaled up. The decoder needs only to upscale the received background coefficients.

MSBShift Method

- **Arbitrarily Shaped ROI Coding:** The MSBShift method not only supports arbitrarily shaped ROI coding without coding the shape, but also enables the flexible adjustment of compression quality in the ROI and background.
- **Multiple ROIs:** Additionally, the new method can efficiently code multiple ROIs with different priorities in an image.

- **Fine Control:** This is the same as in the generic scaling-based method. The MSBShift method can flexibly adjust the relative importance between ROI and BG by using different scaling values.

Coding Algorithm
Steps 1 and 2 of the generic scaling method are used:

- This method (Liu & Fan, 2003) removes all the overlapped bit planes between the ROI and BG coefficients, and relatively modifies the quantization step size of the coefficients. This reduces the final ROI quality.
- We can isolate a certain number of bit planes of the ROI bits in the most signifi-

Figure 8. MSBShift method. Some of the coefficients of ROI-1 and ROI-2 can be raised to different scales. But the MSB of the background is shifted down.

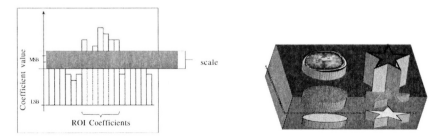

Figure 9. ROIs and coded images using generic scaling method (a) original, (b) and (c) ROIs

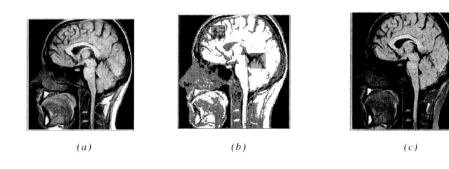

(a)   (b)   (c)

cant bit planes to adjust the importance between the ROI and BG.

- We only need to shift part of the most significant bit planes of the ROI coefficients instead of shifting all of the bit planes of the ROI coefficients as the standard methods do.
- **Complexity and Coding Efficiency:** Since it is not necessary for the MSBShift method to code ROI shapes, the complexity is less than the generic scaling-based method, and the coding efficiency is higher when the same scaling value is used. If the point of lossless coding is reached, the bit rate produced by the MSBShift method is not larger than the Maxshift method because the MSBShift method encodes less or at most the same number of bit planes.

BbBShift Method

- This method (Wang & Bovik, 2002) shifts the bit planes on a bit-plane-by-bit-plane basis instead of shifting them all at once like in the Maxshift method.
- **Finer Control:** The BbBShift method supports arbitrarily shaped ROI coding without coding shape information, and it can offer finer control of the ROI and BG quality than the Maxshift method.

- **No Multiple ROI Coding:** Moreover, the BbBShift method does not support multiple ROI coding.
- **Compression Efficiency:** This is similar to that of the Maxshift method.

Coding Methods: Decoding End

All of the above algorithms cater to the coding schemes at the encoder end. On the decoder end, the operation that is performed is just the reverse of the encoding operation:

- We can exploit the feature of JPEG2000 that enables one to compress once and decompress in many ways according to the user's requirement at the decoder end. The authors have done some research work on these lines, and the results obtained are in the process of publication.
- The encoding operation is done using the baseline algorithm of JPEG2000.
- Using the features of random access to the encoded data, the required region of interest can be progressively decoded.
- Manual data input is required for identifying the location of the likely region of interest.
- This method has applications in the areas of telemedicine, mobile communications, and PDAs (personal digital assistants).

Coding Metrics and Compression Efficiency

- **PSNR at a Given Bit Rate:** Other than subjective judgments, the parameter that measures the coding efficiency is the PSNR in dB (peak signal-to-noise ratio of the reconstructed image) at a given number of bits per pixel.
- **Complexity and Coding Efficiency:** The MSBShift method has less complexity than the generic scaling method as the ROI shape need not be coded for transmission. Coding efficiency is higher when the same scaling is used. The complexity of the MSBShift method is more than Maxshift, but the bit rates achieved are comparable.

CONCLUSION

ROI coding is a very significant and promising research area that can benefit many medical computing applications. The generic scaling and Maxshift methods are popular amongst image-processing communities and are well established. This article has limited scope and is only an introduction for curious developers. The details can be explored and expanded further based on the references given.

REFERENCES

Bhaskaran, V., & Konstantinides, K. (1997). *Image and video compression standards: Algorithms and applications* (2nd ed.). Boston: Kluwer Academic Publishers.

Burak, S., Tomasi, C., Girod, B., & Beaulieu, C. (2001). Medical image compression based on region of interest with application to colon CT images. *IEEE EMBS Proceedings* (pp. 2453-2456).

Christopoulos, C., Askelöf, J., & Larsson, M. (2000). Efficient methods for encoding regions of interest in the upcoming JPEG 2000 still image coding standard. *IEEE Signal Processing Letters, 7*(9), 247-249.

Christopoulos, C., Skodras, A., & Ebrahimi, T. (2000). The JPEG 2000 still image coding system: An overview. *IEEE Transactions on Consumer Electronics, 46*(4), 1103-1127.

Clunie, D. A. (n.d.). Lossless compression of grayscale medical images: Effectiveness of traditional and state of the art approaches. SPIE, *Proceedings, Medical Imaging, 3980,* 74-84. Retrieved from http://www.dclunie.com

Grimes, S. L. (2004). Clinical engineers: Stewards of healthcare technologies. *IEEE EMBS Magazine, 23*(3), 56-58.

Kalawsky, R. S. (2000). The validity of presence as a reliable human performance metric in immersive environments. *Proceedings of the Third International Workshop on Presence,* Delft, Netherlands.

Liu, L., & Fan, G. (2003). A new method for jpeg2000 region of interest image coding: Most significant bitplanes shift. *IEEE Signal Processing, 10*(2), 35-39.

Marcellin, M. W., Gormish, M., Bilgin, A., & Boliek, M. (2000). An overview of JPEG 2000. *Proceedings of IEEE Data Compression Conference,* Snowbird, UT.

Wang, Z., & Bovik, A. C. (2002). Bitplane-by-bitplane shift (BbBShift): A suggestion for JPEG2000 region of interest coding. *IEEE Signal Processing Letters, 9*(5), 160-162,

INTERNET REFERENCES:

http://www.dclunie.com

http://www.nema.org

http://www.rsna.org

http://www.wikipedia.org

KEY TERMS

Color Transform: The RGB components in natural images are more correlated than the components in a luminance-chrominance space. Color transform from one space to the other (typically from RGB space to YCrCb or luminance-chrominance space) is to decorrelate the components, reduce the redundancy, and thereby achieve energy compaction. This is a standard approach for compression.

Data Compression (Encoder and Decoder): It is the process of encoding information using fewer bits (information-bearing units) than a detailed representation through the use of specific encoding schemes to optimize the data. The follow-up compressed-data communication can work when both the sender (encoder) and receiver (decoder) of information share and understand the coding scheme.

Digital Imaging and Communications Medicine (DICOM): Digital Imaging and Communications in Medicine is an imaging standard that allows the exchange of data between different hosts and equipment across the network in a heterogeneous environment. It includes a file format definition and a network communication protocol that uses TCP/IP (transmission-control protocol/Internet protocol) to communicate between systems.

Entropy Coding: It is a coding scheme that assigns codes to symbols so as to match code lengths with the probabilities of the symbols. Three of the most common entropy encoding techniques are Huffman coding, range encoding, and arithmetic encoding.

Hospital or Radiology Information System (HIS or RIS): While PACS applications manage images, HIS and RIS applications manage patients, studies, and results.

Image Coding: A definition of a set of rules to map one set of image data onto another set to make the image or signal more suitable for an intended application. To suit the application, the image-coding scheme may optimize an image for transmission, improving transmission quality and fidelity, modifying the image for providing error detection and/or correction, providing data security, and so forth. Different coding schema may have different sets of advantages and disadvantages.

Image Compression: The application of data compression on digital images. In effect, the objective is to reduce the redundancy of the image data in order to be able to store or transmit data in an efficient form.

Picture Archiving and Communication System (PACS): The Picture Archiving and Communication System is an image-based information system for the acquisition, storage, communication, archiving, display, and manipulation of medical digital images and other relevant data.

Quantization: It is the process of approximating continuous data or signals by a set of discrete symbols and values rather than continuous representation.

Telemedicine: In Greek, *tele* means *far*. Telemedicine is the delivery of medicine or clinical care to remote individuals with the use of modern telecommunication and information technologies.

Teleradiology: A method of distributing digital diagnostic radiological information such as images using radiological systems based on x-rays, ultrasound, magnetic resonance, and other related information through local area or wide area networks between remotely located facilities.

Wavelet Transform: Wavelets in general are functions that can be used to efficiently represent other functions. The discrete wavelet transform is set of filter coefficients obtained over the set of basis wavelets functions. These are localized in scale and in time, as well as in frequency. The frequency is derived from the scale. These functions are scaled and convolved with the function being analyzed all over the time axis to get to transform space inviting compression.

Chapter XL
Imaging the Human Brain with Functional CT Imaging

Sotirios Bisdas
Johann Wolfgang Goethe University Hospital, Germany

Tong San Koh
Nanyang Technological University, Singapore

ABSTRACT

Recent advances in multi-detector computed tomography (CT) have revitalized its role in the clinical routine. In the field of cerebral perfusion, CT provides a rapid, low-cost functional imaging, which by the utilization of a suitable tracer kinetic analysis can provide valuable information in many clinical applications, like acute stroke, cerebrovascular reserve capacity, vasospasm after subarachnoidal hemorrhage, cerebral trauma, tumor imaging, and brain death diagnosis. The limitations of the existing commercially available post processing software are discussed and a new distributed-parameter tracer kinetic model for generating more accurate perfusion parametric maps is introduced.

INTRODUCTION

Recent advances in multidetector computed tomography (CT) have resulted in subsecond volumetric patient scanning, revitalizing the role of CT in the clinical routine. Such quantum technological laps combined with the availability and turnaround efficiency of CT have had a notable impact on the imaging paradigms of the critically ill such as stroke and trauma patients and those under intensive care. CT perfusion is a brilliant example of a protocol that has undergone significant improvements bearing considerable impact on patient care in the acute setting.

In the field of cerebral perfusion, CT overcomes other imaging modalities (e.g., magnetic resonance imaging [MRI], xenon computed tomography, positron-emission tomography [PET], and single-photon-emission computed tomography [SPECT]) through the rapid, low-cost generation of meaningful images and available user-friendly postprocessing software that interprets the data in a clinically relevant manner. The theory behind perfusion CT is a tracer kinetic analysis of the rapidly intravenously injected contrast material.

The purpose of this chapter is to revisit the assessment of perfusion CT imaging in many clinical applications, to suggest new clinical fields (e.g., brain-death diagnosis) for possible future applications of perfusion CT, and to emphasize the pitfalls of the method, suggesting a new distributed-parameter (DP) kinetic model for generating more accurate perfusion parametric maps.

IMAGING TECHNIQUES, INDICATORS, AND TRACER KINETICS MODELS

The measurement of cerebral perfusion relies on a triad including an imaging technique, an indicator, and a model. In the case of CT imaging, the sequential acquisition of cerebral sections (one or more sections per second) is performed during the rapid (6 mL/sec in our clinical protocol) intravenous administration of an iodinated contrast agent (50 mL of a 400 mg/dL non-ionic iodinated contrast material in our protocol).

The iodinated contrast agent is restrained in the cerebral vascular bed, at least at first pass and in healthy cerebral tissue. Tracer kinetic-analysis methods for estimating microcirculatory parameters can generally be grouped under two classes (Larson, Markham, & Raichle, 1987; Lee, 2002): (a) model-independent approaches that include numerical deconvolution-based methods and (b) model-dependent or parametric-fitting approaches. In the model-dependent approach, the tracer kinetics models

used for parametric fitting of the dynamic imaging data are usually linear compartmental models that can be further classified as conventional compartmental (CC) or DP models.

Three main models have been used for model-independent approaches including the maximum-slope model, the equilibring-indicator model, and the central-volume principle. The maximum-slope model requires very short injection times, which are not always tolerable by the patients, and tends to underestimate the cerebral blood flow (BF). Moreover, there is no general consensus regarding the reference arterial input function, which is necessary for the calculation of the perfusion parameters. On the other hand, the equilibring-indicator model and the central-volume model require a mathematical operation called deconvolution (Axel, 1981; Ostergaard et al., 1996). Deconvolution can be realized in two ways. The first method to solve the deconvolution problem is a parametric method in which supplemental hypotheses regarding the anatomical structure or the behaviour of the indicator are taken into account. The second method, called nonparametric, can be performed with single-value deconvolution and involves less source hypotheses. Deconvolution-based CT perfusion offers a fast and robust analysis of neurovascular disorders and has been an important strategy to assess stroke and to characterize intracranial tumors.

On the other side, comprehensive studies have indicated that linear compartmental models could allow a more complete analysis of the kinetic parameters. Also, as illustrated in various works, DP models possess more realism than CC models (Koh, Cheong, Hou, & Soh, 2003). The reason for this is that the tracer concentration gradients within compartments are taken into account in DP models, while in CC models, tracer concentration gradients are assumed to be zero at all times and thus the tracer is assumed to distribute instantaneously on arrival in each compartment.

CLINICAL APPLICATIONS

Acute Stroke

Unenhanced CT, which provides morphologic information about brain parenchyma, has long been the cornerstone for evaluating acute stroke. A normal CT scan of the brain excludes almost always intracranial hemorrhage, which, in evidence of an acute infarction, would herald the need for rapid medical therapy and potentially intravascular intervention. Nevertheless, the alteration of the brain morphology due to cytotoxic edema is not evident until some significant time after the stroke onset, leading many authors to advocate the use of diffusion MRI to evaluate acute infarctions. Perfusion CT has been stratified to assess acute cerebral ischemia, and threshold infarcted and non-infarcted tissue, and to predict tissue and clinical condition outcome (Bisdas et al., 2004). In contrast to other imaging modalities, like PET and MRI, it is well tolerated by patients with acute stroke symptoms and delivers quantitative results. Nevertheless, as aforementioned, the maximum-slope model may deliver unreliable results, and together with deconvolution-based analysis, it is extremely robust and, thus, is not realistic.

With our proposed DP tracer kinetic model, we calculate the perfusion (F); vascular mean transit time (MTT; t1), accounting for the mean transit time of the contrast agent in the intravascular compartment; and intravascular volume (v1). Secondly, we introduce in perfusion CT the use of lag time (tlag), which estimates the delay of the peak of the tissue residue function, aiming at the rapid identification of areas with varying degrees of hypoperfusion. Tlag is user unbiased and is supposed to overcome the problem arising from the individual determination of the arterial input function (AIF), for which no consensus exists regarding the most appropriate location.

Identifying the volume of the dead brain tissue has important prognostic value, but identifying the volume of the potentially salvageable brain tissue could improve the course and aggressiveness of acute–stroke treatment even more. The proposed DP model peers into the cellular biology of the infarcted brain and, in the case of a substantial tracer leakage from the vessels, quantifies the extravascular volume (v2) and the permeability surface product (PS).

The loss of integrity of the blood-brain barrier (BBB) resulting from ischemia or reperfusion is believed to be the precursor to hemorrhagic transformation and poor outcome. Since two major therapy strategies for acute stroke are strongly related to the hazardous effect of hemorrhagic transformation, namely, anticoagulation and thrombolysis, PS values can serve as a tool for selecting treatment paradigms. Recent retrospective observations using MRI showed an early disruption of the BBB in acute stroke, whereas CT can only confirm it at a later stage, missing the initial signs of microbleeding or BBB disruption (Latour et al., 2004).

Furthermore, in tracer kinetic models in which numerical deconvolution is used, the MTT is calculated as the area under the time-density curve, and blood volume (BV) is the convolution of BF and MTT. The potential PS disorders are not accounted for in this case, and MTT corresponds to t1 in our model while BV is equal to v1. Undoubtedly, at the presentation of BBB disruption, BV parametric maps based on numerical deconvolution or conventional compartment models cannot be used to indicate low perfusion. Thus, our DP model can provide valuable and precise physiologic data (Figure 1).

Figure 1. DP-model analysis of functional CT data obtained from a patient with a sudden onset (<2h) of right hemiparesis

a.

b.

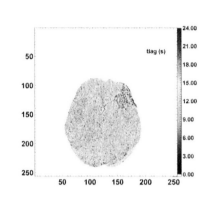

c.

d.

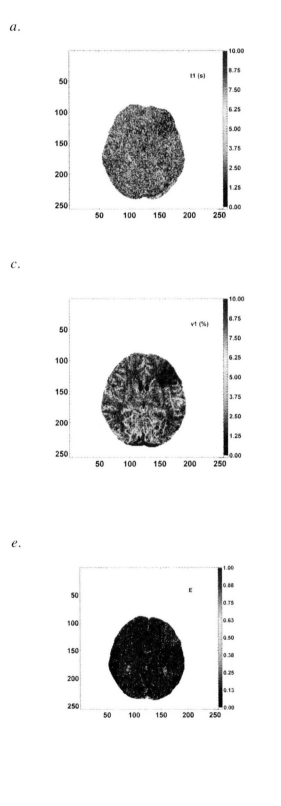

e.

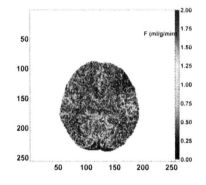

a. The perfusion t1 parametric map shows a time delay of the contrast agent's arrival in the anterior portion of the middle cerebral-artery territory on the right side.

b. The time delay is better recognized in the tlag map, which is independent of the subjectively determined AIF.

c. The v1 parametric map demonstrates reduced intravascular volume, reflecting the ischemic lesion margins.

d. The delineation of the ischemic lesion is also recognized in the F parametric map.

e. Subtle permeability surface product abnormalities are demonstrated in the PS map, indicating a disturbance of the brain-blood barrier's integrity.

Cerebrovascular Reserve Capacity

Patients with chronic steno-occlusive disease of the extracranial carotid represent a complex subgroup of patients with few proven therapeutic options. Neurological symptoms, produced by thromboembolic stroke and by altered cerebral hemodynamics, are very common in these patients. In fact, collateral supply, mostly via the circle of Willis, by extracranial-to-intracranial collaterals and leptomeningeal anastomoses maintains normal perfusion in patients with carotid stenosis. Nevertheless, a percentage of patients have an insufficient collateral supply, which leads to hemodynamic compromise (Derdeyn, Grubb, & Powers, 1999). The impaired cerebral hemodynamics can be identified by demonstrating an impaired vasodilatatory response after acetazolamide challenge-perfusion studies. The acetazolamide test is a reliable predictor of critically reduced cerebral perfusion and may unmask cerebrovascular reserve deficits even in patients with asymptomatic carotid stenosis who have hemodynamic compromise.

The status of cerebrovascular autoregulatory control has been examined with xenon, PET, single-photon-emission, and perfusion CT; perfusion-weighted MRI; and transcranial Doppler ultrasonography. Recent studies on perfusion CT have demonstrated significant correlation between the measured perfusion values and the estimated cerebrovascular reserve with PET measurements (Kudo et al., 2003; Bisdas et al., 2006). With our proposed DP model, the evaluation of the cerebrovascular response as (a) a less-than-expected augmentation relative to the contralateral side, (b) an absent augmentation, or (c) a paradoxical reduction in flow (steal phenomenon) could be easily performed. Thus, the visualization of cerebral perfusion symmetry and the obtained quantitative perfusion results can substantially assist in selecting the patients undergoing bypass surgery and can also be used to evaluate the efficacy of revascularization procedures postoperatively.

Vasospasm

Vasospasm is a frequent complication in the early course of subarachnoidal hemorrhage (SAH). A progression to infarction occurs in approximately half of the symptomatic cases; thus, measurements of cerebral blood flow can be useful in identifying patients at increased risk of cerebral infarction by guiding therapeutic decisions and monitoring responses to therapy. PET, SPECT, xenon CT, and transcranial Doppler sonography have already been employed for this purpose. Perfusion CT offers a rapid and reliable measurement of blood flow as well as of BV and MTT, increasing thus the understanding of the impairment of the brain autoregulation. ROI analysis in our patients with SAH demonstrated prolonged times of t1 and F values under 12 mL/min/100g of tissue (Nabavi et al., 2001). Nevertheless, the presence of massive subarachnoidal blood in the brain cisterns did not allow perfusion measurements of large brain territories as the volume averaging of pathologic tissue and subarachnoidal blood led to false increased F values. In this case, t1 values are more reliable and useful for therapy monitoring.

Traumatic Cerebral Contusions

Patients with traumatic brain injury frequently exhibit cerebral contusions, which may swell and cause increased intracranial pressure with secondary ischemia. It is still controversial whether traumatic contusions represent irreversibly infarcted focal lesions and how their presence can predict outcome in patients with severe head trauma. Conventional CT at admission usually underestimates the extent and severity of the cerebral parenchymal lesions, while initial experience with perfusion measurements, in terms of blood flow, showed the irreversibly damaged zone and the potential viability of tissue in the pericontusional zone (von Oettingen, Bergholt, Gyldensted, & Astrup, 2002). In our clinical setting, we were able to acquire absolute perfusion values of acute traumatic contusions and to predict later infracted areas. Analogously to the peri-infarction penumbral zones in acute ischemic stroke, the pericontusional tissue damage was outlined and the infarction risk was assessed.

Tumors

Expansive masses in the brain are readily recognized with CT imaging in the case of perifocal oedema and contrast-enhancement patterns that are also used to differentiate different types of brain tumours. The use of perfusion CT in this field offers a numerically solid basis for differential diagnosis and assessment of the tumor characteristics beyond that of visual assessment (Roberts, Roberts, Lee, & Dillon, 2002). In terms of BF and BV values, cerebral perfusion assesses the increased tumor-inherent angiogenic activity and neovascularization. The hyperpermeability related to the immature vessels can also be assessed by the PS parametric maps. PS measurements need a perfusion-CT technique modification in the case of the central-volume models in order to account for the extravasation of contrast material due to the disrupted BBB. The use of DP models offers the additional advantage of measuring the extravascular blood volume as well as the first-pass extraction ratio of the tracer into the extravascular extracellular space from the intravascular space (E). A significant correlation between the v2 and E parameters with tumour growth is still not observed as it is demonstrated with the PS values. The latter provide a means

of tumor mitotic monitoring, visualization of the most malignant tumour portions, and therapy response. Apart from the patient radiation exposure during the perfusion CT imaging, a possible limitation of the method is the limited anatomic coverage. The latter results in an inadequate estimation of the tumor volume (in case of large tumors) and a possibly insufficient arterial input function since a large vessel is not in the examined slab of brain tissue. The introduction of 64-detector multislice CT units may solve the problem of anatomic coverage and provide reliable tumor perfusion measurements.

Brain-Death Diagnosis

The diagnosis of brain death must be certain to allow organ transplantation and the discontinuation of artificial ventilation. Brain death is present when all functions of the brain stem have irreversibly ceased. Clinical and electrophysiological criteria may be misinterpreted due to drug intoxication, hypothermia, or technical artefacts. Thus, if clinical assessment is suboptimal, reliable early confirmatory tests may be required for demonstrating the absence of intracranial blood flow. Cerebral angiography, MRI, CT imaging after the inhalation of stable xenon, electroencephalography, brain-perfusion SPECT measurements, and scintigraphy are possible methods for providing brain-death diagnosis in comatose patients (Bonetti, Ciritella, Valle, & Perrone, 1995, Kurtek, Lai, & Kay-Yin, 2000). Perfusion CT proved to be a reliable, safe, and cost-effective method for defining brain death in five patients in our institute. Perfusion CT was easily carried out and interpreted in the comatose patients with brain damage without discontinuing therapy. Brain death was diagnosed by recognizing the absence of brain perfusion, as shown by no intracranial arrival of the contrast material or by extremely prolonged MTT and low BF incompatible with life. The possibility of performing subsequent perfusion measurements, applying each time a new contrast-agent bolus, offers the advantage of greater anatomic coverage, although it should be considered that the used contrast material may damage the harvested organs.

REFERENCES

Axel, L. (1981). A method of calculating brain blood flow with a CT dynamic scanner. *Advanced Neurology, 30*, 67-71.

Bisdas, S., Donnerstag, F., Ahl, B., Bohrer, I., Weissenborn, K., & Becker, H. (2004). Comparison of perfusion computed tomography with diffusion-weighted magnetic resonance imaging in hyperacute ischemic stroke. *Journal of Computer Assisted Tomography, 28*, 747-755.

Bisdas, S., Nemitz, O., Berding, G., Weissenborn, K., Ahl, B., Becker, H., et al. (2006). Correlative assessment of cerebral blood flow obtained with perfusion CT and positron emission tomography in symptomatic stenotic carotid disease. *European Radiology* (in press).

Bonetti, M. G., Ciritella, P., Valle, G., & Perrone, E. (1995). 99mTc HM-PAO brain perfusion SPECT in brain death. *Neuroradiology, 37*, 365-369.

Derdeyn, C. P., Grubb, R. L., Jr., & Powers, W. J. (1999). Cerebral hemodynamic impairment: Methods of measurement and association with stroke risk. *Neurology, 53*, 251-259.

Koh, T. S., Cheong, L. H., Hou, Z., & Soh, Y. C. (2003). A physiologic model of capillary-tissue exchange for dynamic contrast enhanced imaging of tumour microcirculation. *IEEE Transactions on Biomedical Engineering, 50*, 159-167.

Kudo, K., Terae, S., Katoh, C., Oka, M., Shiga, T., Tamaki, N., et al. (2003). Quantitative cerebral flow measurement with dynamic perfusion CT using the vascular-pixel elimination method: Comparison with $H_2^{15}O$ positron emission tomography. *American Journal of Neuroradiology, 24*, 419-426.

Kurtek, R., Lai, K., & Kay-Yin, B. S. (2000). Tc-99m hexamethylpropylene amine oxime scintigraphy in the diagnosis of brain death and its implications for the harvesting of organs used for transplantation. *Clinical Nuclear Medicine, 25*, 7.

Larson, K. B., Markham, J., & Raichle, M. E. (1987). Tracer kinetic models for measuring cerebral blood flow using externally detected radiotracers. *Journal of Cerebral Blood Flow Metabolism, 7*, 443-463.

Latour, L. L., Kang, D. W., Ezzeddine, M. A., et al. (2004). Early blood-brain barrier disruption in human focal brain ischemia. *Ann Neurol, 56*, 468-477.

Lee, T. Y. (2002). Functional CT: Physiological models. *Trends Biotechnol, 20*(8), S3-S10.

Nabavi, D. G., Le Blanc, L. M., Baxter, B., et al. (2001). Monitoring cerebral perfusion after subarachnoidal hemorrhage using CT. *Neuroradiology, 43*, 7-16.

Ostergaard, L., Sorensen, A. G., Kwong, K. K., et al. (1996). High resolution measurement of cerebral blood flow using intravascular tracer bolus passages: Part I. Mathematical approach and statistical analysis. *Magn Reson Med, 36*, 715-725.

Roberts, H. C., Roberts, T. P., Lee, T. Y., & Dillon, W. P. (2002). Dynamic contrast-enhanced CT of human brain tumors: Quantitative assessment of blood volume, blood flow, and microvascular permeability-report of two cases. *American Journal of Neuroradiology, 23*, 828-832.

Von Oettingen, G., Bergholt, B., Gyldensted, C., & Astrup, J. (2002). Blood flow and ischemia within traumatic cerebral contusions. *Neurosurgery, 50*, 781-790.

KEY TERMS

Acetazolamide Test: Test to determine the inherent vasodilatatory activity of the brain vasculature. Acetazolamide, a carbonic anhydrase inhibitor, has been shown to increase cerebral perfusion in healthy subjects.

Arterial Input Function (AIF): The input arterial concentration of the contrast agent in a reference artery needed for the deconvolution process in the central-volume-based perfusion model.

Central-Volume Principle: General perfusion model that assumes an arterial input and a venous output of the injected tracer. The deconvolution of the measured parenchymal and arterial time-curve concentrations gives the mean transit time of the tracer in the vascular bed and subsequently the other perfusion parameters.

Cerebral Contusions: Bruises on the brain, usually caused by a direct, strong blow to the head.

Convolution and Deconvolution: In mathematics and in particular functional analysis, convolution is a mathematical operator that takes two functions f and g and produces a third function that in a sense represents the amount of overlap between f and a reversed and translated version of g. Deconvolution is a process used to reverse the effects of convolution on recorded data. The concept of deconvolution is widely used in the techniques of signal processing and image processing. Since these techniques are in turn widely used in many scientific and engineering disciplines, deconvolution finds many applications. In general, the object of deconvolution is to find the solution of a convolution equation of the form $f * g = h$. Usually, h is some recorded signal, and f is some signal that we wish to recover but has been convolved with some other signal g before we recorded it. The function g might represent the transfer function of an instrument or a driving force that was applied to a physical system. If we know g, or at least know the form of g, then we can perform deterministic deconvolution.

Equilibring-Indicator Model: Perfusion model that applies mainly to diffusible indicators (e.g., those used in nuclear medicine and in xenon CT) and considers a balance of the indicator concentrations between blood and cerebral tissue.

Extravascular Volume (v2): Fractional contrast-agent (tracer) distribution volume in extravasular space.

Intravascular Volume (v1): Fractional contrast-agent (tracer) distribution volume in intravascular space.

Iodinated Contrast Agent: Under normal conditions and in healthy subjects, it is a nondiffusible, iodinated non-ionic tracer whose concentration in the tissue is linearly proportional to the tissue enhancement, the X-ray attenuation, and the intensity of the CT image (expressed as Hounsfield units).

Lag Time (tlag): The delay of the peak of the tissue residue function between different brain regions.

Maximum-Slope Model: Perfusion model that considers a complete extraction of the tracer at first pass. Perfusion is proportional to the total amount of tracer accumulated in a given area as well as to the rate of accumulation (slope of the accumulation curve).

Neovascularization: A newly formed tumor may induce the formation of new capillaries and start to invade the surrounding tissue. The newly developed tumor vessels often display an abnormal architecture, characterized by collapsing or poorly differentiated fragile and leaky vessels, which are frequently unable to meet the rapid growth of tumor cells, resulting in local hypoxia and necrosis. The neovascularization of a primary tumor increases the possibility that cancer cells will enter the blood stream and spread to other organs, and is also necessary for the growth of metastases in distant organs.

Perfusion (F): A constant flow of contrast-enhanced blood that is assumed to supply the intravascular space (unit of measure is mL per 100g tissue•min).

Permeability Surface Area Product (PS): Transfer (diffusion) of the contrast agent (tracer) between the intravascular space and the extravascular extracellular space (unit of measure is mL per 100g tissue•min).

Tissue Residue Function: Function that describes the elimination of a theoretically unique and instantaneous unit bolus of contrast agent once it has entered the vascular system.

Vascular Mean Transit Time (t1): The mean time taken by the contrast (tracer) to traverse the intravascular space (units of measure are minutes and seconds).

Vasospasm: A dangerous side effect of subarachnoid hemorrhage that irritates the blood vessels on the surface of the brain, causing them to constrict erratically, cutting off blood flow.

Section X
Signal Processing Techniques

In digital signal processing, numerous powerful algorithms, both linear and nonlinear, have been developed during the past three decades. These have given rise to tremendous progress in speech and image processing. But digital signal processing is not restricted to communications and information processing. It also plays a leading role in such diverse fields as measurement, automatic control, robotics, medicine, biology, and geophysics, to mention just the more important ones. New signal-processing techniques for use in medicine are clearly presented in this section.

Chapter XLI
Nonlinear Signal Processing Techniques Applied to EEG Measurements

Christos L. Papadelis
Aristotle University of Thessaloniki, Greece

Chrysoula Kourtidou-Papadeli
Greek Aerospace Medical Association and Space Research, Greece

Panagiotis D. Bamidis
Aristotle University of Thessaloniki, Greece

Nicos Maglaveras
Aristotle University of Thessaloniki, Greece

ABSTRACT

The electrical activity of the brain is sensitive to its oxygen supply, and electroencephalography (EEG) has been proposed as a suitable measurement to detect brain activity alterations induced by hypoxia. Since, linear processing techniques that have been used so far in hypoxia studies are based on false linearity assumptions about the generation of the EEG signal, there is a definite need for nonlinear approaches to be applied on EEG data derived from hypoxic conditions. The aim of the present study is to compare nonlinear techniques' effectiveness to identify significant variations in EEG due to hypoxia. EEG data from two channels were derived from ten healthy subjects participated in the present study. Oxygen and nitrogen mixture was used to simulate hypoxic conditions that correspond to an altitude of 25.000 feet. Non-linear measurements such as correlation dimension, approximate entropy, Lyapunov exponent and detrended fluctuation analysis (DFA) parameters were estimated for EEG signals. The results of the present study confirm the effectiveness of nonlinear techniques to identify significant variations in EEG, which reflect alterations in cerebral function induced by cerebral hypoxic conditions.

INTRODUCTION

It has been well over a century since it was discovered that the mammalian brain generates a small but measurable electrical signal (Gloor, 1969). The technique of measuring this electrical activity, called electroencephalography (EEG), is a sensitive but nonspecific measure of brain function, and it is widely applicable in the clinical diagnosis of brain disorders and in brain physiological processes research. Nevertheless, in most of the applications used so far, the EEG recordings result in long traces with marked interobserver variability (Williams, Luders, Brickner, Goormastic, & Klass, 1985). The need for more specific, compact, and reliable medical information derived from EEG has been partially satisfied by quantitative EEG analysis (qEEG). This technique has been confined to feature analysis, conventional power spectrum analysis, parametric description of EEG, or frequency analysis (Geocadin et al., 2000). The theory of linear stochastic processes had led to the development of a collection of tools and techniques for the analysis of EEG. Basically, these were tools for a precise description of the deterministic and stochastic aspects of given time series, and, unfortunately, were based on very simple assumptions about the system (brain) that produced the EEG signal (linearity assumption). Although linear techniques contribute a lot in EEG applicability in clinical practice, the brain's electrical activity presents aperiodic waveforms that suggest its origin in chaotic dynamics (Galka, 2000).

One of the most important mathematical discoveries of the past few decades is that random behaviour can arise in deterministic nonlinear systems with just a few degrees of freedom. The broad spectra and aperiodic oscillations that are observed in recordings of brain activity have suggested to many researchers the possibility that this activity is generated by nonlinear dynamic systems governed by chaotic attractors (Henry, Lovell, & Camacho, 2001). The contribution of models derived from deterministic chaotic systems, such as the Lorentz, Rössler, and Chua attractors, was of fundamental importance for the development of nonlinear signal-processing techniques.

Nonlinear dynamics help us to understand that irregular and seemingly unpredictable time evolutions do not necessarily have to be a result of pure randomness, but on the contrary, can be the result of completely deterministic and fairly simple (low-dimensional) dynamical systems. Moreover, the unpredictability of these systems can be explained as their dynamics are strongly dependent on the starting condition (Lorenz, 1963). The theoretical description of this dynamic behaviour is called deterministic chaos (Signorini & Cerutti, 1999).

The essential problem in deterministic chaos is to determine whether or not a given time series is a deterministic signal from a low-dimensional dynamical system. Grassberger and Procaccia (1983) provided a simple algorithm for the estimation of the correlation dimension from time series. Since then, many scientists have presented a large number of studies reporting low dimension in EEG measurements (Babloyantz & Destexhe, 1986; Babloyantz, Salazar, & Nicolis, 1985). It has also been supported that a chaotic and rather high-dimensional EEG characterizes the healthy state of the brain, whereas a reduction of dimension and a tendency toward nonchaotic, periodic dynamics is characteristic of present or imminent pathologies (Galka, 2000). However, the reports of finite dimension in EEG recordings were and are still received with scepticism by several authors working in the field of nonlinear time-series analysis. First, it is hard to believe that a highly complex system as the brain should exhibit as little complexity as, for example, the Lorentz system (Kantz &

Schreiber, 1995). The second reason for scepticism comes from the fact that the dimension estimators that produced the finite estimates were simplified (Grassberger, 1986; Procaccia, 1988). Moreover, most of the nonlinear parametric measurements (such as correlation and information dimensions, Lyapanov exponents, etc.) are noise sensitive, and the stationarity requirement is not fulfilled.

The aim of the present study is to compare nonlinear techniques' effectiveness to identify significant variations in EEG, which reflect alterations in cerebral function induced by hypoxia. Cerebral hypoxia is caused by the failure of the human body's systems to deliver adequate oxygen to the brain (Marianai & Wright, 1998), and it is a significant clinical condition, especially in intensive-care units.

MATERIAL AND METHODS

Participants, Equipment, and Experimental Protocol

Ten healthy, drug-free people (six men, four women) participated in the study. Their ages ranged from 22 to 27 years old (mean age was 24.3). An oxygen and nitrogen mixture was used to simulate an altitude of 25 feet (10.9% oxygen and 89.1% nitrogen). Neither the participant nor the observer was aware of the gas mixture. The mixture was administered to the participants by an aviation mask (type MBU-2OP Gentex) completely sealed for any leaks; a control valve was connected to the mixture bottles for the right selection of oxygen and nitrogen content.

The Biologic-Brain Atlas III was used for the EEG recordings, connected to the ECI Electro-Cap Electrode system. Two Ag-AgCl electrodes were positioned on the scalp sites C3 and C4 according to the 10-20 international

system. The active sites on the scalp were referenced to linked mastoids. Oxygen saturation (SaO_2) was recorded with a polarographic pulse oximeter, which was placed in one of the fingers of the left hand. The target SaO_2 for the mixture was 70.

At sea level, participants performed a motor task as a warm-up. The motor task was also performed in three conditions of 100% oxygen, hypoxia (gas mixture), and recovery at 25 feet. Each session lasted 3 minutes. The participants were seated in front of a computer screen, a response keypad, and a tracking-control joystick.

During the experimental period, EEG and EOG were monitored via Ag-AgCl electrodes. The EOG electrodes were positioned above and below the left eye and at the outer canthus of both eyes. EOG signals were filtered at 1 to 13 Hz and amplified by Grass P511 amplifiers. During recording periods, qualified personnel monitored the signals on screen to ensure that any controllable artifacts from participant movements or eye blinks could be eliminated.

Artifacts Rejection

EEG recordings were first band-pass filtered (low pass was 0.5 Hz, high pass was 35 Hz), and then the Infomax independent component analysis (ICA) technique was applied in order to remove artifacts from the data, including eye movements, eye blinks, cardiac signals, and muscle noise (Jung et al., 2000). ICA decomposition was performed on EEG measurements using EEGLAB software coded in Matlab (available from http://sccn.ucsd.edu/eeglab; Delorme & Makeig, 2004). Components contaminated by artifacts were rejected, and the remaining components were mixed and projected back onto the scalp channels. A more detailed description of the method followed can be found in Jung et al.

State-Space Reconstruction

The precondition of a successful reconstruction of the state space of the underlying EEG generation process is typically required for the analysis of possible deterministic properties of a time series (Galka, 2000). For discretely sampled data, all approaches to state-space reconstruction can be regarded as variants of the central technique of time-delay embedding. It is possible to perform an analysis of the underlying process, starting from the evaluation of an observed time series $x(n)$, $(n = 1, 2, ..., N)$ of length N (Parker & Chua, 1987). According to the time-delay embedding theory, we obtain multivariate vectors in an m-dimensional space, each defined as:

$$y(n) = \{x(n), x(n+\tau),...,x(x+(m-1)\tau)\},$$
$$n = 1, N - (m-1)\tau, \tag{1}$$

where τ is an appropriate time lag and m is the embedding dimension (Abarbanel, Brown, Sidorowich, & Tsimiring, 1993).

Theoretically, any time delay τ will yield an embedding (Signorini & Cerutti, 1999). However, if we have only finite precision, both too small and too large values of τ cause failures of the reconstruction. If the time delay is small, the values $x(t)$ and $x(t + \tau)$ will be almost equal, the system did not have time to change its state significantly, and there is little gain of information between them. Due to the little gain of information between consecutive components, the impact of noise will be large (redundancy). If τ is large and the dynamical system is chaotic, the reconstruction attractor becomes a largely featureless mess since the reconstruction vectors contain components with hardly any dynamical correlation (overfolding effect).

There have been various proposals for choosing an optimal delay time for topological properties based on the behaviour of the autocorrelation function. These include the earliest time τ at which the autocorrelation drops to a fraction of its initial value (Albano, Muench, Schwartz, Mees, & Rapp, 1988) or has a point of inflection (Fraser & Swinney, 1986).

The methodology of finding an optimal embedding dimension has been provided by Sauer, Yorke, and Casdagli (1994). An embedding dimension of $m \geq 2D_o + 1$, where D_o is the box-counting dimension of the attractor, is sufficient to ensure that the reconstruction is a one-to-one embedding. In an alternative approach, if the attractor has a correlation dimension D_2, then an embedding dimension of $m \geq D_2$ is sufficient to measure the correlation dimension from the embedding. More recently, Cao (1997) proposed a method for the optimal embedding dimension that is based on the property of chaotic attractors in that their orbits should not intersect or overlap with each other. Such an intersection or overlap may result when the attractor is embedded in a dimension lower than the sufficient one stated by the delay-embedding theorem.

Correlation Dimension

The estimation of the fractal dimension for experimental data sets can be performed using the correlation-dimension parameter D_2. D_2 provides an interior bound for the fractal dimension D of the system attractor. The Grassberger-Procaccia algorithm has been proposed for the estimation of the correlation dimension (Grassberger & Procaccia, 1983). This algorithm is based on the assumption that the probability that two points of the set are in the same cell of size r is approximately equal to the probability that two points of the set are separated by a distance ρ less than or equal to r (Henry et al., 2001). Thus, the correlation dimension is approximately given by:

$$C(r) \approx \frac{\sum_{i=1,j>1}^{N} \Theta(r - \rho(\vec{x}_i, \vec{x}_j))}{\frac{1}{2} N(N-1)}, \qquad (2)$$

where the distance τ is typically measuring the Euclidian metric

$$\rho(\vec{x}_i, \vec{x}_j) = \sqrt{\sum_{k=1}^{m} (x_i(k) - x_j(k))^2}, \qquad (3)$$

and the Heaviside function is defined as

$$\Theta(s) = \begin{cases} 1 & if \quad s \geq 0 \\ 0 & if \quad s < 0 \end{cases}. \qquad (4)$$

The precise calculation of the correlation dimension is performed in the limit $N \to \infty$. However, this limit cannot be realized in practical applications. Grassberger and Procaccia (1983) propose the approximate evaluation of $C(r)$ over a range of values of r, and then deduce D_2 from the slope of the straight line of best fit in the linear scaling region of a plot of $logC(r)$ vs. $logr$.

There have been several estimates of the minimum number of data points N_{min} required for estimates of D to be reliable using the Grassberger-Procaccia algorithm. Ruelle (1990) has proposed one of them:

$$N_{min} = 10^{(D/2)}. \qquad (5)$$

Lyapunov Exponents

Lyapunov exponents (LE) describe system dynamics, giving a quantitative measure of the attractor stretching and folding mechanism (Eckmann & Ruelle, 1985). It is a quantitative measure of the sensitive dependence on the initial conditions, and it defines the average rate of divergence of two neighboring trajectories. A sufficient condition to recognize a chaotic system is the presence of at least one positive exponent (Signorini & Cerutti, 1999). A negative exponent implies that the orbits approach a common fixed point. A zero exponent means the orbits maintain their relative positions; they are on a stable attractor.

The algorithm proposed by Wolfe, Swift, Swinney, and Vastano (1985) is used to get the largest LE (LLE) estimation from EEG data. In order to calculate Lyapunov exponents from a time series, an appropriate embedding of the experimental time series has to be constructed by using the time-delay embedding methodology. The EEG time series $x(t)$ for an m-dimensional phase space with delay coordinate τ that is a point on the attractor is given by

$$\{x(t), x(t + \tau), ..., x(t + (m-1)\tau)\}. \qquad (6)$$

The nearest neighbor to the initial point should also be located:

$$\{x(t_o), x(t_o + \tau), ..., x(t_o + (m-1)\tau)\}. \qquad (7)$$

The distance between these two points is denoted as $L(t_o)$. At a later time t_1, the initial length will evolve to length $L'(t_1)$. The mean exponential divergence of two initially close orbits is characterized by:

$$\lambda = \frac{1}{t_M - t_o} \sum_{k=1}^{M} \log_2 \frac{L'(t_k)}{L'(t_{k-1})}. \qquad (8)$$

The set of numerical parameters m, τ, T, S_{max}, and S_{min} has to be chosen, where m is the embedding dimension, T is the evaluation time, and S_{max} and S_{min} are the maximum and minimum separations of the replacement point, respectively. According to Das, Das, and Roy (2002), an embedding dimension between 5 to

20 and a delay of 1 should be chosen when calculating LE for EEG data.

Approximate Entropy

Approximate entropy (ApEn) is a statistic that can be used as a measure to quantify the complexity (or irregularity) of a signal. It was first proposed by Pincus (1991a) and was then used mainly in the analysis of heart-rate variability (Huikuri, Makikallio, & Perkiomaki, 2003; Pincus, 1991b, 1994), endocrine-hormone release pulsatility (Pincus, 1996), and EEG (Burioka et al., 2005; Natarajan, Acharya, Alias, Tiboleng, & Puthusserypady, 2004).

ApEn presents salient features that make it attractive for use in biomedical signal processing. A robust estimator of ApEn can be obtained by using shorter data (in the range of 100 to 5,000 points); it is highly resistant to short transient interference, and the influence of noise can be suppressed by properly choosing the relevant parameter in the algorithm.

Two parameters m and r must be chosen prior to the computation of ApEn, where m specifies the pattern length and r is the effective filter. Assuming that the original data are $\langle x(n) \rangle = x(1), x(2), ..., x(N)$, where N is the total number of data points, the correlation integral $C^m(r)$ (with the embedding dimension m and time lag 1) should be estimated. The approximate entropy measure is finally obtained as follows:

$$ApEn(m,r,L) = \frac{1}{L-m} \sum_{i=1}^{L-m} \log C_i^{m+1}(r) - \frac{1}{L-m+1} \sum_{i=1}^{L-m+1} \log C_i^m(r).$$

$$(9)$$

The ApEn quantifies the likelihood that sets of patterns that are close remain close on the next incremental comparison. For the present study, m is set to 2 and r is set to 25% of the standard deviation of each time series.

Detrend Fluctuation Analysis

The detrend fluctuation analysis (DFA) technique (Peng, Havlin, Stanley, & Goldberger, 1995) is a modification of the root-mean-square analysis of a random walk for nonstationary data (Walleczek, 2000). DFA was proposed for the investigation of correlation properties in nonstationary time series and was applied to the studies of heartbeat (Peng, Havlin, et al.), DNA nucleotides (Peng, Buldyrev, Havlin, Simons, Stanley, & Goldberger, 1994), and EEG (Watters, 1998).

According to Hwa and Ferree (2002), the EEG time series $y(t)$ is divided into B subsets of independent segments of the same size k. Within each subset labelled b, perform a least-square fit of EEG time series $y(t)$ by a straight line $\bar{y}_b(t)$, which is the semilocal trend for the bth subset. Combine $\bar{y}_b(t)$ for all B subsets and denote the B straight segments by:

$$\bar{y}(k,t) = \sum_{b=1}^{B} \bar{y}_b(t)\theta(t-(b-1)k)\theta(bk-t)$$

$$(10)$$

for $1 \leq t \leq kB$. Define

$$F^2(k) = \frac{1}{kB} \sum_{t=1}^{kB} [y(t) - \bar{y}(k,t)]^2,$$

$$(11)$$

where $F(k)$ is the root-mean-squared fluctuation from the semilocal trends in B subsets each having k time points, and is also a measure of the fluctuation in each subset averaged over B subsets. The study of the dependence of $F(k)$ on the subset size k is the essence of DFA (Peng, Buldyrev, et al., 1994; Peng, Havlin, et al., 1995).

If there is a power-law dependence:

$$F(k) \propto k^a,$$

$$(12)$$

then the scaling exponent a is an indicator of the power-law correlations of the fluctuations in EEG (Hwa & Ferree, 2002).

Figure 1. The autocorrelation function vs. the time lags for the experimental data of the 100%-oxygen session (Participant 3, channel C3). The horizontal green line is the value of 1/e.

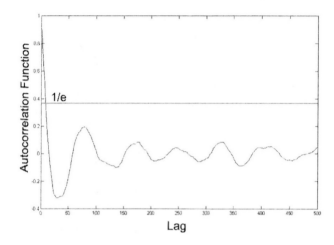

RESULTS

In order for the precondition of a successful reconstruction of the state space of the underlying EEG generation process to be satisfied, the optimal time delay τ and the optimal embedding dimension were estimated. The analysis of the optimal time delay and embedding dimension was performed for the EEG measurements of each participant and each channel for the three experimental sessions. For the optimal time-delay selection, the criterion of the earliest time τ at which the autocorrelation drops to 1/e of its initial value was used (Figure 1). Thus, the autocorrelation function analysis revealed that the optimal time delay ranged from five to nine samples. For the purpose of comparison between attractors estimated for a large number of different segments, it would not be advisable to readjust the time delay for each epoch. Thus, the fixed value of $\tau=8$ samples was used in the present study as the optimal delay time for all EEG segments. For the optimal embedding-dimension estimation, Cao's (1997) technique was used in the present study (Figure 2). From Cao's methodology, an em-

bedding dimension ranging from 4 to 7 was revealed, and a fixed embedding dimension of $d=5$ was used, which also satisfies uelle's (1990) criterion of Equation 5.

A statistically significant decrease of the mean value of the correlation dimension for all participants was observed during the hypoxia session compared to the 100%-oxygen session for both channels (Figure 3): channel C3 (p=0.0418, df=9, t=1.943) and channel C4 (p=0.029, df=9, t=2.175). No statistically significant differences were observed between the recovery session and the 100%-oxygen session, neither for channel C3 (p=0.1162, df=9, t=1.7378) nor for channel C4 (p=0.1822, df=9, t=-1.445). Analysis of variance (ANOVA) did not reveal significant differences between the three experimental sessions for both channels: channel C3 (F=1.225, df=2, p=0.309) and channel C4 (F=2.111, df=2, p=0.14).

Although, Das et al. (2002) have proposed a time delay of 1 for the LE calculation of EEG data, in the present study, a time delay of 8 has been used for the LE estimation. A decrease, but not statistically significant, of the largest Lyapunov exponent for all participants was

Figure 2. Cao's (1997) method was used for the optimal embedding-dimension estimation with a delay time of 8, a maximal dimension of 10, three nearest neighbors, and 1,000 reference points. The correlation dimension vs. embedding dimension for the experimental data of the 100%-oxygen session (Participant 3, channel C3) are presented here.

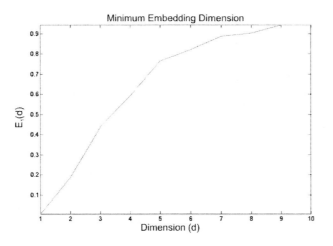

Figure 3. Mean value of D_2 correlation-dimension estimation for all participants. Although a statistically significant decrease of D_2 was observed during the hypoxia session for channel C3, an increase of the corresponding correlation dimension was observed for channel C4.

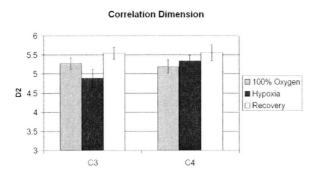

observed during the hypoxia session compared to the 100%-oxygen session for both channels—channel C3 (p=0.0668, df=9, t=-1.123) and channel C4 (p=0.0796, df=9, t=1.671)—as well as between the recovery session and the 100%-oxygen session for channel C3 (p=0.4162, df=9, t=2.7348) and for the channel C4 (p=0.4822, df=9, t=1.332). ANOVA did not

reveal significant differences between the three experimental sessions for both channels: channel C3 (F=2.225, df=2, p=0.122) and channel C4 (F=2.554, df=2, p=0.0972).

The approximate entropy was estimated for segments with 5-second duration (500 samples). The parameter m was set to 2 and r was set to 25% of the standard deviation of each time

Figure 4. Time trends of approximate entropy for electrodes C3 and C4 for all participants. The 100%-oxygen session corresponds to segments 1 to 36, the hypoxia session at a simulated altitude of 25 feet to segments 37 to 72, and the recovery session to segments 73 to 108. The red line represents a regression polynomial trend line of order 6.

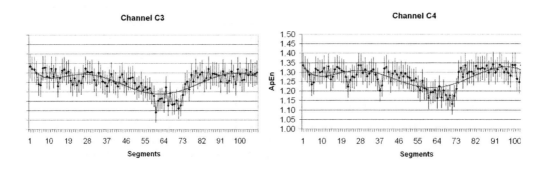

Figure 5. Mean values of approximate entropy for the experimental sessions of 100% oxygen, hypoxia, and recovery for all participants and for both EEG channels C3 and C4. A statistically significant decrease of ApEn was observed during hypoxia.

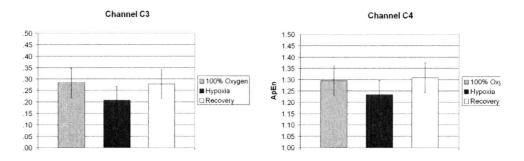

series. Time trends for the ApEn of all participants during all sessions—100% oxygen, hypoxia, and recovery—were evaluated, and the mean value and standard deviation of the ApEn for each EEG segment were calculated at 25. Time trends for electrodes C3 and C4 with the mean values of all participants are presented in Figure 4. Paired t-tests between the 100%-oxygen session and the hypoxia session revealed a statistically significant decrease of ApEn during the hypoxia session for C3 (p=0.0321, df=9, t=2.10837) and C4 (p=0.0418,

df=9, t=1.9438; Figure 5). A linear regression analysis of the ApEn time trend was performed for each experimental session and for all participants, and the slope of each trend line was estimated. ANOVA between the slopes of the three experimental conditions revealed statistically significant differences for C3 (F=5.849, df=2, p=0.007753) and for C4 (F=4.3299, df=2, p=0.0233).

For the DFA, the values of $F(k)$ were calculated for all participants and for all experimental sessions. The value of k ranged from 3 to 7. The

Figure 6. F(k) vs. k of EEG channel C3 for the mean values of the three experimental sessions

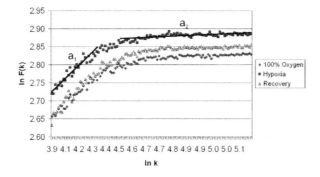

Figure 7. Scatter plot of a_2 vs. a_1 for all participants and for the three experimental sessions. The left panel corresponds to EEG channel C3 and the right one to the EEG channel C4.

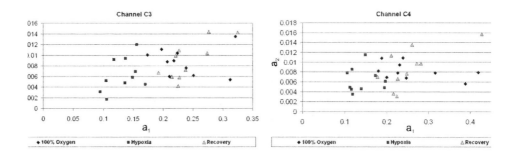

corresponding values of $F(k)$ for the channel C3 are shown in the log-log plot in Figure 6. Evidently, the striking feature is that there are two scaling regions with a discernible bend when the two slopes in the two regions are distinctly different. This feature was found in both channels for all participants. In order to quantify the scaling behaviour, we perform a linear fit in the region for $3.8 < \ln k < 4.4$ and denote the slope by a_1, and similarly for $4.5 < \ln k < 5.2$ with the slope denoted by a_2. The slopes a_1 and a_2 for all participants and for the three experimental sessions are estimated and the results of this analysis are presented in Figure 7 for both channels C3 and C4. We observed a

statistically significant decrease of the a_1 slope during the hypoxia session compared to the 100%-oxygen session for channels C3 ($p<0.001$, df=9, t=6.17) and C4 ($p=0.0017$, df=9, t=3.9363). No statistically significant differences were observed between the recovery session and the 100%-oxygen session for both channels. ANOVA of the slope a_1 between the three experimental sessions revealed statistically significant differences for both channels: for C3 (df=2, F=25.467, $p<0.001$) and for C4 (df=2, F=10.674, $p<0.001$). No statistically significant differences were observed for the slope a_2.

CONCLUSION

The results confirm the effectiveness of nonlinear techniques to identify significant variations in EEG, which reflect alterations in cerebral function induced by cerebral hypoxic conditions. Parameters measuring the dimension of the state space, like the correlation dimension and the Lyapanov exponents, confirm the presence of a low-dimensional system, even if corrupted by a large amount of noise. Statistical analysis revealed a decrease of the correlation dimension during the hypoxia session compared to the 100%-oxygen session, which returned to its initial levels in the recovery session. It is well known that the dimension of EEG time series is closely related to the cognitive activity of the brain (Bruce, 1990). The correlation dimension increases with the degree of cognitive activity. Nonlinear analysis of EEG signals during different mental tasks revealed a decrease of the correlation dimension during reflexological stimulation, indicating that the brain is not involved in cognitive tasks or thinking rigorously, meaning that the brain is in a stoic, stolid, passive state of relaxation (Natarajan et al., 2004). Moreover, a reduction of dimension and a tendency toward nonchaotic behaviour has been presented as a characteristic of present or imminent pathologies (Galka, 2000). This notion is also supported by the present study, in which hypoxia can be characterized as a pathological condition that leads to EEG correlation-dimension decrease. Although, the dimension decrease was statistically significant during hypoxia, ANOVA for D_2 and Lyapanov exponents did not reveal significant differences between the three experimental conditions. Thus, these two nonlinear measurements did not reach significance to distinguish the different experimental conditions. This could be attributed to the small number of data processed in the present study.

Dimension measurements and Lyapanov exponents require a sufficient number of data to process and considerable computation time. Moreover, these measurements are also sensitive to the influence of noise. From the statistical analysis of the present study, approximate entropy and DFA seem to overcome these difficulties. ANOVA between the slopes of the three experimental conditions for ApEn and DFA revealed the effectiveness of the scaling exponents of DFA to identify EEG variations induced by hypoxia.

We conclude that the parameters arisen from nonlinear signal-processing techniques and obtained from the EEG measurements may be effectively employed for the advanced monitoring of cerebral function. The statistical analysis also suggests that complexity measurements such as approximate entropy and detrend fluctuation analysis present the highest effectiveness to identify EEG variations induced by hypoxia.

REFERENCES

Abarbanel, H. D. I., Brown, R., Sidorowich, J. J., & Tsimiring, L. S. (1993). The analysis of observed chaotic data in physical systems. *Reveiws Modern Physics, 65*, 1331-1392.

Albano, A. M., Muench, J., Schwartz, C., Mees, A. I., & Rapp, P. E. (1988). Singular-value decomposition and the Grassberger-Procaccia algorithm. *Physical Review A., 38*, 3017.

Babloyantz, A., & Destexhe, A. (1986). Low-dimensional chaos in an instance of epilepsy. *Proceedings of the National Academy of the Scinces, 83*, 3513-3517.

Babloyantz, A., Salazar, J. M., & Nicolis, C. (1985). Evidence of chaotic dynamics of brain activity during the sleep cycle. *Physical Letters A, 111*, 152-156.

Bruce, J. W. (1990). *Fractal physiology and chaos in medicine.* London: World Scientific Press.

Burioka, N., Miyata, M., Cornelissen, G., Halberg, F., Takeshima, T., Kaplan, D. T., et al. (2005). Approximate entropy in the electroencephalogram during wake and sleep. *Clinical EEG and Neuroscience, 36*(1), 21-24.

Cao, L. (1997). Practical method for determining the minimum embedding dimension of a scalar time series. *Physica D, 120*, 43-50.

Das, A., Das, P., & Roy, A. B. (2002). Applicability of Lyapunov exponents in EEG data analysis. *Complexity International, 9*, 1-20.

Delorme, A., & Makeig, S. (2004). EEGLAB: An open source toolbox for analysis of single-trial EEG dynamics including independent component analysis. *Journal of Neuroscience Methods, 134*, 9-21.

Eckmann, J. P., & Ruelle, D. (1985). Ergodic theory of chaos and strange attractors. *Reviews of Modern Physics, 57*, 617-656.

Fraser, A. M., & Swinney, H. (1986). Independent coordinates for strange attractors from mutual information. *Physical Review A., 33*, 1134-1139.

Galka, A. (2000). *Topics in nonlinear time series analysis: With implications for EEG analysis.* London: World Scientific Press.

Geocadin, R., Ghodadra, R., Kimura, K., Lei, H., Sherman, D., Hanley, D., et al. (2000). A novel quantitative EEG injury measure of global cerebral ischemia. *Journal of Clinical Neurophysiology, 111*, 1779-1787.

Gloor, P. (1969). Hans Berger on the electroencephalogram of man. *Electroencephalography and Clinical Neurophysiology, 28*, 1-36

Grassberger, P. (1986). Do climatic attractors exist? *Nature, 323*, 609-612.

Grassberger, P., & Procaccia, I. (1983). Characterization of strange attractors. *Physical Review Letters, 50*, 346-349.

Henry, B., Lovell, N., & Camacho, F. (2001). Nonlinear dynamics time series analysis. In M. Akay (Ed.), *Nonlinear biomedical signal processing: Vol. 2. Dynamic analysis and modelling* (pp. 71-78). Upper Saddle River, NJ: John Wiley and Sons.

Huikuri, H. V., Makikallio, T. H., & Perkiomaki, J. (2003). Measurement of heart rate variability by methods based on nonlinear dynamics. *Journal of Electrocardiology, 36*(1), 95-99.

Hwa, R. C., & Ferree, T. C. (2002). Fluctuation analysis of human electroencephalography. *Nonlinear Phenomena in Complex Systems, 5*(3), 302-307.

Jung, T. P., Makeig, S., Humphries, C., Lee, T. W., Mckeown, M. J., Iraqui, V., et al. (2000). Removing electroencephalographic artifacts by blind source separation. *Psychophysiology, 37*, 163-178.

Kantz, H., & Schreiber, T. (1995). Dimension estimates and physiological data. *Chaos, 5*, 143-154.

Lorenz, E. N. (1963). Deterministic non-periodic flow. *Journal of Atmospheric Science, 20*, 130-141.

Marianai, J. J., & Wright, L. A. (1998). Acute respiratory failure. In G. L. Baum et al. (Eds.), *Textbook of pulmonary diseases* (6th ed., Vol. 1, pp. 919-940). Philadelphia: Lippincott-Raven.

Natarajan, K., Acharya, U. R., Alias, F., Tiboleng, T., & Puthusserypady, S. K. (2004). Nonlinear analysis of EEG signals at different mental states. *Biomedical Engineering Online, 3*(1), 7.

Parker, T. S., & Chua, L. O. (1987). Chaos: A tutorial for engineers. *Proceedings of IEEE, 75*(8), 982-1008.

Peng, C. K., Buldyrev, S. V., Havlin, S., Simons, M., Stanley, H. E., & Goldberger, A. L. (1994). Mosaic organization of DNA nucleotides. *Physical Review E, 49*, 1685-1689.

Peng, C. K., Havlin, S., Stanley, H. E., & Goldberger, A. L. (1995). Quantification of scaling exponents and crossover phenomena in nonstationary heartbeat time series. *Chaos, 5*, 82-87.

Pincus, S. M. (1991a). Approximate entropy as a measure of system complexity. *Proceedings of the National Academy of Sciences of the United States of America, 88*, 2297-2301.

Pincus, S. M. (1991b). Heart rate control in normal and aborted-SIDS infants. *American Journal of Physiology, 33*, R638-R646.

Pincus, S. M. (1994). Quantification of evolution from order randomness in practical times series analysis. *Methods in Enzymology, 240*, 68-89.

Pincus, S. M. (1996). Older males secrete luteinizing hormone and testosterone more irregularly and joint more asynchronously, than younger males. *Proceedings of the National Academy of Sciences of the United States of America, 93*, 14100-14105.

Procaccia, I. (1988). Complex or just complicated? *Nature, 333*, 498-499.

Ruelle, D. (1990). Deterministic chaos: The science and the fiction. *Proceedings of the National Academy of the Sciences, 427*, 241-248.

Sauer, T., Yorke, J., & Casdagli, M. (1994). Embedology. *Journal of Statistical Physics, 65*, 579-616.

Signorini, M. G., & Cerutti, S. (1999). Nonlinear properties of cardiovascular time series. In M. Di Rienzo, G. Mancia, G. Parati, A. Pedotti, & A. Zanchetti (Eds.), *Methodology and clinical applications of blood pressure and heart rate analysis* (pp. 282-287). Amsterdam: IOS Press.

Walleczek, J. (Ed.). (2000). Fractal mechanisms in neuronal control: Human heartbeat and gait dynamics in health and disease. In *Self-organized biological dynamics and nonlinear control* (pp. 66-96). Cambridge, UK: Cambridge University Press.

Watters, P. A. (1998). Fractal structure in the electroencephalogram. *Complexity International, 5*. Retrieved from http://www.complexity.org.au/ci/vol05/watters/watters.html

Williams, G. W., Luders, H. O., Brickner, A., Goormastic, M., & Klass, D. W. (1985). Interobserver variability in EEG interpretation. *Neurology, 35*, 1714-1719.

Wolfe, A., Swift, J. B., Swinney, H. L., & Vastano, J. A. (1985). Determining Lyapunov exponents from a time series. *Physica D, 16*, 285-317.

KEY TERMS

Electroencephalography (EEG): The recording of electric currents created in the brain by using electrodes placed on the scalp or surface of the brain.

Cerebral Hypoxia: The pathological condition that is caused by the failure of the human body's systems to deliver adequate oxygen to the brain.

Dynamical System: Any system that evolves over time. Dynamical systems whose behaviour changes continuously over time are mathematically described by a coupled set of first-order autonomous, ordinary differential equations.

Entropy: The degree of randomness or disorder in a system.

Fractal Dimension: It is any dimension measurement that allows noninteger values.

Nonlinear: A property of a system whose output is not proportional to its input. It behaves in an erratic and unpredictable fashion and is unstable.

Phase Space: An abstract mathematical space spanned by the dynamical variables of a system.

Section XI
Use of New Technologies in Biomedicine

Medical technology is a science discipline that has been rapidly growing over the last decades. It is characterized by a constant flow of innovations and a high level of research and development. Many technological achievements have changed dramatically the way that medicine diagnoses and treats human disease. Improved healthcare technology has presented many revolutionary medical devices that reduced mortality and morbidity. New various technologies applied in biomedicine are presented in this section.

Chapter XLII
Medical and Biomedical Devices for Clinical Use

Evangelos K. Doumouchtsis
National and Kapodistrian University of Athens, Greece

ABSTRACT

Medical technology has been rapidly growing over the last decades. It is characterized by a constant flow of innovations and a high level of research and development. Many medical and biomedical devices have changed dramatically the way that medicine diagnoses and treats human disease, such as getting three-dimensional images of the internal human body. This chapter describes medical and biomedical devices, the regulatory framework about them, as well as the most active areas of research of medical technology. It also discusses the future trends of the medical industry and biosciences that constantly provide new possibilities of improving health care and patient quality of life.

INTRODUCTION

Medical technology is a science discipline that has been rapidly growing over the last decades. It is characterized by a constant flow of innovations and a high level of research and development. Many technological achievements have changed dramatically the way that medicine diagnoses and treats human disease. For example, the invention of computed tomography (CT), a noninvasive diagnostic technique, allowed clinicians to get three-dimensional images of the inside of the human body, and thus they can detect early many diseases that were

impossible to detect before. Improved healthcare technology has presented many revolutionary medical devices that have reduced mortality and morbidity.

Medical devices range from simple ones like first-aid bandages to more sophisticated ones like positron-emission tomography (PET) scanners. Their main purpose is to improve the health status of patients and to support the prevention, diagnosis, and treatment of disease.

There are thousands of medical and biomedical devices, and this number is rapidly increasing. Therefore, a regulatory framework is essential to ensure the safety and efficiency of the medical devices. In Europe, three directives have been applied by the European Commission in order to provide the guidelines for the development of new medical devices. These are the 93/42/EE directive on medical devices (MDD), the 90/385/EEC directive on active implantable medical devices (AIMDD), and the 98/79/EC in vitro diagnostic medical-device directive (IVDMDD).

SOME EXAMPLES OF MEDICAL DEVICES

The 93/42/EEC directive defines a medical device as:

[a]ny instrument, apparatus, appliance, material or other article, whether used alone or in combination, including the software necessary for its proper application intended by the manufacturer to be used on human beings for the purpose of:

- *diagnosis, prevention, monitoring, treatment or alleviation of disease,*
- *diagnosis, monitoring, treatment, alleviation or compensation for an injury or handicap,*
- *investigation, replacement or modification of the anatomy or of a physiological process,*
- *control of conception,*

and which does not achieve its principal intended action in or on the human body by pharmacological, immunological or metabolic means, but which may be assisted in its function by such means.

According to the Global Medical Devices Nomenclature (GMDN), the product range includes the following categories:

- Aids for disabled persons, for example, wheelchairs, crutches, standing supports, electrical beds, hearing aids, and stoma appliances
- Active and nonactive implantable devices, for example, stents, cardiac pacemakers, hip implants, neurostimulators, and insulin pumps
- Anaesthetic or respiratory equipment, for example, oxygen masks, anaesthesia breathing circuits, and gas delivery units
- Orthopaedic devices, for example, knee prostheses, orthopaedic shoes, and spinal corsets
- Dental devices, for example, dentistry tools and drills, alloys and resins, dental floss, and toothbrushes
- Electromedical and imaging equipment, for example, x-ray machines, scanners, electrocardiographs, monitors, lasers, and microscopes
- In vitro diagnostics, for example, devices for clinical chemistry, microbiology, immunology, and genetic tests
- Ophthalmic devices, for example, contact lenses, optometers, optical lenses, eye glasses, and ophthalmoscopes
- Surgical instruments, for example, scalpels, surgical drills, forceps, tubes, drains, sutures, and masks
- Biotechnological products, for example, tissue-engineered bones, cartilage, and skin
- medical disposables, for example, bandages, dressing, and syringes

An active implantable medical device (AIMD) according to the 90/385/EEC directive is a medical device as defined above that is at the same time both active and implantable.

A medical device is active if it "relies for its functioning on a source of electrical energy or any source of power other than that directly generated by the human body or gravity." This includes, for instance, devices activated by means of pressure, unless this effect is achieved by energy resulting from the body of the patient. The definition implies that the function of the device involves using a source of power to perform useful work. The mere transmission of heat, light, pressure, or vibration does not mean that a device is active.

An active medical device is defined as implantable if it is "totally or partly introduced, surgically or medically, into the human body or by medical intervention into a natural orifice, and which is intended to remain after the procedure."

Examples of AIMDs are as follows:

- Implantable pulse generator for pacing including an electrode
- Implantable pulse generator without an electrode
- An electrode
- Implantable drug-administration device with or without a catheter
- Catheter for implantable drug-administration device

An in vitro diagnostic medical device is any medical device that is a reagent, reagent product, calibrator, control material, kit, instrument, apparatus, piece of equipment, or system, whether used alone or in combination, intended by the manufacturer to be used in vitro for the examination of specimens, including blood and tissue donations derived from the human body, solely or principally for the purpose of providing information related to the following:

- Concerning a physiological or pathological state
- Concerning a congenital abnormality
- To determine the safety and compatibility with potential recipients
- To monitor therapeutic measures (98/79/EC)

AREAS OF MEDICAL DEVICES: NEW TECHNOLOGIES

The most active areas of medical-device research are given in the following sections.

Diagnostic Imaging

Diagnostic imaging systems such as x-ray and ultrasound have been in use for decades; other systems, including computed tomography, magnetic resonance imaging (MRI), and nuclear or positron-emission tomography, are newer technologies. Recently, a revolutionary four-dimensional CT scanner was developed, and it brings new possibilities to diagnosis and treatment. Three-dimensional technology only provides a static image at one instance in time. However, when dealing with parts of the body that move, such as the abdomen, pelvis, or chest, there is the need for a technology that accounts for time as well. This scanner adds the fourth dimension of time, allowing clinicians to track moving organs almost in real time and, for example, to treat tumors by radiation therapy more precisely while limiting the exposure of healthy tissue to radiation (Fontanazza, 2004).

Cardiology

Cardiovascular disease is a major cause of death across Europe and the USA. Intervention cardiology, such as coronary angiography, coronary stents, arrhythmia, and stroke management, provides an example of the contribution of medical technology to patient care. There has been a continuous trend of innovation in these areas. Advanced techniques, such as cardiac rhythm management (CRM), help to avoid complications and improve the quality of life for patients.

CRM consists of the following three key areas:

- Pacing systems
- Implantable cardiac defibrillators (ICDs)
- Automatic external defibrillators (AEDs)

Pacing systems consist of pacemakers and programmers that are needed to monitor and correct slow heart rhythms. The following pacing-system components work together to relieve symptoms of bradycardia (slow heart rate).

- **Pacemaker:** Implantable device that electrically stimulates the heart to pump blood. It contains an electronic circuit and a battery.
- **Pacing Lead:** An insulated wire that carries a tiny electrical pulse to the heart to initiate heartbeat.
- **Programmer:** Monitors the pacemaker. It is usually kept in the hospital or a clinic.

Implantable Cardiac Defibrillators (ICDs) are a new technology introduced in 2004 (MDDI, 2004). They are similar to pacing systems in that they continuously monitor the heart's rhythm. Specifically, ICDs treat tachyarrhythmia (fast heart beat). If the heart beats too quickly, the ICD issues a lifesaving jolt of electricity to restore the heart's normal rhythm and prevent sudden cardiac death. Like pacing systems, ICDs have similar components, including a defibrillator, lead, and a programmer.

An AED is used to jump-start a heart that has failed due to a heart attack or cardiac arrest. Designed so that even nonexperts can operate them without much difficulty, AEDs are rapidly gaining popularity. They can even be found in public places such as airports, train stations, and airplanes (Altera, http://www.altera.com).

In 2004, the industry provided many other new devices that offer improved clinical utility in cardiology. Drug-eluting coronary stents are one of the most significant technologies of the year. A number of studies showed that drug-

eluting stents may be beneficial to certain high-risk patients (MDDI, 2004).

One trend driving growth in the device industry is the ability to give patients more control over their own healthcare. The FDA (Food and Drug Administration) approved over-the-counter sales of a home defibrillator (Swain, 2005). Another device for home use is a recently developed biosensor that monitors a couple's vital signs as they sleep, notifying one person when it detects abnormal signs in the other (Engel & Cook, 2005).

Endocrinology

Endocrinology is another important area in which medical devices play a vital role in patient care. Devices for diabetes treatment, for example, include insulin-delivery products such as syringes, pens, automatic injectors, insulin patches, and external or implantable pumps. Precise blood glucose monitoring can substantially reduce the risk of developing complications and slow the progression of the disease. Many diabetic patients also rely on sophisticated dialysis equipment (Eucomed Medical Technology, 2004).

A characteristic example is monitoring glucose levels in blood to regulate an infusion of insulin. The FDA approved a hybrid device that included a wireless link between an insulin pump and a blood glucose monitor (Wilson, 2004). This, in combination with an insulin dosing controller, could be described as an artificial pancreas.

Electromedical Devices

The electromedical segment comprises the following three key areas:

- Patient monitoring
- Ventilation and life support
- Anesthesia

Patient-monitoring equipment capture and analyze a patient's vital information for clinical decision makers. Advances in patient monitoring include new form factors that facilitate patient transport.

Ventilation and life support is another important area in the medical sector. These equipment primarily consist of ventilators and drug-delivery systems. These are very tightly integrated with the central monitoring system.

Anaesthesia is a life-critical application that needs the utmost human attention, especially while delivering it to the patient. Technology plays a key role in anaesthesia-delivery equipment by delivering the precise dosage to the patient (Altera, http://www.altera.com).

Life-Science and Hospital Equipment

Life-science and hospital equipment such as spectrometers, centrifuges, protein analyzers, powered beds, surgical instruments, radiation equipment, and endoscopes are some examples of medical devices that are used in healthcare.

Wireless Technologies

Many new medical devices use more and more wireless technologies, such as Bluetooth. Several device manufacturers have already implemented Bluetooth technologies and received FDA approval. Some examples are a wireless defibrillator and monitor that allows the transmittal of vital-sign reports to a PDA (personal digital assistant), a pulse oximeter that offers patient mobility within 10 meters of the monitoring device, and a wireless device that is used for monitoring patient weight and blood pressure in the home while data is transmitted to a home gateway for remote retrieval and review. All these technologies provide amazing possibilities for improving healthcare and patient quality of life (Albrecht, 2004).

THE FUTURE OF MEDICAL DEVICES

The field of research on medical technology constantly expands. There are already hundreds of revolutionary medical devices under development. Some examples of the medical devices of the future, expected to open new horizons to medicine, are listed as follows:

- Neurostimulation devices
- Nanoscale biosensors
- Tissue-engineered components
- Less invasive hip replacements
- Advanced biomaterials
- Ultrahigh-resolution imaging systems
- Drug-device hybrids
- Biosensors
- Nanodevices
- Virtual reality
- Biorobotics
- Brain-machine interfaces
- The computerization of medicine (Bronzino, 2004)

CONCLUSION

Devices of the future will incorporate information technology, nanotechnology, and biosciences. In the near future, a convergence between engineering and biology is expected. Medical technology should develop new skills in molecular and cell biology in order to correspond to the demands of medical science. As industry trends move toward smaller, lower power, sensor-driven devices, new sciences such as protein-based therapies present new targets and new opportunities (Conroy, 2005).

REFERENCES

Albrecht, M. (2004). *Bluetooth and medical devices*. Breakthrough Technologies, LLC. Retrieved from http://www.breaktech.com/content.php?article.60

Bronzino, J. (2004). *The medical device industry in Southern New England's I-91 corridor: Potential for growth and the role of Beacon*. Retrieved from http://www.cbia.com/business/Presentations/2004/Sept/bronzio%20presentation.ppt

Conroy, S. (2005). Devices of the future must incorporate nanotech and biotech. *Medical Device & Diagnostic Industry, 32.* Retrieved from http://www.devicelink.com/mddi/archive/05/01/028.html

Directive 98/79/EC of the European Parliament and of the Council on *in vitro* diagnostic medical devices: L 331/5. (1998). *Official Journal of the European Communities, 331,* 5.

Dorland's pocket medical dictionary. (1998). W. B. Saunders Company.

Engel, D., & Cook, C. (2005). Biosensor platform offers real-time monitoring of vital signs. *European Medical Device Manufacturer.* Retrieved from http://www.devicelink.com/emdm/archive/05/01/002.html

Eucomed Medical Technology. (2004). *Medical technology brief.* Retrieved from http://www.eucomed.be/docs/Brief%202004%20Final.pdf

European Commission DG Enterprise Directorate G. (1994). *Unit 4: Pressure equipment, medical devices, metrology. Guidelines relating to the application of the council directive 90/385/EEC on active implantable medical devices: The council directive 93/42/EEC on medical devices.*

Fontanazza, M. (2004). Imaging technology moves to the fourth dimension. *Medical Device & Diagnostic Industry, 26.* Retrieved from http://www.devicelink.com/mddi/archive/04/12/010.html

IBM. (n.d.). *Medical technology equipment modality definitions/glossary.* Retrieved from http://www-1.ibm.com/financing/pdf/us/igf4-a042.pdf

MDDI. (2004). Focus on technology: Providing improved utility at reduced costs. *Medical Device & Diagnostic Industry.* Retrieved from http://www.devicelink.com/mddi/archive/04/12/016.html

Swain, E. (2005). Making news in 2004. *Medical Device & Diagnostic Industry, 63.* Retrieved from http://www.devicelink.com/mddi/archive/05/02/004.html

Wilson, D. (2004). *MedEdge 2004: Convergence of life sciences and medical devices.* Breakthrough Technologies, LLC. Retrieved from http://www.breaktech.com/content.php?article.63

KEY TERMS

Computerized Tomography: A CT scan is an x-ray procedure that is enhanced by a computer. This results in a three-dimensional view (referred to as a slice) of a particular part of the body. Typical applications include viewing the chest, abdomen, and spinal cord.

Coronary Stent: A coronary stent is an artificial support device that is inserted in the coronary artery to keep the vessel open.

Defibrillator: An electronic apparatus used to counteract atrial or ventricular fibrillation by the application of a brief electroshock to the heart, either directly or through electrodes placed on the chest wall.

MRI Scanner: Magnetic resonance imaging is an imaging technique used primarily in medical settings to produce high-quality images of the inside of the human body. MRI produces images that are the visual equivalent of a slice of the anatomy, and it is also capable of producing those images in an infinite number of projections through the body. To produce its images, MRI uses radio frequencies, a computer, and a large magnet that surrounds the patient.

PET Scanner: PET stands for positron-emission tomography and is a method of body scanning that detects radioactive compounds that have been injected into the body to provide information on function rather than structure, and to help differentiate normal tissue from cancer.

Pulse Oximeter: An oximeter that measures the oxygen saturation of arterial blood by passing a beam of red and infrared light through a pulsating capillary bed, the ratio of red to infrared transmission varying with the oxygen saturation of the blood; because it responds only to pulsatile objects, it does not detect nonpulsating objects like skin and venous blood.

Chapter XLIII
Artificial Intelligence in Medicine and Biomedicine

Athanasios Zekios
National and Kapodistrian University of Athens, Greece

Dimitra Petroudi
National and Kapodistrian University of Athens, Greece

ABSTRACT

Man has always strived to augment his abilities by inventing tools. Artificial intelligence in medicine (AIM), has taken up the challenge of creating and distributing advanced tools, utilising technical developments aimed at augmenting man's reasoning. Increasing quality healthcare needs and advances in medical and pharmaceutical sciences, yet restrictions on physicians' time for learning while practicing, indicate these tools will prove invaluable in effecting changes (i.e. Simpler organising, storing, and retrieving of important medical facts/ new findings) especially when treating difficult cases; continual availability of same for learning purposes; assisting with appropriate diagnostic, prognostic and therapeutic decisions/ decision making techniques, using databases, flowcharts and decision theory. Proof of these tools' indispensability through actual trials, is pending.

INTRODUCTION

Men and women strive to augment their abilities by building tools. From the invention of the club to lengthen their reach and strengthen their blows to the refinement of the electron microscope to sharpen their vision, tools have extended humans' ability to sense and to manipulate the world about them. Today we stand on the threshold of new technical developments that will augment people's reasoning; the computer and the programming methods being devised for this are the new tools to effect this change.

Medicine and biomedicine are fields in which the help of such tools is critically needed. Our increasing expectations of the highest quality healthcare and the rapid growth of ever more detailed medical knowledge leave the physician without adequate time to devote to each case and struggling to keep up with the newest developments in the field. There is also another huge problem. Continued training and recertification procedures encourage the physician to keep more of the relevant information constantly in mind, but fundamental limitations of human memory and recall coupled with the growth of knowledge assure that most of what is known cannot be known by most individuals. Currently, there is the opportunity for new computer tools to help organize, store, and retrieve appropriate medical knowledge needed by the practitioner in dealing with each difficult case, and to suggest appropriate diagnostic, prognostic, and therapeutic decisions and decision-making techniques.

A field that is now taking up the challenge of creating and distributing the tools mentioned above is artificial intelligence in medicine (AIM).

ARTIFICIAL INTELLIGENCE

What is artificial intelligence in medicine? One introductory textbook defines artificial intelligence this way: "Artificial Intelligence is the study of ideas which enable computers to do the things that make people seem intelligent. The central goals of Artificial Intelligence are to make computers more useful and to understand the principles which make intelligence possible." This is a rather straightforward definition, but it embodies certain assumptions about the idea of intelligence and the relationship between human reasoning and computation, which are, in some circles, quite controversial.

Historically, researchers in AI have had to defend this linkage against humanist attacks on the reduction of the human intellect to computational steps. The debate has sometimes been heated, as exemplified by the following quote

from the introduction to an early collection of AI papers.

Is it Possible for Computing Machines to Think?

If one defines thinking as an activity peculiarly and exclusively human then the answer is no. Any such behaviour in machines, therefore, would have to be called thinking-like behaviour. If someone postulates that there is something in the essence of thinking which is inscrutable, mysterious, and mystical then the answer is again no. But it the opposite answer if one admits that the question is to be answered by experiment and observation, comparing the behaviour of the computer with that behaviour of human beings to which the term "thinking" is generally applied.

ARTIFICIAL INTELLIGENCE IN MEDICINE

AIM is AI specialized to medical applications. Researchers in AIM need not engage in the controversy introduced above. Although we employ humanlike reasoning methods in the programs we write, we may justify that choice either as a commitment to a human-computer equivalence sought by some or as a good engineering technique for capturing the best-understood source of existing expertise on medicine: the practice of human experts. Most researchers adopt the latter view.

Another currently much smaller use of computers in medicine is their application to the substance rather than the form of healthcare. If the computer is a useful manager of billing records, it should also maintain medical records, laboratory data, data from clinical trials, and so forth. And if the computer is useful to store data, it should also help to analyze, organize, and retrieve it. Three main approaches to this second type of medical computing have so far been used.

Flowcharts

A flowchart is conceptually the simplest decision-making tool. It encodes, in principle, the sequences of actions a good clinician would perform for any one of some population of patients.

Databases

Large databases of clinical histories of patients sharing a common presentation or disease are now being collected in several fields. The growth of data capture and storage facilities and their co-occurring decline in cost make attractive the accumulation of enormous numbers of cases, both for research and clinical uses.

Decision Theory

Decision theory is a mathematical theory of decision making under uncertainty. It assumes that one can quantify the a priori and conditional likelihoods of existing states and their manifestations, and can similarly determine an evaluation (utility) of all contemplated outcomes.

SYSTEMS REFER TO AIM

The Present Illness Program (PIP) is able to infer that if a patient passed a military physical or a life-insurance company's health examination, then neither blood, sugar, nor protein was present at that time in the urine. This is a widely known heuristic among physicians, being one of the many ways that past data can be inferred in the absence of definitive reports.

The CASNET system, developed at Rutgers University, in its major incarnation is a diagnos-

tic and therapeutic program for glaucoma and related diseases of the eye that describes EXPERT, a somewhat simpler and more widely applied system that is being used in the analysis of thyroid disorders and in rheumatology. CASNET identified the fundamental issue of causality as essential in the diagnostic and therapeutic process.

The MYCIN system was developed at Stanford University originally for the diagnosis and treatment of bacterial infections of the blood and later extended to handle other infectious diseases as well. The fundamental insight of the MYCIN investigators was that the complex behaviour of a program, which might require a flowchart of hundreds of pages to implement as a clinical algorithm, could be reproduced by a few hundred concise rules and a simple recursive algorithm (described in a one-page flowchart) to apply each rule just when it promised to yield information needed by another rule.

INTERNIST-I uses a problem-formulation heuristic to select from among all its known diseases the set that should be considered as competing explanations of the currently known abnormal findings in a case. A distinction is made between the tasks of formulating such a differential problem and of solving it. Formulating the problem is what might be called an ill-structured task, similar to the problem of making up an interesting mathematical theorem or designing a house; solving the differentiation problem once formulated is well structured, inviting the application of numerous conventional methods. The simple heuristic of INTERNIST-1 is seen to do well in many complex cases, but falters in cases requiring an analysis from several different viewpoints, for example, an interaction between the causal mechanism of the disease and the organ systems involved in it. Based on such deficiencies, a new, extended method of medical knowledge representation and problem formulation is presented that is intended to form the basis for CADU-CEUS, the second-generation follow-up to IN-TERNIST-1.

PROBLEMS

The significant questions facing the field of artificial intelligence in medicine are "Who is an appropriate user of a healthcare-related computer application?" and "How and when should computers be used in clinical practice?"

Perhaps one of the more difficult questions to answer is "Who should use a healthcare-related computer application?" One of the early papers on ethical issues in informatics reported that the potential users of informatics systems included physicians, nurses, physicians' assistants, paramedical personnel, students of the health sciences, patients, and insurance and government evaluators. As discussed among the major groups of people involved in medical-informatics ethics, other groups that should be included are nurse practitioners, pharmacists, managers, administrators, scientists, researchers, applied computer professionals, other ancillary healthcare personnel, and patients and their employers.

Trying to determine who should be allowed to use a healthcare-related computer application will be an ethical challenge, one that is already under way. Use by physicians in practice, and medical and nursing students seems plausible. However, before using a diagnostic decision-support system, the user must be able to recognize when there is an error and when it is providing accurate information.

The key problems encountered when using clinical computer programs to determine policy or aid in practice are the following.:

1. Human cognition is still superior to machine intelligence.
2. Decisions about whether to treat a given patient are often value laden and must be made relative to treatment goals.
3. Applying computational operations on aggregate data to individual patients runs the risk of including individuals in groups they resemble but to which they do not actually belong.

In regard to the last problem, clinicians run the risk of including individuals in the wrong groups all the time. It is a long-standing logic challenge, trying to infer correctly that an individual belongs in a particular set, group, or class. Computers have not been able to solve this problem, yet.

FUTURE OF ARTIFICIAL INTELLIGENCE IN MEDICINE

The field of artificial intelligence in medicine has been slow to make its mark on medicine; however, this may soon change. With the emphasis in medicine shifting to more evidence-based practice, the increasing reliance on computers, the increasing volume of information for clinicians to assimilate, and the many pressures to practice medicine more efficiently, those in the field of AIM may find themselves thrust into the forefront of medicine as they will be providing computer-based solutions for this ever-changing field.

POTENTIAL OF ARTIFICIAL INTELLIGENCE IN MEDICINE

The potential of AI in medicine has been expressed by a number of researchers. The potential of AI techniques in medicine are as follows: (a) They provide a laboratory for the examination, organization, representation, and cataloguing of medical knowledge, (b) produce new tools to support medical decision making, training, and research, (c) integrate activities in medical, computer, cognitive, and other sciences, and d) offer a content-rich discipline for future scientific medical specialties.

CONCLUSION

We must realize that although current AIM programs already give quite impressive demonstrations of the success of the techniques used and of the dedication of the investigators, none of the programs reported on here or developed by other similar efforts is in current clinical use. Perhaps, as it has been argued, programs will only be clinically accepted once their indispensability is established, and only when successful demonstrations exist that physicians or other medical personnel working with such programs are more successful than those working without them. Alternatively, social and administrative mechanisms may be more responsible for the ultimate utilization or abandonment of these tools.

REFERENCES

Bleich, H. L. (1972). Computer-based consultation: Electrolyte and acid-base disorders. *Amer. J. Med., 53,* 285.

Coiera, E. W. (1996). Artificial intelligence in medicine: The challenges ahead. *J Am Med Inform Assoc, 3,* 363-366.

Doyle, J. (1978). A truth maintenance system. *Artificial Intelligence, 12,* 231-272.

Gorry, G. A., Silverman, H., & Pauker, S. G. (1978). Capturing clinical expertise: A computer program that considers clinical responses to digitalis. *Amer. J Med, 64,* 452-460.

Morris, A. H. (2000). Developing and implementing computerized protocols for standardization of clinical decisions. *Ann Intern Med., 132,* 373-383.

Pauker, S. G., Gorry, G. A., Kassirer, J. P., & Schwartz, W. B. (1976). Toward the simulation of clinical cognition: Taking a present illness by computer. *Amer. J Med, 60,* 981-995.

Schwartz, W. B. (1970). Medicine and the computer: The promise and problems of change. *New Engl. J. Med., 283,* 1257-1264.

Shortliffe, E. H., et al. (1979). Knowledge engineering for medical decision making: A review of computer-based clinical decision aids. *Proceedings of the IEEE, 67*(9), 1207-1224.

Slack, W. V., & Van Cura, L. J. (1968). Patient reaction to computer-based medical interviewing. *Comput. Biomed Res, 1,* 527-531.

Szolovits, P., & Pauker, S. G. (1978). Categorical and probabilistic reasoning in medical diagnosis. *Artificial Intelligence, 11,* 115-144.

Szolovits, P., & Pauker, S. G. (1979). Computers and clinical decision making: Whether, how, and for whom? *Proceedings of the IEEE, 67*(9), 1224-1226.

Tautu, P., & Wagner. G. (1978). The process of medical diagnosis: Routes of mathematical investigations. *Meth, Inform. Med., 7*(1).

URL REFERENCES

http://compubiosys.medsch.ucla.edu/AI/

http://www.abcnews.go.com/ABC2000/abc2000tech/geek38.html

http://www.coiera.com/ailist/list.html

http://www.coiera.com/aimd.html

http://www.cs.washington.edu/research/jair/home.html

http://www.csd.abdn.ac.uk/research/ai_in_medicine.html

http://www.elsevier.com/locate/artmed

http://www.hi-europe.info/files/2002/9980.htm

http://www.journeyofhearts.org/jofh/jofh_old/minf_528/ai.htm

http://www.medg.lcs.mit.edu/ftp/psz/AIM82/ch1.html#c1_definitions

http://www.openclinical.org/aiinmedicine.html

KEY TERMS

Artificial Intelligence: A collection of mathematical and computing methods for predicting complex real-world processes, such as the behaviour of complicated games, like chess; the behaviour of experts, who might predict future real-estate values, render medical diagnoses, or translate foreign languages; the behaviour of complex biological systems; or ordinary human behaviour, such as perceiving objects visually or auditorily.

Biomedicine: The branch of medical science that applies biological and physiological principles to clinical practice.

Clinical Decision-Support System: Active knowledge systems that use two or more items of patient data to generate case-specific advice.

Database: An organized body of related information.

Decision Theory: A branch of statistics concerning strategies for decision making in nondeterministic systems. Decision theory seeks to find strategies that maximise the expected value of a utility function measuring the desirability of possible outcomes.

Expert System: Computer programs that use artificial-intelligence strategies such as symbolic representation, inference, and heuristic search to perform sophisticated tasks once thought possible only for human experts.

Flowchart: A diagram of the sequence of operations in a computer program.

Chapter XLIV
Comparative Genomics and Structure Prediction in Dental Research

Andriani Daskalaki
Max Planck Institute of Molecular Genetics, Germany

Jorge Numata
Free University, Germany

ABSTRACT

Since the completion of the Human Genome Project (HGP) in 2003, the 3.2 billion basepairs which make up the human genome have been sequenced. These sequences contain the plan for the mechanisms controlling the behavior of each cell. The small variations in the DNA sequence that lead to different characteristics, such as facial features, or color, are known as polymorphisms, which also can cause oral diseases. Periodontitis is a chronic infective disease of the gums caused by bacteria present in dental plaque. Severaazl techniques have been developed to regenerate4 periodontal tissues including guided tissue regeneration (GTR), and the use of enamel matrix derivative (EMD). EMD is an extract of enamel matrix and contains amelogenins. This is evidence to show that amelogenins are involved not only in enamel formation, but also in the formation of the periodontal attachment during tooth formation. Comparative sequence analysis is an approach for detecting functional regions in genomic and protein sequences. Motifs, conserved domains, secondary structure characteristics, and functional sites of proteins related to oral health may be compared, revealing the degree of sequence conservation during vertebrate evolution. Secondary and tertiary structures are important in understanding the function of a protein. In a comparative sequence analysis, the most well-known bioinformatics tools that are used are: basic local-alignment search tool (BLAST), multiple-sequence alignment software (ClustalW), and PROSITE, a database of proten families and domains. The PROSITE database consists of biologically significant sites, patterns, and profiles that help to reliably identify to which known protein family a sequence belongs. Phylogeny Inference Package (PHYLIP) can be used for building phylogenetic trees and a Python-enhanced molecular graphics program (PyMOL) for 3D visualization of proteins.

INTRODUCTION

Dental researchers collaborating with bioinformaticians have achieved advances in oral-health research by actualizing the impact of genetics in oral health. With the help of bioinformatics, a spectrum of questions in dentistry can be addressed.

Comparative genomics approaches are used to identify the functional domains of a protein and suggest similarities for assigning 3-D structures by homology modeling. It is then possible to use classical molecular dynamics simulations to account for the dynamic behavior in protein function. Multiple-sequence analysis of proteins in different species reveals the degree of sequence conservation at the nucleotide and protein levels. Motifs, conserved domains, secondary structure characteristics, and functional sites of proteins related to oral health may be compared, revealing the degree of sequence conservation during vertebrate evolution.

Three-dimensional structure predictions developed by the modeling of conserved domains of proteins support a key role for specific residues in processes like mineralization.

COMPARATIVE GENOMICS

Comparative sequence analysis is an approach for detecting functional regions in genomic and protein sequences. It facilitates the identification of conserved domains, motifs, and distantly related sequences of different organisms, and provides evolutional insights into the underlying biology of organisms (Rubin et al., 2000).

The extracellular matrix of dentin primarily consists of Type I collagen, noncollagenous matrix proteins, and proteoglycans.

Amelogenin and osteocalcin are noncollagenous matrix proteins secreted by the ameloblasts and odontoblasts, respectively. These proteins primarily function in enamel mineralization.

Krishnaraaju et al. (2003) have used bioinformatics tools for multiple-sequence analysis of these proteins in different species.

Phylogenetic analysis using sequence data is used to study sequence relatedness.

STRUCTURE PREDICTION

Secondary and tertiary structures are important in understanding the function of a protein. Frequently, however, such information is not available because neither crystallographic nor nuclear magnetic resonance (NMR) structure determination has been carried out. In this case, structure-prediction methods may help. Homology-based methods are not perfect, and depend on the following:

1. One or more known crystal or NMR 3-D structures
2. Strong sequence similarity of the unknown structures (>25%)

The secondary structure elements may be predicted with good accuracy. However, side-chain rotameters and loop insertions may be far from reality.

Figure 1. Three-dimensional structure of osteocalcin. The graphic was generated by a PyMOL viewer. Calcium (CA) binding with gamma-carboxyglutamic acid (Cgu) is shown. Residues forming the alpha-helices (secondary structure) are highlighted with ribbons.

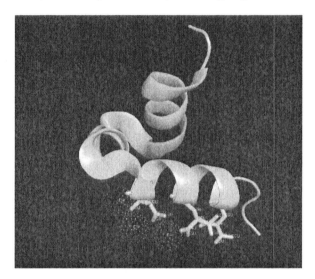

If the sequence or structural similarity is established between the protein of interest and the sequence with a known 3-D structure, it is possible to predict the 3-D structure in the conserved domain database. The 3-D structure (Figure 1) provides evidence that the protein osteocalcin is involved in mineralization in dental and bone structures by similar mechanisms.

BIOINFORMATIC TOOLS

1. **BLAST:** Basic local-alignment search tool. This tool is used to find protein sequences that are similar to query in the protein database.
2. **CLUSTALW:** Multiple-sequence alignment software. In the alignment, similarity among amino acids can be determined based on specific alignment parameters (for example, BLOSUM matrices).
3. **MEME:** Multiple-expectation maximization for motif elicitation. This tool discovers motifs in the sequence by a search of the protein database.
4. **PROSITE:** It identifies posttranslationally modified sites such as phosphorylation, glycosylation, and N-myristoylation on homologous sequences.
5. **PHYLIP:** Phylogeny Inference Package. A phylogenetic tree can be generated to find the closely related organisms from multiple-sequence alignment.
6. **PyMOL:** PyMOL is a molecular graphics program with an embedded Python interpreter designed for the real-time visualization and rapid generation of high-quality molecular graphics images and animations.

CONCLUSION

Predicting the three-dimensional structures of protein from sequence data by comparative modeling provides information on which experiments can be planned. If the sequence of structural similarity is established between the target (protein of interest) and the template (sequence for which the 3-D structure is known), it is possible to predict the 3-D structure of a protein or domain using publicly available sources (NCBI). Furthermore, methods like energy scoring functions, loop building, homology modeling, and energy minimization can be used.

REFERENCES

Actis, L. A., Rhodes, E. R., & Tomaras, A. P. (2003). Genetic and molecular characterization of a dental pathogen using genome-wide approaches. *Advances in Dental Research, 17,* 95-99.

Altschul, S. F., Gish, W., Miller, W., Myers, E. W., & Lipman, D. J. (1990). Basic local alignment search tool. *Journal of Molecular Biology, 215,* 403-410.

Bailey, T. L., & Elkan, C. (1995). The value of prior knowledge in discovering motifs with MEME. *Proceedings of the International Conference on Intelligent Systems and Molecular Biology, 3,* 21-29.

Krishnaraju, R. K., et al. (2003). Comparative genomics and structure prediction of dental matrix proteins. *Adv Dent Res, 17,* 100-103.

Moradian-Oldak, J. (2001). Amelogenins: Assembly, processing and control of crystal morphology. *Matrix Biology, 20,* 293-305.

Rubin, G. M., Yandell, M. D., Wortman, J. R., Gabor Miklos, G. L., Nelson, C. R., Hariharan, I. K., et al. (2000). Comparative genomics of the eukaryotes. *Science, 287,* 2204-2215.

Sebastiani, P. (2003). Bayesian machine learning and its potential applications to the genomic study of oral oncology. *Adv Dent Res, 17,* 104-108.

Sigrist, C. J., Cerutti, L., Hulo, N., Gattiker, A., Falquet, L. Pagni, M., et al. (2002). PROSITE: A documented database using patterns and profiles as motif descriptors. *Brief Bioinformatics, 3,* 265-274.

LINKS

http://en.wikipedia.org

http://meme.sdsc.edu/meme/meme-intro.html

http://pymol.sourceforge.net/

http://www.dhgp.de/info/lexica/dictionary.html

http://evolution.genetics.washington.edu/phylip/general.html

http://lectures.molgen.mpg.de/Algorithmische_Bioinformatik_WS0405/material/Steinke_lecture_19_1.pdf

http://www.ncbi.nlm.nih.gov/Education/BLASTinfo/glossary2.html

KEY TERMS

Alignment: The process of lining up two or more sequences to assess the degree of similarity and homology.

BLAST (Basic Local-Alignment Search Tool): A sequence-comparison algorithm optimized for speed and used to search sequence databases for optimal local alignments to a query.

Conservation: A high degree of similarity in the structure of homologous proteins amongst various phyla. This is seen as an indication of its importance in cellular function.

Domains: Portions of a protein assumed to fold independently and possessing their own functions.

Glycosylation: Process or result of the addition of saccharides to proteins and lipids. The process is one of four principal posttranslational modification steps in the synthesis of membrane and secreted proteins.

Homologous: Two or more structures are said to be homologous if they are alike because of shared ancestry from a common ancestor (evolutionary), or because they are from the same tissue in embryonal development (developmental ancestry).

MEME: A software tool for discovering motifs in a group of related DNA (deoxyribonucleic acid) or protein sequences. MEME uses statistical modeling techniques to automatically choose the best width, number of occurrences, and description for each motif.

Motif: A sequence pattern that occurs repeatedly in a group of related proteins or genes.

Myristoylation: A posttranslational protein modification. It is catalyzed by the enzyme N-myristoyltransferase and occurs on glycine residues exposed during cotranslational N-terminal methionine removal.

Nuclear Magnetic Resonance (NMR): A physical phenomenon based upon the magnetic property of an atom's nucleus. NMR spectroscopy can provide detailed information on the exact three-dimensional structure of biological molecules in a solution.

Phosphorylation: The addition of a phosphate (PO_4) group to a protein or a small molecule.

PHYLIP: The *Phyl*ogeny *I*nference *P*ackage is a package of programs for inferring phylogenies (evolutionary trees). Methods available in the package include parsimony, distance matrix, likelihood methods, bootstrapping, and consensus trees.

Posttranslational Modification: Chemical modification of a protein after its translation.

Protein: A protein consists of amino-acid chains. Proteins play a key role in most biologic processes.

PyMOL: A molecular visualization system.

Sequence: A sequence defines the order of nucleotides in the DNA or RNA (ribonucleic acid), or the order of amino acids in a protein.

Chapter XLV
Genomic Databanks for Biomedical Informatics

Andrea Maffezzoli
Politecnico di Milano, Italy

Marco Masseroli
Politecnico di Milano, Italy

ABSTRACT

In the area of medical informatics, the recent ICT (information and communication technology) tools and systems supporting knowledge on sciences involved in the study of genes, chromosomes, and protein's expression level in various organisms, that is genomics and proteomics, are becoming necessary to develop new prospects for the comprehension of mechanisms lying at the base of biological processes which cause a disease. This can allow more effective diagnostic and treatment methods and also personalized pharmacological therapies. At this purpose, the mutual intervention of different sciences, such as biology, medicine, engineering, informatics and mathematics, becomes an indispensable step: The development of a science embracing all these fields is identified in bioinformatics, which was conceived for the analysis, storage and processing of huge amount of biological data. The achievement of all the aforementioned operations involves the creation of the so-called genomic or proteomic databanks, which represent a major source of information on nucleotide sequences, as well as biological, clinical, physiological and bibliographical annotations related to singular sequences. There are different types of databanks based on their peculiar characteristics and features (such as primary and derivative or specialized databanks), and several ways to access data stored in these databanks; there are also specific bioinformatics databank-based tools developed to perform searching operations and to extract significant information, in order to summarize and compare gene annotations related to the causes of a disease and finally to identify a list of the most significant genes as cause of disease.

MEDICAL INFORMATICS AND E-HEALTH IN THE POST-GENOMIC ERA

The subject of medical informatics (MI) plays a very important role among the several branches of bioengineering because it deals with the practical and theoretical issues of the implementation of ICT in a wide range of solutions in the medical field, as well as in the more general health sector.

The constant evolution and improving of the technologies involved make it possible to guess that medical informatics will become increasingly important in the years to come. Consequently, in the last years, the complexity of medical-informatics solutions causes them to always be referred to as belonging to the so-called e-health field. This term hints at a wider role and groups all the numerous activities arising from MI applications.

E-health responds to growing demands for quality health services, patient mobility, data recording and processing, and finally for the more rational management of the economic resources and human efforts destined to these services.

E-health tools and applications can provide fast and easy access to electronic health records at the point of need: They can support diagnosis by noninvasive imaging-based systems, they support surgeons in planning clinical interventions using patient-specific digital data, and they provide access to specialized resources for education and training. Digital data transfer enables more effective networking among clinical institutions across the world and the creation of a global network of centers of reference. Electronic health records also enable the extraction of information for research, management, public-health, or other related statistics of benefit to health professionals.

More generally, e-health aims to improve the overall quality, productivity, and efficiency of the sector.

For these purposes, new knowledge and skilled personnel are needed, as well as essential, in order to implement new technologies and gain adequate financial support, from both the private and public sectors. This will carry very important consequences for the industries operating in the field, the so-called e-health industries, which represent today the third industrial force in the European health sector, and which will bring new life to ICT industries.

Examples of the operational capabilities of MI are as follows:

- Communication networks in hospitals
- Medical databases
- Telemedicine services
- MI Web-based portals
- ICT tools and systems dealing with the patient
  - Diagnosis
  - Monitoring
  - Treatment
  - Prevention

In particular, if we refer to the ICT tools and systems (Lacroix, 2002), the related applications can generate new and undiscovered developments, especially if viewed from the perspective of the latter discoveries carried out after human-genome sequencing and in the post-genomic era, with the subsequent developments of genomics, the systematic study of genes, chromosomes, and nucleic acids in an organism, and proteomics, which analyzes the proteins' expression levels in the biological processes of an organism.

In the postgenomic era, the complete sequencing of the human genome has helped to develop new prospects for the comprehension of the many mechanisms existing at the base of biological processes that cause disease.

A new vision of pharmacology has also started, supporting so-called pharmacogenetics and pharmacogenomics, which study how an individual's genetic inheritance affects the body's response to drugs. Pharmacogenomics focuses on a treatment that must be personalized according to the genetic profile of the patient: This could potentially reveal better and safer drugs, undiscovered and related macromolecular targets, new therapies, and new and more effective prevention methods.

It can also be noticed that this new era involves the intervention of different sciences, such as biology, medicine, engineering, informatics and mathematics, and different professional figures corresponding to different stages of analysis and study.

BIOMEDICAL INFORMATICS: A NEW APPROACH FOR GENOMIC RESEARCH

In this renewed scenario, the study of human genomes has marked the need of synergy between two sciences that have stayed distinct and unrelated until now: medical informatics and bioinformatics (BI).

The two sciences have different origins:

- MI was conceived with the introduction of computers in hospitals in order to perform some special applications, such as those for electronic data records, Bayesian systems, online bibliographic databases, and so forth.
- Bioinformatics was developed for the analysis, storage, and processing of huge amounts of biological data coming from laboratories, and it is an interdisciplinary research area interfacing between the biological and computational sciences, resulting in a fundamental management information system for molecular biology.

The completion of the human genome project has been greatly facilitated by MI tools and modern computational capabilities. Currently, BI is focused on the following three subjects:

1. Structural bioinformatics, which studies the prediction of molecular structure
2. Sequence analysis
3. Macromolecular databases

In bioinformatics, computers are used for all types of data useful for biological and macromolecular research, and consequently, the methods peculiar to information and communication technology are applied to forecast and analyze the molecular structures taken into account.

The ultimate goal of BI is to uncover the richness of biological information hidden in the mass of data and to obtain clearer insight into the fundamental biology of organisms.

From the synergy of BI and MI, biomedical informatics (BMI) was created, born for the development and sharing of biomedical knowledge coming from MI and BI, and for the support of computational molecular biology, which is the combined performance of mathematical, statistical, informatics, and technological techniques used in molecular-biology research (Martin-Sanchez et al., 2004).

The union of the two sciences means a powerful research method that provides a scientific and technical framework supporting an analysis that is totally personalized according to information available from each patient, consisting of data that were both clinical and genomic. This represents a more dynamic approach, based on the genotype of the patient and able to carry out a predictive analysis, which is an analysis that can provide the application of prevention measures.

Biomedical informatics allows us to focus on small DNA (deoxyribonucleic acid) changes or protein syntheses, and to understand the functioning and regulation of genes in order to discover new diagnosis techniques and to develop specific products in pharmacogenomics, which fight the disease on a molecular level.

BMI is intended to create a point of encounter between the genotypical and phenotypical information of a patient.

The purposes of BMI can be summed as follows (Tavazoie, Hughes, Campbell, Cho, & Church, 1999):

- Development of prevention measures in disease treatment
- Discovery of new therapies and related biological targets to fight the disease
- Efficiency, celerity, and cheapness of biology and pharmacogenomic research

The current state of BMI shows the need for creating comprehensive databases of both clinical data and genomic data, for having standards for the creation of databases and ontologies (Gene Ontology Consortium, 2000; Martucci, Masseroli, & Pinciroli, 2004; Masseroli, Martucci, & Pinciroli, 2004), and for analyses such as DNA microarrays for patient classifications.

The first results of BMI are the so-called biomolecular data banks, which are databases reporting clinical and genomic information together with physiological and environmental data. There are also new informatics tools and Web applications, and even standards to obtain an effective interaction between the different phases of data processing, hardware components, network architectures, and system security technologies.

The following functionalities appear essential to create such a framework:

- The storage of all data and information in special databases located at different sites,

consultable via the Web with different architectures or operating systems
- Performing data-mining analysis including learning algorithms, methods for significant information extraction, decision-support systems, and queries into databases (these methods should preferably be accomplished online)
- Performing text-mining elaboration, such as the extraction of data and information from text, thanks to the latest natural language processing (NLP) capabilities

Nevertheless, some difficulties can arise in such an integrated BMI approach due to different learning and analysis strategies, or to the absence of proper technologies useful to the solutions.

GENOMIC DATA BANKS: FUNCTIONS, PURPOSES, AND THEIR EFFECTIVE USE

Genomic data banks orderly store genomic and proteomic or molecular data, and provide an interface for their querying. Broadly referring to the data they contain, biomolecular data banks is another proper term for them. These data banks represent an integrated environment to manage a great amount of data, and they are able to report heterogeneous structural and functional information on genes and proteins.

Biomolecular data banks represent a major source of information on nucleotide sequences (DNA, RNA [ribonucleic acid], proteins), together with biological, clinical, physiological, and experimental data, and bibliographical annotations related to the enquired genes. Therefore, these data banks can be the information source of biomedical-informatics analysis tools that extract significant information related to the causes of a disease and on its possible treatments.

To look for any piece of information in the large amount of data on molecular sequences and gene annotations collected in genomic data banks, generally some keywords or identifiers have to be used. They enable one to identify stored biomolecular information by gene name or identifier, GenBank accession number, or by controlled terms describing their involvement in biological processes, molecular functions, biochemical pathways, and so forth.

Since 1994, every year the scientific journal *Nucleic Acids Research* (http://nar.oupjournals.org/) publishes a specific review on molecular biology data banks, including a list of open-access data banks together with brief descriptions and related URLs. The 2005 update quotes a list of 719 data banks, 171 more than the previous year (Galperin, 2005).

As of February 2005, sequences for more than 1,200 species, including 973 viruses, 197 bacteria, and 39 eukaryotes, were known, and 207 genomes were completed. The most studied genomes are those of the human, fruit fly (Drosophila melanogaster), mouse, rat, zebra fish, thale cress (Arabidopsis thaliana), escherichia coli, pea, maize, and wheat.

Most of the data stored in biomolecular data banks are public and freely accessible through the Internet, and they are submitted in the following types:

- Nucleotide sequences
- Genomic mapping data
- Expression profiles (2D-SDS PAGE, DNA chips)
- Protein sequences
- 3-D structures of nucleic acids and proteins
- Metabolic data
- Functional annotations
- Bibliographic information

Data Banks' Accessibility

Genomic data banks are accessible in different ways, but at present, all these ways are not functional to efficiently use the provided annotations for easily studying lists of genes.

The ways to access available data are the following:

- **Access through a Web Server (HTML [HyperText Markup Language] or XML [Extensible Markup Language] Pages):** This is the most common provided access, which usually presents unstructured information and heterogeneous Web interfaces, and the related query results on a single biomolecular sequence are mainly returned in HTML format; on the other hand, it requires time to comprehensively query multiple data banks.
- **Access through an FTP (File Transfer Protocol) Server:** It requires one to have significant technological and human resources for locally reimplementing the data bank, and sometimes there are no relations among provided data (ASCII [American Standard Code for Information Interchange] flat file format).
- **Direct Access:** It is rarely allowed due to security issues and because data-bank schemes are heterogeneous and unknown a priori, query languages differ among data banks, and there is a lack of a common vocabulary.
- **Direct HTTP (HyperText Transfer Protocol) Linking:** It is generally available if the data-bank entry identification code is known and each link returns a Web page (usually in HTML format) with all data available in the data bank for the considered entry.

Generally, biomedical researchers need to have an aggregated form of the genomic data in order to browse them easily and perform articulated queries on them. Despite efforts to integrate gene annotations, relevant gene data are still sparsely stored among heterogeneous data banks. Consequently, the increasing amount of information available requires new approaches to summarize, visualize, and compare the gene annotations in order to make it possible to discover new knowledge.

The effective use of the huge amount of data available in genomic data banks presents several difficulties because the storage is accomplished in distinct data banks, and the data banks are heterogeneous in schema and contents, and generally can be interrogated only for a single genomic sequence at a time. Moreover, they are mostly accessible for interrogation via the Web only, and the data retrieved as interrogation results are usually available, not structured, on HTML pages only.

For the data banks with access through FTP servers and the rare ones with direct access, solutions to the interrogation difficulties can include the following:

- Creating local databases (i.e., mirrors) associated with the original data banks; the related drawbacks are keeping the mirrors updated and multiple-database issues
- Designing and using special query languages to access and query data in multiple databases of heterogeneous DBMS, or through the definition and use of metadata
- Automatic mapping of queries to answer the need of performing the same query on several databases

For data banks providing access through a Web server, solutions to the interrogation difficulties reside in creating new tools allowing one to do the following:

- Automatically extract specific data of interest in the HTML or XML pages of different data banks
- Store in aggregate form the extracted data
- Structure the aggregate data to enable the performing of subsequent, specific queries on them

Biomolecular data banks can be classified in different ways according to specific characteristics.

Above all, they can be subdivided into the two following classes:

- Primary data banks
- Derivative or specialized data banks

Primary Data Banks

The primary data banks regard nucleic acids and amino acids, and they only contain the essential information to identify a sequence and its main characteristics. Each sequence introduced in a data bank with its annotation constitutes a so-called entry.

DNA (nucleic acids) data banks include the following:

- GenBank at NCBI (USA, http://www.ncbi.nlm.nih.gov/)
- EMBL at EBI (European Molecular Biology Laboratory, United Kingdom, http://www.ebi.ac.uk/embl.html/)
- DDBJ (Japan, http://www.ddbj.nig.ac.jp/)

Protein (amino acids) data banks include the following:

- Swiss-Prot/TrEMBL (high level of annotation; http://www.expasy.org/sprot/)
- PIR (Protein Identification Resource, http://pir.georgetown.edu/)

- UniProt (Unified Protein Resource, http://www.pir.uniprot.org/)

The first DNA data bank, created in 1980, was the European Molecular Biology Laboratory Data Library. In 1982, the American data bank GenBank was created, followed in 1986 by DDBJ, the Japanese DNA data bank. Data banks concerning proteins and carbohydrates are Swiss-Prot/TrEMBL (http://www.expasy.org/sprot/) and PIR (http://pir.georgetown.edu/).

The EMBL, GenBank, and DDBJ form the International Nucleotide Sequence Database Collaboration, which uses the Taxonomy Project in order to make available a unified taxonomy in all three data banks, and the Feature Table in order to identify a set of information to associate to each sequence and the mechanism of data exchange.

Derivative Data Banks

The derivative or specialized data banks contain both the genomic data of primary data banks and their taxonomic, biological, physiological, or medical annotations; thus, they represent a very useful source of information complementary to primary data banks.

The specialized data banks can be the following:

- Human curated (e.g., Entrez Gene, Swiss-Prot, NCBI RefSeq nRNA)
- Computationally derived (e.g., UniGene)
- A combination of both (e.g., NCBI Genome Assembly)

Specialized databanks can be classified as follows:

- A simple subset of the primary data bank, homogeneous from the biological point of view, and accurately revised and enhanced

with specific biological information inherent to the considered subset. A good example is the PIR Sequence-Structure data bank (PIR-NRL3D, http://www-nbrf.georgetown.edu/; Pattabiraman et al., 1990). PIR-NRL3D is a data bank of proteins, derived from the Protein Information Resource databank, with a known 3-D structure and whose atomic coordinates are recorded in the Protein Data Bank (PDB).

- A set of multi-aligned homologous sequences, such as rRNA (Neefs et al., 1993; http://www.psb.ugent.be/rRNA/index.html/) and tRNAC (Steinberg et al., 1993) data banks.
- A set of specific information complementary to those in the primary data banks, and specific for a well-defined class of sequences. A good example for this class is the Eukaryotic Promoter Databank (EPD, http://www.epd.isb-sib.ch/; Bucher et al., 1996).
- Genomic databanks, representative of the whole set of information derived from mapping and sequencing projects of the human genome and of other genomes selected as model organisms. A good example is the Genome Data Base (GDB, http://gdbwww.gdb.org/).
- Integrational databanks, recently created to collect information dispersedly stored in other specialized data banks. Good examples are the GeneCards (http://bioinformatics.weizmann.ac.il/cards/) and SOURCE (http://source.stanford.edu/) data banks.

Examples of other derivative data banks are the following:

- Unigene (http://www.ncbi.nlm.nih.gov/UniGene/)

- Entrez Gene (http://www.ncbi.nih.gov/ entrez/query.fcgi?db=gene/)

The biomolecular data banks can be also classified in other different and simpler ways, such as in genome data banks or proteome data banks, depending on the type of information they contain, that is, genomic or proteomic data.

Bioinformatic Data-Bank-Based Tools

Several bioinformatic software tools have been developed to perform information extraction and searching operations on database-stored data by using different technologies (Masseroli, Stella, Meani, Alcalay, & Pinciroli, 2004).

Factors that must be taken into consideration when designing these tools are as follows:

- The end user (the biologist) may not be a frequent user of computer technology.
- These software tools must be made available over the Internet given the global distribution of the scientific research community.

A specific type of these bioinformatic tools is represented by database search tools, which are software programs designed for extracting the meaningful information from the mass of data and carrying out the analysis steps.

These database search tools are classified as follows:

- **Sequence-Based Tools:** These database search algorithms are used to compute comparisons between a candidate query sequence and each of the sequences stored within a database in order to find all the pairs of sequences that have similarity

above a defined threshold. There are three principal database search algorithms.
  - Smith-Waterman algorithm (http:// decypher2.stanford.edu/), which uses dynamic programming to compute the most sensitive similarity alignments
  - FASTA (http://www-nbrf.georgetown. edu/pirwww/search/fasta.html/), which is an approximate heuristic algorithm used to compute suboptimal similarity comparisons
  - BLAST (http://www.ncbi.nlm.nih.gov/ BLAST/), which is another approximate heuristic algorithm used to compute suboptimal similarity comparisons, but it is better and faster than FASTA, giving a statistical evaluation of the result's significance
- **Text-Based Tools:** These include SRS6 (http://srs6.ebi.ac.uk/srs6bin/cgi-bin/ wgetz?-page+top/), ENTREZ (http:// www.ncbi.nlm.nih.gov/Entrez/), and DBGET/LinkDB (http://www.genome.jp/ dbget-bin/www_bfind?linkdb/).

CONCLUSION

In the last years, life sciences, such as biology and medicine, and computational sciences, such as informatics, statistics, and engineering, have been merging their efforts to try to reach a very difficult goal in genomics and proteomics: a better knowledge of biological mechanisms and processes, especially those that are the cause of diseases.

The development and application of biomedical informatics in medicine, biology, and healthcare sectors have the objective of searching for new and more effective diagnostic, monitoring, and treatment methods. These are mainly focused on personalized pharmacological therapies developed thanks to pharmacogenomics.

In order to achieve such aims, genomic data banks are fundamental sources of structured biomolecular data and biomedical knowledge, including extremely valuable functional and clinical information.

Recently developed bioinformatics algorithms and tools exploit such relevant information within the heterogeneous and widely distributed databases of biomolecular data banks accessible through Web servers to extract lists of the most significant genes as causes of disease, and to gather and evaluate the relevance of the gene annotations related to them. In the end, genomic data banks and bioinformatic data-bank-based tools are useful to highlight significant biological characteristics and to support a global approach in order to improve the understanding of complex cellular mechanisms and physiological knowledge.

REFERENCES

Bucher, P., Karplus, K., Moeri, N., & Hofmann, K., (1996). A flexible search technique based on generalized profiles. *Computers and Chemistry, 20,* 3-24.

Galperin, M. J. (2005). The molecular biology database collection: 2005 update. *Nucleic Acids Research, 33,* D5-D24.

Gene Ontology Consortium. (2000). Gene ontology: Tool for the unification of biology. *Nature Genetics, 25,* 25-29.

Glynn, D., Jr., Sherman, B. T., Hosack, D. A., Yang, J., Gao, W., & Lane, H. C. (2003). DAVID: Database for annotation, visualization, and integrated discovery. *Genome Biology, 4,* R60.

Lacroix, Z. (2002). Biological data integration: Wrapping data and tools. *IEEE Transactions on Information Technology in Biomedicine,* 6(2), 123-128.

Martin-Sanchez, F., Iakovidis, I., Norager, S., Maojo, V., de Groen, P., Van der Lei, J., et al. (2003). Synergy between medical informatics and bioinformatics: Facilitating genomic medicine for future healthcare. *Journal of Biomedical Informatics, 37,* 30-42.

Martucci, D., Masseroli, M., & Pinciroli, F. (2004). Gene ontology application to genomic functional annotation, statistical analysis and knowledge mining. *Studies in Health Technology Informatics, 102,* 108-131.

Masseroli, M., Martucci, D., & Pinciroli, F. (2004). GFINDer: Genome Function INtegrated Discoverer through dynamic annotation, statistical analysis, and mining. *Nucleic Acids Research, 32,* w293-w300.

Masseroli, M., Stella, A., Meani, N., Alcalay, M., & Pinciroli, F. (2004). MyWest: My Web extraction software tool for effective mining of annotations from Web-based databanks. *Bioinformatics, 20,* 3326-3335.

Neefs, J. M., Van de Peer, Y., De Rijk, P., Chapelle, S., De Wachter, R. (1993). Compilation of small ribosomal subunit RNA structures. *Nucleic Acids Research, 21,* 3025-3049.

Pattabiraman, N., Namboodiri, K., Lowrey, A., Gaver, B. P. (1990). *NRL_3D: A sequence-environment. Protein Sequences Data Analysis, 3,* 387-405.

Steinberg, S., Misch, A., & Sprinzl, M. (1993). Compilation of tRNA sequences and sequences of tRNA genes. *Nucleic Acids Research, 21,* 3011-3015.

Tavazoie, S., Hughes, J. D., Campbell, M. J., Cho, R. J., & Church, G. M. (1999). Systematic determination of genetic network architecture. *Nature Genetics, 22,* 281-285.

KEY TERMS

Bioinformatics: A branch of biology and informatics concerned with the development of techniques for the collection and manipulation of biological data, and the use of such data to make biological discoveries or predictions. It comprehends all computational methods and theories applicable to molecular biology and areas of computer-based techniques for solving biological problems including the manipulation of models and data sets.

Biomedical Informatics: The discipline that studies biomedical information and knowledge, focusing in particular on their structure, acquisition, integration, management, and optimal use. It adopts and applies results from a variety of other disciplines including information science, computer science, cognitive science, business and organization management, statistics and biometrics, mathematics, artificial intelligence, operations research, and basic and clinical health sciences.

Biomolecular Databanks: Structured repositories of biomolecular, genomic, or proteomic data and their related biological, medical, and clinical information.

Computational Molecular Biology: A new discipline bringing together computational, statistical, experimental, and technological methods that is energizing and accelerating the development of new techniques and tools for molecular biology.

E-Health: It refers to the application of information and communications technologies to the whole range of activities related to the health sector.

Genomic Data Banks: They hold, treat, and analyze genomic data, together with biological, clinical, or experimental information.

Genomics: The systematic identification and study of genomes, each of which include all the genetic material of a living organism.

Medical Informatics: The field of information science concerned with the analysis and dissemination of medical data through the application of computer-science technologies to various aspects of healthcare and medicine.

Pharmacogenetics: A branch of genetics that deals with the genetic components of variability in the individual responses to and metabolism of drugs.

Pharmacogenomics: An extension of the established science of pharmacogenetics. The process of treatment is tailored to fit the precise makeup of each individual patient.

Proteomics: The study of all possible proteins (amino-acid sequences) of an organism, translated from different transcripts.

Chapter XLVI
Basic Principles and Applications of Microarrays in Medicine

Andriani Daskalaki
Max Planck Institute of Molecular Genetics, Germany

Athina A. Lazakidou
University of Piraeus, Greece

ABSTRACT

The simultaneous expression of a large number of genes is a critical component of normal growth and development, and the maintenance of health. Microarray technology is used to understand fundamental aspects of growth and development, as well as to explore the underlying genetic causes of many human diseases. Systematic analysis of microarray data will yield insight into molecular biological processes and the functions of thousands of gene products in parallel. This approach allows for better understanding in cellular signaling, disease classification, diagnosis, and prognosis. Microarrays allow scientists to analyze the expression of many genes in a single experiment quickly and efficiently. One important goal of computational analysis of microarrays is to extract clues from microarray data and translate the information into biological understanding diseases in medicine and dentistry. There are different platforms or types of DNA microarrays that are commercially available: Glass DNA microarrays and high-density oligonucleotide microarrays. DNA microarray experiments generate large quantities of genome-wide data. To extract useful information from expression profiles, computational tools that compute, statistically validate and display data can be used. An important step in the computation of microarray data is normalization. The purpose of the normalization prozess is to identify and remove the effects of systematic variation in the measured fluorescence intensities other than differential expressions. There are different methods for the normalization of data: total intensity normalization, regression normalization, normalization using ratio statistics, and variance stabilization (VSN). A major goal of microarray data analysis is to identify differentially expressed genes. Selecting marker genes is an important issue for disease classification based on gene expression data.

The selection of marker genes is critical in tumor classification using gene expression data. Many methods have been proposed to select differentially expressed genes, including parametric and nonparametric tests, and others.

INTRODUCTION

The proper and harmonious expression of a large number of genes is a critical component of normal growth and development, and the maintenance of proper health. Disruptions or changes in gene expression are responsible for many diseases.

Biomedical research evolves and advances not only through the compilation of knowledge, but also through the development of new technologies. Using traditional methods to assay gene expression, researchers were able to survey a relatively small number of genes at a time. The emergence of new tools enables researchers to address previously intractable problems and to uncover novel potential targets for therapies. Microarrays allow scientists to analyze the expression of many genes in a single experiment quickly and efficiently. They represent a major methodological advance and illustrate how the advent of new technologies provides powerful tools for researchers. Scientists are using microarray technology to try to understand fundamental aspects of growth and development, as well as to explore the underlying genetic causes of many human diseases.

Since many genes contribute to normal functioning, research efforts are moving from the search for a disease-specific gene to the understanding of the biochemical and molecular functioning of a variety of genes and how complicated networks of interaction can lead to a disease state, such as oral cancer. With the DNA (deoxyribonucleic acid) microarray-based research, we can look forward to more accurate diagnosis, surgical treatment, and drug-delivery therapy based on an individual patient's genetic profile.

DNA microarray technology has been used for genome-wide gene-expression studies that incorporate molecular-genetics and computer-science skills on massive levels. This technology allows comparisons of gene-expression levels in samples derived from normal and diseased tissues, treated and nontreated tissues, and tissues in different stages of differentiation or development. It uses nucleic-acid hybridization techniques and computers to evaluate the mRNA (messenger ribonucleic acid) expression profile of thousands of genes simultaneously for the purposes of gene discovery, disease diagnosis, improved drug development, and therapeutics tailored to specific disease processes.

DNA microarrays are miniature arrays containing gene fragments that are either synthesized directly onto or spotted onto glass or other substrates. Each spot serves as a highly specific and sensitive detector of the corresponding mRNA. Further computational analysis of microarray data allows the classification of genes by their mRNA expression patterns. Global gene-expression profiles in cells or tissues will provide us with a better understanding of the molecular basis of a phenotype, pathology, or treatment.

Furthermore, there exists an increasing number of applications for protein and antibody microarrays (Feilner et al., 2004) in basic research diagnostics, drug discovery, and in vitro risk assessment of nutrients.

TYPES OF DNA MICROARRAYS

There are currently two platforms or types of DNA microarrays that are commercially available.

1. Glass DNA microarrays that involve the microspotting of prefabricated cDNA (complementary DNA) fragments on a glass slide.
2. High-density oligonucleotide microarrays, often referred to as chips, that involve in situ oligonucleotide synthesis.

However, from a manufacturing point of view, there are fundamental differences between the two platforms in regard to the sizes of printed DNA fragments, the methods of printing the DNA spots on the slide or chip, and also the data images generated.

*   **cDNA Microarrays:** On a glass surface, complementary DNA can be spotted. A high-speed robot is used to spot PCR-amplified cDNA onto a chemically modified (polylysine, aminosilane) glass slide. The DNA-arrayed slides are then hybridized with fluorescently labeled cDNA reverse transcribed from mRNA populations. During this process, the slide is hybridized with two different cDNA samples labeled separately with two distinct fluorescent dyes, such as Cy3 (cyanine 3, green dye) and Cy5 (cyanine 5, red dye; two-color hybridization). The relative intensities of the two fluorescent dyes within a spot represent the relative mRNA expression levels of the gene. For example, if fluorescent labels Cy3 (green) and Cy5 (red) are used to make each sample's cDNA probe, the expression level of a gene will be displayed as green or red when the gene is differentially

Figure 1. GeneChip System 3000Dx

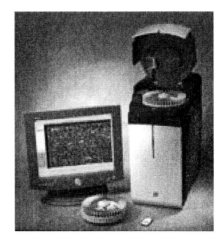

expressed, or yellow when the level is the same in the two samples.

*   **Oligonucleotide Microarrays:** In these arrays, DNA oligonucleotides are synthesized in situ onto the DNA chip using photolabile protecting groups and photolithographic masks to add the selective sequences of nucleotides. They offer a fast, high-throughput alternative for the parallel detection of microbes from virtually any sample. The application potential spreads across most sectors of life sciences, including environmental microbiology and microbial ecology. Each probe consists of 25-base-pair (bp) oligonucleotides (thus called 25-mers) where 20 different oligonucleotide pairs represent one gene. A pair consists of a perfect-match and a mismatch oligonucleotide, in which the 13th nucleotide is verändert. The perfect-match signals are subtracted by the mismatch signals, and the net values are used for the comparisons. In the Affymetrix GeneChip system (Figure 1), in contrast to the cDNA or presynthesized oligonucleotide deposited arrays, only one

Figure 2. Experimental design for a microarray experiment

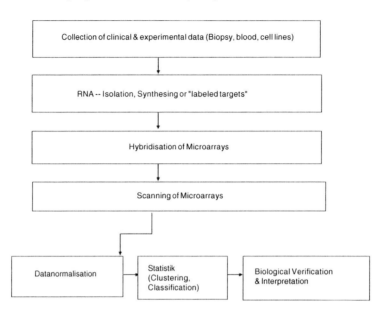

sample is hybridized on to one array (target), and comparisons can be made among multiple arrays (one-color hybridization).

DATA ANALYSIS

The raw data from a cDNA microarray experiment consist of pairs of image files, 16-bit TIFFs, one for each of the dyes. Image analysis is required to extract measures of the red and green fluorescence intensities, R and G, for each spot on the array. In the image analysis, the first step is to estimate the location of the spot centers (addressing). Then pixels have to be classified as foreground (signal) or background (segmentation).

At the end, we have to extract the available information, foreground and background intensities, and quality measures for each spot on the array and each dye. Spots usually vary in size and shape (area, perimeter, circularity). Also, pixel and ratio intensities (uniformity) as well as

brightness (foreground-background ratio) can vary within a spot. Beyond the spot quality (brightness, uniformity, morphology), the slide quality (percentage of spots without signal, range of intensities, distribution of spot signal area) is of importance.

Normalization

The purpose of normalization is to identify and remove the effects of systematic variation in the measured fluorescence intensities other than differential expressions, such as the following:

- Expression, for example, different labeling efficiencies of the dyes.
- Different amounts of Cy3- and Cy5-labeled mRNA. In hybridizations, where the same mRNA sample is labeled with the Cy3 and Cy5 dyes, the imbalance in the red and green intensities is usually not constant across the spots within and be-

tween arrays, and can vary according to overall spot intensity, location, and so forth.

- Different scanning parameters (scanning artifacts).
- Printing.

Normalization is needed to ensure that differences in intensities are indeed due to differential expression. Normalization is necessary before any analysis that involves within- or between-slide comparisons of intensities, for example, clustering and testing.

There are different methods for the normalization of data:

- **Total Intensity Normalization:** This method stands on the assumption that the total quantities of messages from both samples are the same. Under this assumption, a normalization factor can be calculated from the total integrated intensity (in one-color hybridization, for example, in the Affymetrix GeneChip system) or from the total average fold difference of the Cy3 and Cy5 channels (in two-color hybridization, for example, in deposited cDNA arrays) for all the elements in one array. This normalization factor is then used to adjust the scale or fold for each gene in the array.
- **Regression Normalization:** In a scatter plot of both channels in two-color hybridization, the genes would scatter along a straight diagonal line when two closely related samples are compared. Normalization of this data can be performed by calculating the best-fit slope and by applying the regression to adjust the levels of all the genes.
- **Normalization Using Ratio Statistics:** Using all spots on the array would be a problem when many genes are differentially expressed. This method assumes

that a subset of genes, referred to as housekeeping genes, do not change their profiles throughout the experiments. These genes are thought to be constantly expressed across a wide range of biological samples (e.g., GAPDH). The normalization factor calculated from this subset of housekeeping genes is used to adjust experimental variability in the samples being compared.

Alternatively, a set of exogenous controls can be spiked onto the arrays, and mRNA from the set are equally added into the initial RNA samples before labeling. The average expression ratio from these controls should be equal to 1, and this factor is used to normalize the data to identify differentially expressed genes.

- **Variance Stabilization (VSN):** This method builds upon the fact that the variance of microarray data depends on the signal intensity, and that a transformation can be found after the variance is approximately constant. VSN assumes that less than half of the genes on the arrays are differentially transcribed across the experiment.

Clustering

DNA microarray experiments generate large quantities of genome-wide data. To extract useful information from expression profiles, computational tools that cluster and display data can be used. Although there are many ways to analyze gene-expression data, hierarchical clustering (Eisen, Spellman, Brown, & Botstein, 1998) and self-organizing map (SOM) clustering (Tamayo et al., 1999) have been widely used to display the data.

Hierarchical clustering is simple and the results are easily visualized. In hierarchical clustering, the distances between genes are calculated for all of the genes based on their expression pattern, and the closer genes are merged to produce a cluster. The distances between these small clusters are calculated to produce a new cluster. Self-organizing map clustering assigns genes to a series of groups on the basis of expression-pattern similarities. Random vectors are constructed for each group, and a gene is assigned to the closest vector.

APPLICATIONS OF MICROARRAYS

Traditional molecular research tools for gene-expression study are limited to dealing with a small group of genes at a time. Recent advances in the microarray field have enabled the study of large numbers of genes in a single experiment. DNA microarrays not only detect global changes of gene expression, but also have many other potential applications including the identification of polymorphism (Wang et al., 1998), diagnostic tools for diseases, and drug discovery.

The application of microarray technology for microbial diagnostics is a field in the stage of dynamic development, with many options available and advantages and disadvantages associated with each option. One major goal of microarray data analysis is to identify differentially expressed genes. Selecting marker genes for sample classification is also an important issue for disease classification based on gene-expression data. The selection of marker genes is critical in tumor classification using gene-expression data. Many methods have been proposed to select differentially expressed genes, including the two-sample t-tests (Dudoit, Yang, Callow, & Speed, 2002), ANOVA (Kerr, Martin, & Churchill, 2000), SAM (Tusher, Tibshirani, & Chu, 2001), Wilcoxon nonparametric two-sample tests, and others.

MAIN PROBLEMS OF MICROARRAYS

- **Complex Interpretation:** Microarrays obtained from expression profiling are too complex to interpret. The problem of the biological interpretation of gene-expression data occurs when cellular events are mediated in protein levels. mRNA profiling provides us with only the levels of mRNA messages. In addition, the current array data include the transcriptional behaviors of a large portion of, at the moment, uncharacterized genes.
- **Expensive:** Microarray technology is still expensive and requires biological materials that may be difficult to collect. Therefore, most studies perform only a few replicated microarray experiments.
- **Bias in Hybridization:** We need to understand array-specific effects regarding the hybridization behavior of the oligoprobes such as immobilization.
- **Sequence Databases of Less Conserved Markers:** Large sequence databases of less conserved markers are needed. Linking this sequence information to phylogenetic traits (i.e., antibiotic resistance in clinical microbiology) will enable the prediction of these functions, at least at a given level of certainty, from microarray results.
- **Oligoprobe Design:** Oligoprobe design is often limited by the length, GC content, number, and position of diagnostic residues within a diagnostic region.

CONCLUSION

One important goal of computational analysis is to extract clues from microarray data and translate the information into biological understanding. Systematic analysis of microarray data will yield insight into molecular biological processes and the functions of thousands of gene products in parallel. This approach allows for better understanding in cellular signaling, disease classification, diagnosis, and prognosis.

Proteome technologies for monitoring changes in protein abundance and protein modification are important because the correlation between gene and protein expression is variable, and the posttranslational protein modifications are responsible for realizing signaling and information processing. Tissue microarrays (Kononen et al., 1998) and protein microarrays (MacBeath & Schreiber, 2000; Zhu et al., 2001) have been developed in which samples of up to hundreds of tissues or proteins are analyzed simultaneously on one glass slide.

Unfortunately, microarray data are not easily shared due to the variation of standards among experiments. The need for researchers to agree on one particular standard, referred to as a universal standard, is very difficult to achieve. Thus, ongoing efforts to find a common standard sample for all experiments are in progress to facilitate widespread data sharing.

REFERENCES

Bodrossy, L., & Sessitsch, A. (2004). Oligonucleotide microarrays in microbial diagnostics. *Current Opinion in Microbiology, 7*, 245-254. Retrieved from http://www.diagnostic-arrays.com/download/Bodrossy_and_Sessitsch_2004_preprint.pdf

Buhler, J. (2002). Glossary of biotechnology terms. *Anatomy of a comparative gene expression study.* Retrieved May 7, 2005, from http://www.cs.wustl.edu/~jbuhler/research/array/glossary.html#hybridize

Dudoit, S., Gentleman, R., Irizarry, R., & Yang, Y. H. (2002). *Pre-processing in DNA microarray experiments: Bioconductor short course.* Retrieved from http://www.bioconductor.org/workshops/WyethCourse101702/PreProc/PreProc4.pdf

Dudoit, S., Yang, Y. H., Callow, M. J., & Speed, T. P. (2002). Statistical methods for identifying differentially expressed genes in replicated cDNA microarray experiments. *Stat. Sinica, 12*, 111-139.

Eisen, M. B., Spellman, P. T., Brown P. O., & Botstein, D. (1998). Cluster analysis and display of genome-wide expression patterns. *Proceedings of the National Academy of Sciences of the United States of Ameria, 95*, 14863-14868.

Feilner, T., Kreutzberger, J., Niemann, B., Kramer, A., Possling, A., Seitz, H., et al. (2004). Proteomic studies using microarrays. *Current Proteomics, 1*(4), 283-295.

Huber, W. (2003). *Practical DNA microarray analysis.* First Analysis Steps. Retrieved from http://www.bioconductor.org/workshops/NGFN03/qcnorm.pdf

Kerr, M. K., Martin, M., & Churchill, G. A. (2000). *Analysis of variance for gene expression microarray data* [Tech. Rep.]. Bar Harbor, ME: The Jackson Laboratory.

Kononen, J., Bubendorf, L., Kallioniemi, A., Barlund, M., Schraml, P., Leighton, S., et al. (1998). Tissue microarrays for high-throughput molecular profiling of tumor specimens. *Nat Med., 4*, 844-847.

Kuo, W. P., Whipple, M. E., Sonis, S. T., Ohno-Machado, L., & Jenssen, T. K. (2002). Gene expression profiling by DNA microarrays and its application to dental research: Review. *Oral Oncol., 38*(7), 650-656.

MacBeath, G., & Schreiber, S. (2000). Printing proteins as microarrays for high-throughput function determination. *Science, 289,* 1760-1763.

Tamayo, P., Slonim, D., Mesirov, J., Zhu, Q., Kitareewan, S., Dmitrovsky, E., et al. (1999). Interpreting patterns of gene expression with self-organizing maps: Methods and application to hematopoietic differentiation. *Proceedings of the National Academy of Sciences of the United States of Ameria, 96,* 2907-2912.

Tusher, V. G., Tibshirani, R., & Chu, G. (2001). Significance analysis of microarrays applied to the ionizing radiation response. *Proc. Natl. Acad. Sci., 98,* 5116–5121.

Wang, D. G., Fan J.-B., Siao, C-J., Berno, A., Young, P., Sapolsky, et al. (1998). Large-scale identification, mapping, and genotyping of single-nucleotide polymorphisms in the human genome. *Science, 280,* 1077-1082.

Zhong, G., & Hongyu, Z. (2005). A semiparametric approach for marker gene selection based on gene expression data. *Bioinformatics, 21*(4), 529-536.

Zhu, H., Bilgin, M., Bangham, R., Hall, D., Casamayor, A., Bertone, P., et al. (2001). Global analysis of protein activities using proteome chips. *Science, 293,* 2101-2105.

URL REFERENCES

http://dial.liacs.nl/Courses/MicroArrayDataAnalysis/Exercises/Normalization_VSN_R_Course_and_PB.pdf

http://page.mi.fu-berlin.de/~fabioinf/internes/studium/vorlesungen/genetik/lh_genetik_ss02_Glossar1.pdf

http:// www.diagnostic-arrays.com

http://www.ima.umn.edu/talks/workshops/9-29-10-3.2003/huber/whuber-vsn-ima-oct2003.htm

http://www.lshtm.ac.uk/itd/grf/microarray overview.htm

http://www.ncbi.nlm.nih.gov/About/primer/microarrays.html

KEY TERMS

Channel: Data from one color (Cy3, cyanine 3, green dye; Cy5, cyanine 5, red dye).

Hybridization: The process of joining two complementary single-stranded nucleic acids over their complementary bases (C-G and A-T). The microarray holds hundreds or thousands of spots, each of which contains a different DNA sequence. If a probe contains cDNA whose sequence is complementary to the DNA on a given spot, that cDNA will hybridize to the spot, where it will be detectable by its fluorescence (Buhler, 2002).

Microarray: A miniature array containing gene fragments that are either synthesized directly onto or spotted onto glass or other substrates.

Normalization: Data transformation. Its purpose is to identify and remove the effects of systematic variation in the measured fluorescence intensities.

Probe: Immobile substrate (DNA, protein) spotted on the array.

Target: Mobile substrate (DNA, protein) hybridized to the array.

Chapter XLVII
System Patterns of the Human Organism and their Heredity

Manfred Doepp
Holistic DiagCenter, Germany

Gabriele Edelmann
Holistic DiagCenter, Germany

ABSTRACT

The frequency distribution analysis of biological data enables an insight into the regulatory state of the organism. In case of strong or permanent deviations from the balance of the systems (e.g. of the vegetative nervous system) abnormalities and/or diseases will result. They are associated with a tendency either to chaos or to rigidity. We examined in this way families over two or three generations. Similarities in their distribution histogram types are evaluated which confirm a genetic disposition and a heritability of system patterns. Risk profiles are resulting individually and concerning the descendants making possible a systemic prevention therapy or a modification of the life style. The analysis method may be adapted to a lot of medical examinations and represents an objective second opinion concerning health prevention.

INTRODUCTION

Analysis of the human genome goes forward continuously, and the genetic types of many organ functions, dysfunctions, and diseases are meanwhile becoming known. Problems exist concerning genes directing regulatory systems or feedback mechanisms; as for complex purposes, several genes are cooperating (Finch & Tanzi, 1997). In order to study the heritability of closed-loop control-system patterns, the frequency distribution of biological events and/or dates enables an insight into the condition of the organism (Popp, 1987; Rossmann & Popp, 1986; Zhang & Popp, 1996). The lognormal (LN) distribution is considered to represent health, and the normal (N) distribution (bell curve=random) is a suspicion of cancer. This is the state of the art.

The bell curve is the result of an accident and occurs in living beings with a deficit or an absence of regulatory networks and coherence, what is to be referred to as chaos (Doepp & Edelmann, 2004; Zhang & Popp, 1996). In the normality of a high-powered and controlled arrangement, which works in coherence and is in a steady state, an asymmetric=lognormal distribution (Gevelein & Heite, 1950; Sachs, 1969) seems to surrender. Recently, we found that an exaggeration of this results in a tendency of the regulations of the organism toward rigidity (delta distribution). It is accompanied by rigidity biologically as, for example, with Parkinson's or arterial sclerosis (Doepp & Edelmann, 2003).

The basic principle is that the normal state of all controlled systems, for example, the vegetative nervous system, contains a certain variation—an oscillation—around the middle line concerning how it is usually at phase transitions, like the laser threshold (Haken, 1964).

The chaos theory supplies the reason that the best adaptation is guaranteed through conditions changing continuously in the environment due to the inherent order in chaos (Feigenbaum, 1978; Prigogin & Stengers, 1981), or through the deterministic chaos of nonlinear and/or dissipative systems. Pure chaos is too confused and pure order too inflexible, so a combination of both developed in the evolution of living beings.

Synergy comes between all parts of the organism enabled with coherence, with the result of a highly organized entirety. This shows itself equal to the demands and appropriately reactive to exterior stressors and dangers.

The distribution of accelerated electrons and consequently entropy becomes keys for the understanding of the organizational state of the organism. However, there is a difference between animals and mankind: Animals are determined by their instinct. They do not own a higher consciousness and they have low creativity, whereas humans have low instinct and high creativity.

This means that the lognormal distribution is typical for all living beings beside humans, and for humans the golden-section distribution is the typical one. This regulation type is situated at the laser threshold (Table 1), which is the last bastion of the order inside chaos (Type 3). Health is considered to be a wavelike motion, a crest between two terminals: a gentle one and an extreme one.

Order is necessary as a basis for continuity, and lability is the basis for adaptations as well as for all charm-reaction courses of events. These two soft polarities should be sufficient for life; however, extreme terminals are usually taking place that lead to diseases and finally to death. Our analysis is able to detect the actual condition of the organism by distinguishing five types.

There are two chaotic (1 + 2) and two rigid (4 + 5) types, and two soft (2 + 4) and two extreme (1 + 5) types. The soft types lead to dysfunctions and abnormal conditions that are usually reversible by lifestyle modifications. However, in the case of extreme types, more serious consequences will follow like diseases that need treatment in order to be cured. Table 2 demonstrates examples of this.

PROBLEM FORMULATION

Up to now, the theory of chaos and the methods of statistical analysis seemed to be more important than appearances in nature. Previous results (Doepp & Edelmann, 2003, 2004) had led us to the assumption that analysis is not only a question of distinguishing between lognormal and normal distribution, but of distinguishing more patterns. The routine usage of distribution analysis in more than 1,000 cases showed us that distributions with two, three, or more peaks representing the coincidence of different ab-

Table 1. Relationships between physics, system statistics, and medicine: five principally different types

Frequency-Distribution Analysis of Biological Data: Five Types				
open system		health	closed system	
accelerated electrons < 50%		dynamic equilibrium metastable	accelerated electrons > 50%	
integration of influences			emission of influences	
high entropy high adaption high absorption high-frequency modulation low coherence		life at the laser threshold act of balance	low entropy low adaption low absorption low-frequency modulation high coherence	
predominantly coincidental intuition, flexibility Yin			predominantly ordered ratio, reason Yang	
extremely:	lability	centered	stability	*extremely:*
chaos	catabolism creativity	wavelike motion, sine curve, dynamics, evolution	anabolism clearness	**rigidity**
vagotonic			sympathetic	
matrix: increased sol		sol : gel = 50 : 50	matrix: increased gel	
diseases: auto-aggression cancer fatigue syndr.	*abnormal conditions:* sensitivity neurosis allergy	order + coincidence = deterministic chaos	*abnormal conditions:* distress overacidity cramping	*diseases:* depression Parkinson's sclerosis
bell curve: Gaussian	**tendency toward bell curve**	**golden section**	**lognormal**	**delta type**
a : b ≥ 1,0	a : b ≈ 0,8	a : b ≈ 0,618	a : b ≈ 0,45	a : b ≤ 0,3
Type 1	**Type 2**	**Type 3**	**Type 4**	**Type 5**

Notes: a and b are complementary distances on the abscissa in the frequency-distribution histogram. a = distance from the left limit to the maximum, b = distance from the maximum to the right limit

normalities are not so rare. We investigated several families concerning their frequency-distribution patterns in order to find out a possible heritage. In this study, different patterns inside the frequency-distribution histograms should be examined if certain types are to be found in two to three generations of two families, suggesting a heritability of system analysis patterns.

Material and Methods

We use as qualified measured values the skin resistances in the original and/or final points of meridians within the meridian diagnostics and achieve a number of mostly more than 1,600 results per patient. As a result, good statistical processing is guaranteed. The resistance values are converted into their reciprocals of the conductivity since those correspond to the vitality status.

The histograms receive an evaluation of their dates retrospectively by means of chi-square (chi) and Kolmogorov-Smirnov (KS) analysis of their frequency distributions compared with the adapted normal and lognormal curves (Zhang & Popp, 1996). As discussed in earlier publications (Doepp & Edelmann, 2004),

Figure 1. Examples for the five principal frequency distribution types of human beings

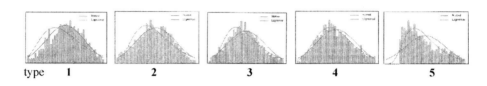

type   1   2   3   4   5

Table 2. Examples of abnormal conditions of the regulation state of the organism and typical diseases

	chaos: Types 1 or 2	rigidity: Types 4 or 5
2 and 4: abnormal states	allergy	distress → cramping
	neurosis	overacidity
	low adrenalin	High adrenalin
1 and 5: diseases	auto-aggression	sclerosis → infarction
	burnout syndrome	multiple sclerosis
	cancer (entodermal)	lymphatism
	chronic fatigue syndrome	Morbus Parkinson

we had found that the addition of the ratios of chi N/LN and KS N/LN revealed the best diagnostic relevance: a sum index (SI; see Table 3).

PROBLEM SOLUTION

Results

Out of several family results with close similarities between relatives, we selected for demonstration two: one with lability-chaos images (Figure 2) and one with a tendency toward

Table 3. Ranges of the calculated sum index

1 - chaos	< 1.9
2 - tendency toward chaos	1.9-2.6
3 - normal range	2.7-5.2
4 - tendency toward rigidity	5.3-8.2
5 - rigidity	> 8.2

rigidity (Figure 3). According to the distribution types of Family A, the following symptoms exist: neurasthenia, different allergies, sensitivities, and dependencies on various alkaloids. Obviously, a chaotic regulation means a predisposition for two, three, or even five peaks. The only person with a different pattern and phenotype is Son 1, who has another father with certainly another genetic type. Impressive is the similarity of Granddaughter 2 and her mother, showing two peaks beside a valley in the central areas of their results. The father of this girl ought to have a chaotic genetic type, too.

According to the genetic type in Family B, no chaos-typical symptoms exist; however, predominantly metabolic diseases like diabetes mellitus, high blood pressure, arterial sclerosis, obesity, and lymphatism do exist. The mother has a lognormal distribution, the father a delta-like distribution.

The children are not yet in the extreme rigidity phase but show clear tendencies. They now have the chance to work against their genetic material by bringing flexibility into their

Figure 2. Family A's frequency-distribution histograms of 12 relatives from three generations: Chaotic

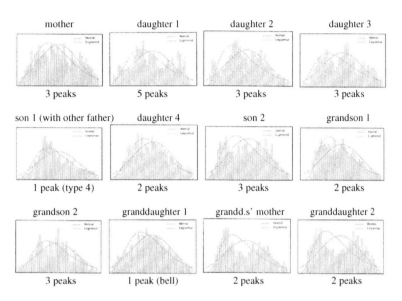

Figure 3. Family B's frequency distribution histograms of five relatives from two generations: Tendency to order and rigidity

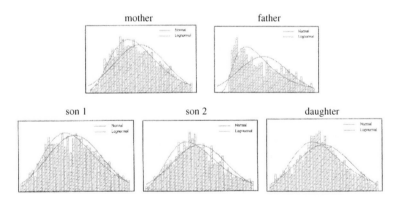

lifestyle in order to keep the genotype from becoming the phenotype as a whole.

Discussion

The two examples demonstrated here let us assume that there is a genetic disposition for a regulatory status within the range between the extreme types 1 and 5. This corresponds to a genetic disposition for the regulation variability of the vegetative nervous system. Not one of the histograms is contradictory to the assumption.

Figure 4. Frequency-distribution histogram (total analysis) of a patient with cardiac dysrhythmia (chaos peak, right) and a cerebrovascular accident (rigidity peak, left)

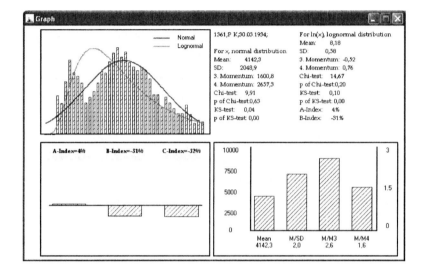

In the last years, classical distribution patterns showing one peak have been becoming rare more and more. However, the tendency toward two or more peaks is higher in persons having a chaotic distribution pattern. It seems that chaos-determining genetic material is a predisposition for bi- or multipolarity of the organism regulation, which is usually accelerated by external influences. Sometimes the psyche and the personality are incorporated by fragmentation or dissociation. Then dependencies and addictions are found according to the genetic disposition (Doepp & Edelmann, 2002). A chaotic tendency usually causes hypotonic blood pressure (low adrenalin), while a rigid tendency causes hypertonic blood pressure (high adrenalin).

In Figure 4, we demonstrate the histogram of a patient with two peaks resulting from a chaos disease (heart arrhythmia) and a rigidity disease (cerebrovascular infarction caused by a thromboembolism). His sum index is 1.0, which means that the chaos is predominant and

that the apoplectic insult is not the effect of a general arterial sclerosis.

It is to be considered, thus, that with the existence of two or more different affecting diagnoses, the frequency distribution in fact shows a superposition of two or more typical peaks. Here, pattern-recognition analysis, which can indicate distribution models characteristic of every illness, should be performed in addition to the mathematical calculation of the SI. Soft regulation abnormalities may exist temporarily and are reversible: Distress leads to rigidity as well as neurosis to chaos. Such functional-abnormal discoveries are not to be interpreted, thus, as illnesses, although they deviate from the normal.

CONCLUSION

The analysis of the frequency distribution of biological data (here, the skin resistance values in the original and final points of the meridians) facilitates a diagnostic insight into the control systems of the organism to be gained easily. The regulatory type can be classified and quantified. With a chaotic or rigid inclination go both conditions and illnesses. In this study, we demonstrate that these results can be used for the recognition of genetic disposition and heritability.

The presented analysis not only has an objective character and an evidence basis, but it can give the therapist information about the existing risks and possible illnesses in the future for the individual and the descendants. In knowledge of this, prevention can be performed successfully. Approximately 80% of the population dies of one of two illnesses: arterial sclerosis (rigid) with the result of an infarct, and cancer (partly chaotic).

Frequency-distribution analysis is not a method on its own, but is a by-product of a lot of clinical investigations of feedback-controlled systems creating adequate numbers of biological data (>500). As a computer program, it may be implemented into several medical routine activities. In each case, the state of the regulation network is determined and the patient may receive well-based recommendations for his or her lifestyle. In many cases, a second opinion is derived in the field of medical decision making. This mathematical-statistical procedure as a system analysis of the human organism has proven to be of high relevance in healthcare.

REFERENCES

Doepp, M., & Edelmann, G. (2002). The switching of the brain as an addiction-like condition: Interference of the meridians by electrosmog? *AKU, 30*(3), 133-139.

Doepp, M., & Edelmann, G. (2003). Clinical evaluation of the frequency distribution analysis of biological data. *Erfahrungsheilkunde, 12*, 818-824.

Doepp, M., & Edelmann, G. (2004). Chaos in human being: An aid for medical decision making. *WSEAS Transactions on Biology and Biomedicine, 4*(1), 403-409.

Feigenbaum, M. J. (1978). Quantitative universality for a class of nonlinear transformations. *Journal of Statistical Physics, 19*, 25.

Finch, C. E., & Tanzi, R. E. (1997). Genetics of aging. *Science, 278*, 407-410.

Gebelein, H., & Heite, H.-J. (1950). About the imbalance of biological frequency distributions. *Klin. Wochenschrift, 28*, 41.

Haken, H. (1964). A nonlinear theory of laser noise and coherence. *Zeitschrift für Physik, 181*, 96-124.

Popp, F.-A. (1987). *New horizons in medicine* (2nd ed.). Heidelberg, Germany: Haug.

Prigogine, I., & Stengers, I. (1981). *Dialog with the nature: New ways of scientific thinking*. Munich, Germany: Piper.

Rossmann, H., & Popp, F.-A. (1986). Statistics of the electro-acupuncture according to Voll. *Ärztezeitschrift für Naturheilverfahren, 1*, 51-59.

Sachs, L. (1969). *Statistical evaluation methods*. Berlin, Germany: Springer.

Zhang, C., & Popp, F.-A. (1996). Log-normal distribution measure of physiological parameters and the coherence of biological systems. In C. Zhang, F.-A. Popp, & M. Bischof (Eds.), *Current developments of biophysics* (pp. 102-111). Hangzhou University Press.

KEY TERMS

Biometric Medicine: The human organism allows the detection of huge amounts of data describing the function of organs, cell populations, and systems. For each of those data collections, mathematical and statistical evaluations may be applied in order to find normal ranges and to control the agreement of a person's results with those of a normal population. Significances are calculated.

Frequency Distribution: Biological data are collected that are generated by a randomized procedure of a measuring principle concerning any system of the organism. There should be more than 500 data. They are plotted in a graph with the measured values on the x-axis and the frequencies on the y-axis, thereby producing a distribution pattern.

Frequency-Distribution Analysis: The distribution pattern is compared with a normal curve (Gaussian) and a lognormal curve. Two mathematical methods are used for this purpose: the chi-square analysis and the Kolmogorov Smirnov analysis. Both are able to analyse the adaption of a person's value distribution by the two curves.

Heredity: It is the process by which mental and physical characteristics are passed by parents to their children. One's genetic type cannot be changed later (up to now); however, one's lifestyle often decides whether or not changes become reality in the phenotype. So, a hereditary risk is not an unchangeable fate but may be compensated for if the person gets to know it early enough and consequently can avoid certain lifestyle mistakes.

Medical Decision Making: Clinical medicine is not a science and does not produce any truth. Every diagnosis and therapy is the result of a probability calculation. For that purpose, all symptoms and digital results are emphasized according to their evidence abilities. The diagnosis with the highest probability is used as a hypothesis. It is also called the first-opinion diagnosis and should be controlled by another independent procedure producing a second opinion. An agreement of both enhances the probability of the diagnosis (and/or a therapy recommendation) in the run of the decision making.

Meridian Diagnostics: The net of meridians is one of the body's regulation systems. According to traditional Chinese medicine (TCM), 12 paired meridians exist in man. In order to determine their functional states, the electrical resistance in the beginning and the end points (Ting points) of those meridians is measured (24 points). The important conductance shows that the energetic state is reciprocal to the resistance. The test runs are performed 20 to 100 times per patient under different and randomized circumstances.

Prevention Therapy: Four hundred years ago, Sir Walter Raleigh said, "Prevention is the daughter of intelligence." This means it is better to stop a negative development from happening rather than try to deal with the problems after it has happened. However, a prevention therapy must be based on the knowledge of an undesirable development. For that purpose, existing functional and regulatory problems may be detected long before a disease becomes obvious. The solution is to use an early detection method that evaluates the state of the regulatory systems of the organism and finds out the individual risk factors.

Systems of the Human Organism: Inside the human organism, several systems exist that are all regulated by feedback mechanisms in order to maintain parameters concerned around its mean value. Some of those controlled systems are the heart rate, blood pressure, perfusion rate, immune system, lymphatic system, hormonal system, breath rate, oxygen supply, meridian system, skin temperature, and so forth. All those systems may be used in order to generate accumulations of biological data.

Chapter XLVIII
Evaluation Methods for Biomedical Technology

Maria Sevdali
Scientific Collaborator of Technological Educational Institution Kalamata, Greece

ABSTRACT

Over the past few years specialized tools for the measurement of the health level have been developed related to the quality of life (health-related quality of life—HRQOL) and in general they include both the objective and subjective criteria of human operation as it is illustrated through a person's individual and social activities. These psychometric tools are addressed either to adults or to children and actually elevate the health services user to a basic assessor of the effectiveness of medical interventions (medication, modern surgical techniques, biomedical equipment, etc.) and generally of the entire health system.

INTRODUCTION

The definition of health has been approached by different points of view. However, the prevailing definition is the one adopted by the World Health Organization (1948), which describes health as a "[s]ituation of complete bodily, mental and social well-being and not simply the absence of illness or infirmity."

Due to the particularity of health, objective difficulties exist in efforts to estimate the health status of an individual. Today, several ways of measuring health exist that reflect the variety of perceptions of health. Thus, if somebody believes that health is good physical condition, it is natural to use indicators of physical condition. If, however, social or sentimental sides of the health definition are also considered, indicators that include also these sides of health would be used.

The process of health measurement is assisted by indicators of mortality, sickliness, and positive health. The latter can be expressed itself as a subjective behavior (indicators of functional ability, general health profiles, indicators of good psychological condition, indicators of social balance, indicators of quality of life) but also as an objective reality (general indicators, indicators of general behavior, environmental indicators, socioeconomic indicators).

The utilisation of the above-mentioned indicators reflects the perception that the benefit of medical care aims at the improvement of quality of life. For that reason, these indicators are also named indicators of quality of life. Consequently, the degree of improvement of life quality for a social team constitutes the control criterion of provided medical care. Thus, such indicators constitute basic elements of the evaluation of health services, different treatments, medical operations, and so forth.

Several standardised models (questionnaires) exist for the measurement of the health status of a population concerning the quality of life (health-related quality of life, HRQOL). These tools produce a depicted plan of prosperity and portray changes of levels of natural and mental health before and after a patient's introduction to the health system.

MODELS OF HRQOL

Basic notions that can be processed by the HRQOL tools are natural and mental health through the evaluation of individual health notions. Health bodies assemble the evaluations of restrictions in individual activities (that is to say, difficulties of implementation and output in a specific activity) but also in social actions (that is to say, insufficient correspondence in the implementation of common activities) with a tool or a health plan (World Health Organization, 1997). More specifically, all the psychometric tools portray health status through a

numerical scale from 0 to 1, with death being 0 and complete health being 1. Thus, death and the quality of life are combined in a single number that can be used at the same time with other methods such as QALYs (qualitatively parked years of life), which can be used for cost-benefit analyses (Bennett & Torrance, 1996).

The HRQOL evaluation methods are subdivided into two categories: (a) adult HRQOL tools and (b) underage HRQOL tools (Tables 1 and 2). However, the sample's age-related composition is not the only application criterion for a medical result evaluation method. The selection of the assessment methods depends on a number of factors such as (a) the process means of the method (i.e., the time required to extract the results), (b) the evaluation method's reliability, possible modifications in time, and process changes, (c) the application features of the tool, and (d) the applicability of the tool content in the particular study (http://ntl.bts.gov/lib/11000/11400/11433/keynote_3.htm).

EVALUATION OF BIOMEDICAL TECHNOLOGY

The presence or absence of health symptoms does not constitute the unique criterion for conclusions with regard to the health level of an individual. The multidimensional tools of the evaluation of health-related quality of life depict the sense of prosperity in a patient through the recording of his or her psychological, social, and natural activity.

In case of the comparison of different surgical methods (a simple day operation compared to a traditionally longer one), a day operation has a limited influence on the mental health of a patient provided that he or she is allowed to return shortly to his or her way of life. It immediately exempts the patient from senti-

Table 1. Examples of generic health status and HRQOL measures for use in biomedical technology (adults)

Measure	Abbreviation	Selected References	Number of Items or Questions	Domains
Medical Outcomes 36-Item Short Form Health Survey	SF-36	Sevdali and Petropoulou (2004)	36/12	Physical functioning, physical role, bodily pain, general health, vitality, social functioning, emotional role, mental health, physical summary score, mental summary score
Quality of Well-Being Scale	QWB	Kaplan and Bush (1982)	107	Mobility, physical activity, social activity, symptom and problem complexes
European Quality of Life Scale	EuroQoL	EuroQoL Group (1990)	15	Mobility, self-care, usual activities, pain or discomfort, anxiety or depression
Functional Capacity Index	FCI	MacKenzie, Dainiano, Miller, and Luchter (1996)	64	Excretion, eating, sexual function, ambulation, bending and lifting, hand and arm movement, visual function, auditory function, speech, cognitive function
Health Utilities Index Mark III	HUI:3	Feeney, Torrance, and Furlong (1996)	45	Vision, hearing, speech, ambulation, dexterity, emotion, cognition, pain
Barthel Index	Barthel	Mahoney and Barthel (1965)	10	Bladder and bowel control, grooming, toilet use, feeding, transfer, mobility, dressing, climbing stairs, bathing
Functional Independence Measure	FIM	Linacare et al. (1994)	18	Self-care, sphincter control, mobility, locomotion, communication, social cognition

ments of pain and probable infections, decreases the cost of hospital care because of his or her short stay, and helps in the decongestion and saving of hospital beds through the benefit of qualitative utility. As far as the evaluation of the contribution of medicines of the same type (with the same degree of effectiveness for certain diseases; e.g., antibiotics) is concerned, the first step is to check the medicines' likely short-term or long-term side effects. Afterward, if the health benefit to a patient is ensured at the highest extent, the one with smaller cost is selected so that resources are guaranteed both at the individual and the sanitary level. Additionally, health plans can be very useful in the drawing of objective conclusions in cases of different estimates for the result of an illness. For example, in incidents of the hospitalisation of individuals with cerebral episodes that came back from comatose situations with residues of

Table 2. Examples of generic health status and HRQOL measures for use in biomedical technology (children and adolescents)

Measure	Abbreviation	Selected References	Number of Items or Questions	Domains
Functional Status II-Revised	FSII(R)	Stein and Jessop (1990)	43/14	Physical, psychological, intellectual, and social behavioral, manifestations of illness that interfere with age-appropriate activities
Child Health and Illness Profile	CHIP	Starfield et al. (1993)	175	Activity, comfort, satisfaction with health (perceived well-being), disorders, achievement, resilience
Pediatric Quality of Life Inventory	PedsQL	Varni, Seid, and Rode (1999)	30	Physical functioning, emotional functioning, social functioning, school functioning, well-being, global perception of overall health status
Child Health Questionnaire	CHQ	Landgraf and Abetz (1996)	50/28	Physical functioning, self-esteem, mental health, general health perceptions, behavior, bodily pain, social-physical role, social-emotional-behavioral role, parental impact and time, parental impact and emotion, family activities, family cohesion

infirmity, this situation is recorded as improvements in their medical files; however, the patients consider that they henceforth experience lower levels of quality of life, with impacts on their natural and mental health (Sevdali and Petropoulou, 2004).

CONCLUSION

Therefore, deductively we would say that the evaluation of health levels with the use of psychometrics indicators investigates the promotion of health as good and contributes to the objective evaluation of sanitary programs and health systems. HRQOL tools can cover cases in which conflicts exist between the patient and medical science. They give multifaceted dimension in health and bring the patient as a basic factor in the collection of information about the degree of the effectiveness of each therapeutic method, pharmaceutical education program, and piece of biomedical equipment in the quality of life. Their usefulness is unquestioned since they provide possibilities for applications at various levels, such as (a) microscopically at a clinic or hospital level, as in a database with elements that concern the natural, psychological, and mental health of patients with particular diseases before and after their submission in therapies, and (b) macroscopically (e.g., evaluation of the utility of patients in two or more stages due to the issuing of medicines for the confrontation of certain illnesses in combination with their cost) for the mapping out of effective health policy.

REFERENCES

Bennett, K. J., & Torrance, G. W. (1996). Measuring health state preferences and utilities: Rating scale, time trade-off, and standard gamble techniques. In B. Spilker (Ed.), *Quality of life and pharmacoeconomics in clinical trials* (2nd ed.) (pp. 253-265). Philadelphia: Lippincott-Raven Publishers.

DeBruin, A. F., De Witte, L. P., Stevens, F., & Diederiks, J. P. M. (1992). Sickness impact profile: The state of the art of a generic functional status measure. *Social Science Medicine, 35*(8), 1003-1014.

EuroQol Group. (1990). EuroQol: A new facility for the measurement of health-related quality of life. *Health Policy, 16,* 199-208.

Feeny, D. H., Torrance, G. W., & Furlong, W. J. (1996). Health utilities index. In B. Spilker (Ed.), *Quality of life and pharmacoeconomics in clinical trials* (2nd ed.) (pp. 239-252). Philadelphia: Lippincott-Raven Publishers.

Kaplan, R. M., & Bush, J. W. (1982). Health-related quality of life measurement for evaluation research and policy analysis. *Health Psychology, 1,* 61-80.

Landgraf, J. M., & Abetz, L. N. (1996). Measuring health outcomes in pediatric populations: Issues in psychometrics and application. In B. Spilker (Ed.), *Quality of life and pharmacoeconomics in clinical trials* (2nd ed.) (pp. 793-802). Philadelphia: Lippincott-Raven Publishers.

Linacre, J. M., Heinemann, A. W., Wright, B. D., Granger, C. V., & Hamilton B. B. (1994). The structure and stability of the functional independence measure. *Arch Phys Med Rehabil, 75,* 127-132.

MacKenzie, E. J., Dainiano, A., Miller, T., & Luchter, S. (1996). The development of the functional capacity index. *Journal of Trauma, 41,* 799.

Mahoney, F. I., & Barthel, D. W. (1965). Functional evaluation: The Barthel index. *Maryland State Medical Journal, 14,* 56-61.

Sevdali, M., & Petropoulou, M. (2004). *Measurement of health levels using the evaluation method sf36: Comparative study of 2 hospital units* (pp. 11-15). Patra, Greece: Helenic Open University.

Staffield, B., Reiley, A., Green, B., Ensminger, M., Ryan S., Kelleher, K., et al. (1997). The adolescent child health and illness profile: A population-based measure of health. *Medical Care, 33,* 553-566.

Stein, R. E. K., & Jessop, D. J. (1990). Functional status II(R): A measure of child health status. *Medical Care, 28,* 1041-1055.

Varni, J. W., Seid, M., & Rode, C. A. (1999). The PedsQL: Measurement model of the pediatric quality of life inventory. *Medical Care, 37,* 126.

World Health Organization (1948). *World Health Organization constitution.* Geneva, Switzerland: Author.

World Health Organization. (1997). *The international classification of impairments, activities and participation: A manual of dimensions of disablement and functioning. Beta-1 draft for field trials.* Geneva, Switzerland: Author.

Section XII
Ergonomic and Safety Issues in Computerized Medical Equipment

As the cost of microcomputer technology continues to drop, computers are also now increasingly being used in medical systems and equipment such as ventilators and pacemakers, sometimes with safety-critical results. Ergonomic user-interface design, alarm design, and safety issues in computerized medical equipment are clearly presented and discussed in this section.

Chapter XLIX
Ergonomic User Interface Design in Computerized Medical Equipment

D. John Doyle
Cleveland Clinic Foundation, USA

ABSTRACT

Current statistics suggest that preventable medical error is a common cause of patient morbidity and mortality, being responsible for between 44,000 and 98,000 deaths annually, and resulting in injuries that cost between $17 billion and $29 billion annually. An important approach to tackling this problem is to apply system design principles from human factors engineering (ergonomics). By doing so, systems and equipment become easier for people to work with, ultimately reducing the frequency of errors. In particular, in the case of medical equipment, the design of the user interface can impact enormously on its successful use. In this chapter we consider some of the elements of good and bad medical equipment design, using examples drawn from the literature and elsewhere. The concept of ecological interface design is also discussed, and some practical design guidelines are provided.

INTRODUCTION

American statistics suggest that preventable medical error is the eighth leading cause of death, being responsible for between 44,000 and 98,000 deaths annually, and resulting in injuries that cost between $17 billion and $29 billion annually (Kohn, Corrigan, & Donaldson, 1999). Experts have often stated that an impor-

tant approach to improving patient safety is to apply system design principles from human-factors engineering (ergonomics; Kohn et al.; Leape, 1994). Human-factors engineering is a relatively young scientific discipline that focuses on those factors that affect the performance of individuals using systems or equipment (Kroemer, 2001). The product may be as simple as a spoon or an office chair, or as complex as an aircraft carrier, but in all cases the goal is to design products to conform to human nature rather than merely expect people to adapt to technology. By doing so, systems and equipment become easier for people to work with, ultimately reducing the frequency of errors.

In the case of medical equipment, the design can impact enormously on its successful use. In particular, errors in operating such equipment are often caused, at least in part, by the design of the user interface. Of course, such errors can not only hamper patient care, but in some cases can even lead to injury or death. It is obviously important that medical equipment be designed with special consideration given the impact of design on safe operation. Thus, the user interface for medical equipment should be straightforward and intuitive: If its operation is excessively complex or counterintuitive, safety can be compromised. Human-factors techniques have been applied to other industries, such as nuclear power and aviation, and have been very successful in reducing error and improving safety in these contexts. Note also that in addition to increasing safety, an added benefit of using good ergonomic design practices is the likelihood that training costs will be reduced.

BAD DESIGN EXAMPLES

Examples of perplexing, arcane, and hazardous designs produced in violation of ergonomic principles are not hard to find. For instance, Michael J. Darnell's Web site www.baddesigns.com offers a collection of frequently humorous examples. But when bad designs in medical equipment lead to injury or death, the situation can be far from amusing. This is sometimes the case for computerized medical equipment.

In one case reported on the U.S. Food and Drug Administration Web site (http://www.fda.gov), a patient was overdosed after a nurse read the number 7 as a 1 in the drug-infusion pump display. Because the flow-rate display was recessed, the top of the 7 was blocked from view at many viewing angles.

In another case report from the same source, a physician treating a patient with oxygen set the flow-control knob between 1 and 2 liters per minute, not realizing that the scale numbers represented discrete, rather than continuous, settings. Unbeknownst to the physician, there was no oxygen flow between the settings, even though the knob rotated smoothly, implying that intermediate settings were available. The patient, an infant, became hypoxic before the error was discovered. One solution could have been a rotary control that snaps into discrete settings.

In yet another case, a patient on a ventilator died following the accidental detachment of the ventilator tubing from the humidifier. Unfortunately, an alarm did not sound because the pressure-limit alarm setting had been set so low that it was essentially nonfunctional.

Finally, Figure 1 illustrates a less hazardous example drawn from personal experience.

A series of reports from the laboratory of Dr. Kim Vicente of the University of Toronto have looked at user-interface issues for patient-controlled analgesia (PCA) equipment (Lin, Isla, Doniz, Harkness, Vicente, & Doyle, 1998; Lin, Vicente, & Doyle, 2001; Vicente, Kada-Bekhaled, Hillel, Cassano, & Orser, 2003). PCA is a computer-based medical technology used to treat severe pain via the self-administration of analgesic agents such as morphine. Potential benefits include superior pain control, automatic documentation, and improved utilization of nursing resources.

Unfortunately, however, one of these units (Abbott Lifecare 4100 PCA Plus II) has been linked to a number of overdose deaths. This machine is easily set up incorrectly by

Figure 1. The user interface for medical equipment should be straightforward, friendly, and intuitive. Also, rarely is the operating manual available to the end user, which makes the labeling of the controls especially important. Consider then the user controls shown for this operating-room table in use at the author's facility. The top and bottom left-hand controls lower the head and feet, respectively, while the right-hand controls raise the head and feet. But what if the entire operating table is to be raised or lowered, which is by far the most common request from the surgeon? It turns out that the entire table is raised by pushing both right-hand buttons, while the entire table is lowered by pushing both left-hand buttons. This arrangement makes sense if one thinks about it for a while, but an intuitive interface should not require a lot of thinking. Furthermore, there is plenty of space available on the control panel to add two extra buttons.

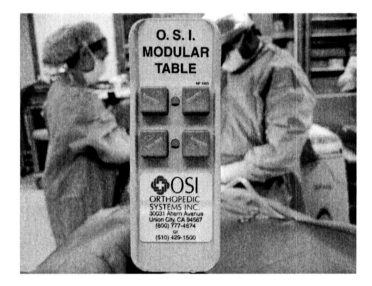

caregivers, who must manually enter the PCA parameters, and a number of patients have received drug overdoses as a result of user errors when using this product: the insertion of a 5 mg/mL morphine cartridge when the machine is expecting a 1 mg/mL concentration, or the acceptance of the default (initial) drug concentration when the correct action is to scroll up to the correct value, among other errors. In the latter case, when nurses program the drug concentration, the Lifecare 4100 display shows a particular concentration (e.g., 0.1 mg/mL). Nurses can either accept this initially displayed value or modify it using the arrow controls. The critical flaw in the design is that in this situation, the Lifecare 4100 offers the minimal drug concentration as the initial choice. If nurses mistakenly accept the initially displayed minimal value (e.g., 0.1 mg/mL) instead of changing it to the correct (and higher) value (e.g., 2.0 mg/mL), the machine will run as if the drug is less concentrated than it really is. As a result, it will pump more liquid, and thus more of the drug, into the patient than is desired.

Aware of the dangers of the Lifecare 4100, Lin, Isla, et al. (1998) and Lin, Vicente, et al. (2001) studied the unit using cognitive task-analysis techniques. Based on this analysis, the interface was then redesigned "to include a dialog structure with fewer steps, a dialog overview showing the user's location in the programming sequence, better command feedback, easier error recovery, and clearer labels and messages " (Lin, Isla, et al., 1998, p. 253). Studies of the new interface showed significantly faster programming times, lower mental workload, and fewer errors compared to the manufacturer's original interface. Regrettably, the improved interface design was not used by the manufacturer.

DESIGN GUIDELINES

The U.S. Food and Drug Administration has offered a number of guidelines to help with the design of medical equipment, such as the following (adapted from http://www.fda.gov):

- Make the design consistent with user expectations; both the user's prior experience with medical devices and well-established conventions are important.
- Design workstations, controls, and displays around the basic capabilities of the user, such as strength, dexterity, memory, reach, vision, and hearing.
- Design well-organized and uncluttered control and display arrangements. Keys, switches, and control knobs should be sufficiently apart for easy manipulation and placed in a way that reduces the chance of inadvertent activation.
- Ensure that the association between controls and displays is obvious. This facilitates proper identification and reduces the user's memory load.

- Ensure that the intensity and pitch of auditory signals and the brightness of visual signals allow them to be perceived by users working under real-world conditions.
- Make labels and displays so that they can be easily read from typical viewing angles and distances.
- Use color and shape coding to facilitate the identification of controls and displays. Colors and codes should not conflict with industry conventions.

ECOLOGICAL INTERFACE DESIGN

Ecological interface design (EID) is a conceptual framework developed by Vicente and Rasmussen (1990, 1992) for designing human-machine interfaces for complex systems such as are often found in process-control applications or in computer-based medical equipment. The primary goal of EID is to aid operators, especially knowledge workers, in handling novel or unusual situations. Studies suggest that the use of EID methods can improve operator performance when compared with classical design approaches (Vicente, 2002). The basis for EID is Rasmussen's (1986) skills-rules-knowledge model of cognitive control, and in this model, critical incidents can result from errors at any of the skills-rules-knowledge levels of human cognition.

The first form of incident includes skill-based errors involving the faulty execution of an otherwise correct plan. Here, behavior is unconscious, nonverbal, and automatic. An example would be inadvertently turning on the wrong switch. Even the most experienced clinicians are prone to skill-based errors as they often occur during highly routine procedures such as in reading a drug label or adjusting a control.

A second category is rule-based errors and involves the failure to apply a rule, such as stopping at a stop sign when driving a car, or not administering a drug to which the patient is allergic. At this level, one step up in Rasmussen's (1986) cognitive model, people use stored (or precompiled) rules acquired with training or with experience on the job.

Lastly, there are knowledge-based errors in which the initial intention is itself wrong, often due to inadequate knowledge or experience. A clinical example would be administering 10 mg of morphine to an infant. This corresponds to Rasmussen's (1986) highest cognitive level, and is most suited for unfamiliar environments where prior experience is unavailable to provide a system of rules, such as troubleshooting a new piece of medical equipment for the first time.

Under Rasmussen's (1986) skills-rules-knowledge model, human behavior moves along a ladder as experience increases. Early on, when one is placed in an unfamiliar environment, problem-solving behavior will be at the knowledge level. As experience is gained so that rules can be formed, the rules level takes over. In some situations, further experience may lead to even further automation (skills level).

For each of the three cognitive levels, the way in which information and environmental cues are perceived differs. Signals guide skill-based behavior, while symbols apply to knowledge-based behavior. Signals supply time-space information only; they have no meaning at higher levels, and they cannot be verbalized. Signs may trigger rules (stop, start, etc.) or may indicate the state of the system (valve open or closed), but they do not express functional relationships (e.g., the consequences of an open valve). Finally, symbols refer to concepts that support analytical reasoning, such as mod-eling the system to allow one to determine the consequences of an open valve.

What does all this have to do with avoiding human error when operating complex medical equipment? The answer lies in the following. Rasmussen's (1986) three levels of cognition can be grouped into two broader categories: (a) analytical-based behavior (knowledge-based behavior) and (b) perceptual-based behavior (rule and skill based). Such a categorization is helpful because perceptual processing has important advantages over analytical-based behavior: Analytical behavior is slow, demanding, and serial in nature, whereas perceptual behavior is fast, effortless, parallel, and less error prone. Thus, the goal of design should be to help people avoid situations requiring them to work at the knowledge-based level, while supporting the use of analytical problem solving for use in unfamiliar situations. And, as emphasized above, design guidelines that match the environment to the people involved is known as ecological interface design.

REFERENCES

Kohn, L. T, Corrigan, J. M., & Donaldson, M. S. (1999). *To err is human: Building a safer health system.* Washington, DC: National Academy Press.

Kroemer, K. H. E. (2001). *Ergonomics: How to design for ease and efficiency* (2nd ed.). Upper Saddle River, NJ: Prentice Hall.

Leape, L. L. (1994). Error in medicine. *The Journal of the American Medical Association, 272,* 1851-1857.

Lin, L., Isla, R., Doniz, K., Harkness, H., Vicente, K. J., & Doyle, D. J. (1998). Applying human factors to the design of medical equipment: Patient-controlled analgesia. *Journal of Clinical Monitoring and Computing, 14,* 253-263.

Lin, L., Vicente, K. J., & Doyle, D. J. (2001). Patient safety, potential adverse drug events, and medical device design: A human factors engineering approach. *Journal of Biomedical Informatics, 34*, 274-284.

Rasmussen, J. (1986). *Information processing and human-machine interaction: An approach to cognitive engineering.* New York: North-Holland.

Vicente, K. J. (2002). Ecological interface design: Progress and challenges. *Human Factors, 44*, 62-78.

Vicente, K. J., Kada-Bekhaled, K., Hillel, G., Cassano, A., & Orser, B. A. (2003). Programming errors contribute to death from patient-controlled analgesia: Case report and estimate of probability. *Canadian Journal of Anaesthesia, 50*, 328-332.

Vicente, K. J., & Rasmussen, J. (1990). The ecology of human-machine systems II: Mediating "direct perception" in complex work domains. *Ecological Psychology, 2*, 207-250.

Vicente, K. J., & Rasmussen, J. (1992). Ecological interface design: Theoretical foundations. *IEEE Transactions on Systems, Man and Cybernetics, 22*, 589-596.

KEY TERMS

Cognitive Task Analysis (CTA): A family of methods and tools for understanding the mental processes central to observable behavior, especially those cognitive processes fundamental to task performance in complex settings. Methods used in CTA may include knowledge elicitation (the process of obtaining information through in-depth interviews and by other means) and knowledge representation (the process of concisely displaying data, depicting relationships, etc.).

Ecological Interface Design (EID): A conceptual framework for designing human-machine interfaces for complex systems such as computer-based medical equipment. The primary goal of EID is to aid operators, especially knowledge workers, in handling novel or unanticipated situations.

Ergonomics: A synonym for human-factors engineering, especially in the European literature.

Human-Factors Engineering (HFE): The branch of engineering devoted to the study of the interactions between humans and systems, especially complex systems, with the goal of designing systems that are safe, comfortable, effective, and easy to use.

Patient-Controlled Analgesia (PCA): A computer-based medical technology used to treat severe pain via the self-administration of analgesic agents such as morphine.

Skills-Rules-Knowledge Model: A multilevel model of cognitive control developed by Rasmussen that is especially helpful in examining human error and critical incidents.

User Interface: The components of a system that the operator uses to interact with that system. For example, in the case of a computer, the operator interacts with it using the monitor, keyboard, mouse, and so forth.

Chapter L
Safety Issues in Computerized Medical Equipment

D. John Doyle
Cleveland Clinic Foundation, USA

ABSTRACT

Computers now are being used increasingly in safety-critical systems like nuclear power plants and aircraft and, as a consequence, have occasionally been involved in deadly mishaps. As microcomputer technology continues to proliferate, computers are also now increasingly being used in medical equipment such as ventilators and pacemakers, sometimes with safety-critical results. This chapter discusses some of the special concerns that arise when computer technology is introduced into medical equipment, using two case studies as examples: the Therac-25 radiation therapy unit and Abbott's patient controlled analgesia machine. Also discussed are some of the regulations that have been proposed by the (American) Food and Drug Administration (FDA) to help tackle the special problems that can arise when developing software-based medical equipment.

INTRODUCTION

Computers are now increasingly being introduced into safety-critical systems like nuclear power plants and aircraft, and, as a consequence, have occasionally been involved in deadly mishaps. As the cost of microcomputer technology continues to drop, computers are also now increasingly being used in medical systems and equipment such as ventilators or pacemakers, sometimes with safety-critical results. This article illustrates some of the special concerns that arise when computer technology is introduced into medical equipment using two case studies as examples. Also discussed are some of the regulations that have been proposed by the (American) Food and Drug Administration (FDA) to help tackle the special problems that can arise when developing software-based medical equipment.

THE CASE OF THE THERAC-25 RADIATION THERAPY UNIT

In 1986, two cancer patients died when they received lethal doses of radiation from a Therac-25 radiotherapy unit. An investigation revealed that one contributor to this catastrophe was the failure of the design team to recognize a race condition: a miscoordination between concurrent tasks. This error resulted in individuals being overradiated (to death in two cases) in Texas and Georgia while receiving cancer therapy using the Therac-25 system (Leveson & Turner, 1993).

Although the technical details of the failure remain secret as a result of a legal settlement, experts have come up with the following account as the most likely accident scenario. A modern radiation-therapy machine is based on a linear accelerator that produces a high-energy electron beam. One may direct the electrons directly into the patient, or, to produce X-rays, one places a heavy metal target in the electron beam so that when the electron beam hits the target, X-rays come out from the other end. The target is moved in and out of the beam automatically under software control, depending on whether an electron beam or an X-ray beam is selected to treat the patient. Also, the current in the electron beam is programmed to be much greater in the X-ray mode because of energy losses that result when the target is used in making X-rays.

However, in the overdose cases, because of a software-design error, the computer ran as if it was in X-ray made rather than in electron mode, resulting in excessive radiation. The problem was a subtle error that no one had detected during the extensive testing the machine had undergone before being introduced into clinical use. In fact, the error surfaced only when an operator happened to use a specific, unusual combination of keystrokes to instruct the machine about the radiation parameters to be used. Srpecifically, if an extremely fast-typing operator inadvertently selected the X-ray mode instead of the electron-beam mode, and then used an editing key to correct the command to select the electron-beam mode instead, it was possible for the computer to lag behind the orders. The result was that the device appeared to have made the correction but in fact still had incorrect settings.

How could this happen? Experts speculate that the software developer might not have considered it necessary to guard against this failure mode or might not have even imagined it since radiation-therapy designers have traditionally used electromechanical interlocks to ensure safety in this setting. Also, analysts reviewing the case noted that the unit should have been programmed to discard unreasonable readings, as the injurious setting presumably would have been. Finally, there should have been no way for the computer's verifications on the video screen to become unsynchronized from the keyboard commands.

ERGONOMIC ISSUES

Ergonomics is the art and science of matching equipment design and job procedures to the worker, usually with a view to reducing error and improving productivity. Ergonomics may additionally be defined as the study of the interaction between people and machinery, and the factors that influence that interaction. Also known as human factors, ergonomics is a relatively new discipline, but one that has led to enormous improvements in equipment design as the principles of good ergonomic design have become discovered and refined over time (Kroemer, 2001; Vicente, 2004). As a result, equipment ranging from automobiles and photocopiers to nuclear power plants have all seen improvements in design from the application of ergonomic principles.

Still, examples of confusing, baffling, and even dangerous designs produced in violation of ergonomic principles are not hard to find. For instance, Michael J. Darnell's Web site www.baddesigns.com offers a collection of frequently amusing examples. But when bad designs lead to injury or death, the situation can be far from entertaining. This is sometimes the case for computerized medical equipment.

THE CASE OF THE ABBOTT PATIENT-CONTROLLED ANALGESIA MACHINE

In the case of the Therac-25 system, the unit did not operate as the designers intended. However, the poor ergonomic design of complex medical equipment can lead to patient morbidity and mortality even while still operating correctly. The following case study illustrates this situation.

Patient-controlled analgesia (PCA) is a computer-based medical technology now used extensively to treat postoperative pain via the self-administration of analgesic agents such as morphine (Ferrante, Ostheimer, & Covino, 1990). Potential benefits include superior pain control, automatic electronic documentation, and improved utilization of nursing resources. Unfortunately, however, analgesics are also a frequent cause of adverse drug events, usually related to respiratory depression (Bates et al., 1995; Classen, Pesotnik, Evans, & Burke, 1991).

A typical PCA machine contains an embedded computer programmed to give, for instance, 1 mg of morphine intravenously every time the patient pushes a button on the end of a cable. To help prevent excessive drug administration, the onboard computer ignores further patient demands until a lockout period (usually

set for 5 to 10 minutes) has passed. In addition, 1-hour or 4-hour cumulative limits also are available in some models.

Despite such safety features, numerous reports of respiratory depression and death associated with PCA pumps have appeared (Baxter, 1994; Etches, 1994; Geller, 1993; Kwan, 1995). One particularly notorious unit is the Abbott Lifecare 4100 PCA Plus II machine. This machine is easily misprogrammed by caregivers, who must manually enter the PCA parameters, and is in need of a more sensible and forgiving user interface (Lin, Isla, Doniz, Harkness, Vicente, & Doyle, 1998). A number of patients have received drug overdoses as a result of PCA errors when using this product: the insertion of a 5 mg/mL morphine cartridge when the machine is expecting a 1 mg/mL concentration, or the acceptance of the default (initial) drug concentration when the correct action is to scroll up to the correct value, among other errors (Doyle, 2003; Lin, Vicente, & Doyle, 2001; Vicente, Kada-Bekhaled, Hillel, Cassano, & Orser, 2003).

In 1997, ECRI (Emergency Care Research Institute, 1997) documented three deaths that occurred while patients were connected to the Lifecare 4100. In at least two of the cases, the alleged reasons for the deaths were the same. In the mode of operation in use, when nurses program the drug concentration, the Lifecare 4100 display shows a particular concentration (e.g., 0.1 mg/mL). Nurses can either accept this initially displayed value or modify it using the arrow controls. The critical flaw in the design is that in this situation, the Lifecare 4100 offers the minimal drug concentration as the initial choice. If nurses mistakenly accept the initially displayed minimal value (e.g., 0.1 mg/mL) instead of changing it to the correct (and higher) value (e.g., 2.0 mg/mL), the machine will run as if the drug is less concentrated than it really is. As a result, it will pump more liquid, and thus more of the drug, into the patient than is desired.

One potentially important consideration in the case of the Abbott PCA machine is that the device operates exactly as specified in the technical and operations manuals: The problem is primarily one of the unwise selection of user defaults. This makes the situation different from design flaws such as those in the Therac-25 where the flawed unit operates in a manner differently than the design specifications require. While some individuals might argue that there is no design flaw present in the Abbott PCA unit in the sense that it operates exactly as the designers intended, it should be clear that where an alternative design exists that is safer and no more costly or difficult to implement, the original design must be considered to be inferior, flawed, or defective.

FDA REGULATIONS FOR MEDICAL SOFTWARE DEVELOPMENT

Concerns such as those identified above raise the issue of whether a certification process for the development and testing of medical software should be in place. Interested parties include all medical software developers, medical equipment manufacturers, the Food and Drug Administration, Canada's Health Protection Branch, and, of course, a variety of standards agencies (ANSI, ASTM, CEN, CSA, IEEE, ISO, UL). Most efforts emphasize good software-development practices and special safety measures appropriate to the clinical setting.

In recent years, at least partly as a result of patients injured or killed due to medical software defects, the FDA has taken a special interest in computer and software issues as they relate to the clinical domain. In particular, the 1990 Medical Device Amendments to the

Food and Drug Act have led to significant changes in the regulation of medical software. This act now places special emphasis on quality issues and the need to incorporate validation criteria in design from the very beginning of system development. The act also replaces the prior emphasis on a premarket approval process with a focus on postmarket surveillance, and users are now required to report to the FDA and the manufacturer any defects that cause injuries or death. A number of reports dealing with these and related issues have been published (Coppess, Miller, Zipes, & Groh, 1999; Crumpler & Rudolph, 1997; Martensson, 1993; Murfitt, 1990; Schnider, 1996; Trimbach, 1995). In addition, the FDA itself has placed some excellent didactic materials on the Web (FDA, 2005a, 2005b, 2005c). These resources would be expected to be valuable to all workers in mission-critical domains.

Medical software can be defined as a set of instructions that enables a computer to monitor or control a medical device. Their regulations for medical software developers would require a software developer to show that the algorithm, or mathematical technique, used in the computer program has been correctly implemented in software. The FDA also requires assurance through a risk analysis that any software failure could not injure a patient. How that assurance can be provided in general is still unclear since any risk analysis is necessarily linked to the specifics of the application. For instance, clinicians will instantly recognize that software errors in controlling a sodium nitroprusside infusion are far more likely to result in patient injury than, say, a real-time phonocardiographic monitoring system designed to detect the new onset of cardiac murmurs in coronary care unit patients (for example, with suspected ischemia of the mitral valve musculature). Techniques for evaluating software safety are relatively new, drawn in part from the aviation and nuclear industries as well as from academia. Who does the checking, how much evidence is enough, and whether the FDA or other authority can perform an independent check of the software are important regulatory and cost issues. Furthermore, software developers may be wary of submitting complete listings of their computer programs because of concerns that competitors might get a look at the source code via a request under the (American) Freedom of Information Act.

One advocated approach to this challenge is to begin with the idea that not all computer errors are equally serious, as with the example given above where drug-controller systems are seen to be riskier than, say, a simple monitor. Thus, risk-analysis techniques would require more exhaustive safeguards in software developed for risky applications as compared to applications that are inherently safer. Software developers must also continue to improve the methods they use for documenting, writing, testing, and maintaining medical computer programs. The need for software-development methods that insure that programs are written in a consistent, easily understood, and reliable way must be seen to be paramount. Too often, programmers include a description of what each part of their program does (the documentation) only as an afterthought rather than starting their software writing from specifications provided in a carefully developed design document.

As with buggy commercial software, in the rush to the marketplace, when delays can put a company at a competitive disadvantage, software testing may lose out. This can happen even in the medical environment. Delays in releasing a software package to allow additional testing must be balanced against the possibility of failing to detect any errors. When financial losses or injury result from software defects, the situation can lead to lawsuits. Software is clearly a product, and if it is defec-

tive and injures a consumer or a patient, then the manufacturer may be liable. To many medical-device producers, the threat of litigation may be even more effective than government regulations for assuring the quality of medical software products.

REFERENCES

Bates, D. W., Cullen, D. J., Laird, N., Petersen, L. A., Small, S. D., Servi, D., et al. (1995). Incidence of adverse drug events and potential adverse drug events: Implication for prevention. *The Journal of the American Medical Association, 274*, 29-34.

Baxter, A. D. (1994). Respiratory depression with patient-controlled analgesia. *Canadian Journal of Anaesthesia, 41*, 87-90.

Classen, D. C., Pesotnik, S. L., Evans, R. S., & Burke, J. P. (1991). Computerized surveillance of adverse drug events in hospital patients. *The Journal of the American Medical Association, 266*, 2847-2851.

Coppess, M. A., Miller, J. M., Zipes, D. P., & Groh, W. J. (1999). Software error resulting in malfunction of an implantable cardioverter defibrillator. *Journal of Cardiovascular Electrophysiology, 10*, 871-873.

Crumpler, E. S., & Rudolph, H. (1997). FDA software policy and regulation of medical device software. *Food and Drug Law Journal, 52*, 511-516.

Doyle, D. J. (2003). Programming errors from patient-controlled analgesia. *Canadian Journal of Anaesthesia, 50*, 855-856.

Emergency Care Research Institute (ECRI). (1997). Abbott PCA Plus II patient-controlled analgesia pumps prone to misprogramming resulting in narcotic overinfusions. *Health Devices, 26*, 389-391.

Etches, R. C. (1994). Respiratory depression associated patient-controlled analgesia: A review of eight cases. *Canadian Journal of Anaesthesia, 41*, 125-132.

Ferrante, F. M., Ostheimer, G. W., & Covino, B. G. (1990). *Patient-controlled analgesia.* Boston: Blackwell Scientific Publications.

Food and Drug Administration (FDA). (2005a). *Design control guidance for medical device manufacturers.* Retrieved from http://www.fda.gov/cdrh/comp/designgd.html

Food and Drug Administration (FDA). (2005b). *Do it by design: An introduction to human factors in medical devices.* Retrieved from http://www.fda.gov/cdrh/humfac/doit.html

Food and Drug Administration (FDA). (2005c). *Guidance for industry: General principle of software validation.* Retrieved from http://www.fda.gov/cdrh/comp/guidance/938.html

Geller, R. J. (1993). Meperidine in patient-controlled analgesia: A near-fatal mishap. *Anesthesia and Analgesia, 76*, 655-657.

Kroemer, K. H. E. (2001). *Ergonomics: How to design for ease and efficiency* (2nd ed.). Upper Saddle River, NJ: Prentice Hall.

Kwan, A. (1995). Overdose of morphine during PCA. *Anaesthesia, 50*, 919.

Leveson, N., & Turner, C. (1993). An investigation of the Therac-25 accidents. *Computer, 26*, 18-41.

Lin, L., Isla, R., Doniz, K., Harkness, H., Vicente, K. J., & Doyle, D. J. (1998). Applying human factors to the design of medical equipment: Patient-controlled analgesia. *Journal of Clinical Monitoring and Computing, 14*, 253-263.

Lin, L., Vicente, K. J., & Doyle, D. J. (2001). Patient safety, potential adverse drug events, and medical device design: A human factors engineering approach. *Journal of Biomedical Informatics, 34*, 274-284.

Martensson, K. (1993). Prevalidation of computer systems regulating medical device manufacturing processes. *Medical Device Technology, 4*, 22-25.

Murfitt, R. R. (1990). United States government regulation of medical device software: A review. *Journal of Medical Engineering and Technology, 14*, 111-113.

Schnider, P. (1996). FDA & clinical software vendors: A line in the sand? *Healthcare Informatics, 13*, 100-106.

Trimbach, J. (1995). FDA regulation of clinical software: What does this mean for the industry? *Healthcare Informatics, 12*, 10-14.

Vicente, K. J. (2004). *The human factor: Revolutionizing the way people live with technology.* New York: Routledge.

Vicente, K. J., Kada-Bekhaled, K., Hillel, G., Cassano, A., & Orser, B. A. (2003). Programming errors contribute to death from patient-controlled analgesia: Case report and estimate of probability. *Canadian Journal of Anaesthesia, 50*, 328-332.

KEY TERMS

ECRI: Formerly the Emergency Care Research Institute, ECRI is an independent, nonprofit health-services research agency that conducts research on patient safety issues. They maintain an online presence at http://www.ecri.org.

Ergonomics: A synonym for human-factors engineering, especially in the European literature.

Food and Drug Administration (FDA): A branch of the American government concerned with safety in medical equipment (among other things). Their Web site (http://www.fda.gov) provides a variety of useful resources for equipment designers.

Human-Factors Engineering (HFE): The branch of engineering devoted to the study of the interactions between humans and systems, especially complex systems, with the goal of designing systems that are safe, comfortable, effective, and easy to use.

Medical Device Software: Software internal to medical devices such as pacemakers, ventilators, anesthesia machines, and so forth. Software written for medical devices should be written to higher standards of safety and reliability than ordinary software.

Patient-Controlled Analgesia (PCA): A computer-based medical technology used to treat severe pain via the self-administration of analgesic agents such as morphine.

Chapter LI
Alarm Design in Computerized Medical Equipment

D. John Doyle
Cleveland Clinic Foundation, USA

ABSTRACT

Alarms are frequently employed in safety-critical environments such as in aviation and nuclear power plants. Now that microcomputer technology has revolutionized the design of patient monitors for use in modern hospital operating rooms (ORs) and intensive care units (ICUs), alarms are used in countless medical products ranging from infusion pumps to ventilators. This is especially true in anesthesia/surgical and critical care environments. In this chapter we examine the use of alarms in the acute care clinical environment, focusing on their strengths and limitations in the setting of patient monitoring equipment.

INTRODUCTION

Alarms are frequently employed in safety-critical environments such as in aviation and nuclear power plants. Now that microcomputer technology has revolutionized the design of patient monitors for use in modern hospital operating rooms (ORs) and intensive-care units (ICUs), alarms are used in countless medical products ranging from infusion pumps to ventilators. This is especially true in anesthesia or surgical and critical-care environments. In this brief review, we examine the use of alarms in the acute-care clinical environment, focusing on its strengths and limitations in the setting of patient-monitoring equipment.

ALARM DESIGN

For a clinical alarm system to be helpful when an adverse clinical situation occurs, an alarm must be sounded, the problem identified and corrected, and the patient treated. The earlier that an alarm occurs, the easier it is for the clinician to take actions to prevent patient injury (Schreiber & Schreiber, 1989).

Alarm systems in medical equipment should also be easy to (temporarily) silence, should offer power-on default settings to prevent the inadvertent use of settings meant for a previous patient, and should incorporate a display that enables the operator to detect problems or trends in its early stages. Also, the physical composition of auditory alarms should be designed to convey a sense of urgency that matches the actual urgency of the triggering clinical situation. Finally, the alarm should be nonstartling, instantly recognizable to the trained respondent, and designed such that it would not generally lead to anxiety in others, such as patients and their families (Quinn, 1989).

Alarms in medical equipment may be as straightforward as a simple threshold alarm such as an alarm that is activated when a patient's heart rate exceeds 120 beats per minute. Such simple alarm designs have the potential to be enhanced in several interesting ways. First, a duration condition might be added, such as the requirement that a patient's heart rate exceed 120 beats per minute for a period of, say, 30 seconds before alarm activation occurs. Note that such an arrangement has the potential to reduce the frequency of false alarms, but may also delay the detection of some important clinical events.

Second, the heart-rate data used for such an alarm system might be drawn from multiple sources, again in an effort to reduce the frequency of false alarms (sensor fusion). As an example, an alarm system might require that both the heart rate obtained from the electrocardiogram and the heart rate obtained from an alternate data source (e.g., pulse oximeter device, arterial catheter) exceed (or fall below) a particular number. (As a bonus, when the sources of information fail to provide similar numbers, the clinician can be informed that there is a data-quality problem, such as might result from movement artifacts or from other causes.)

New developments in intelligent or knowledge-based alarm technology have also been introduced commercially and experimentally with the hope of improving patient safety (Koski, Sukuvaara, Makivirta, & Kari, 1994; Westenskow, Orr, Simon, Bender, & Frankenberger, 1992). Such smart alarms combine expert-system techniques with alarm technology either to provide more informative alarms, to reduce the frequency of false alarms, or to provide initial suggestions about how to deal with the problem that triggered the alarm. These systems may offer the ability to change alarm priority with elapsed time (cascading alarms), or suppress secondary alarms that are the consequence of a primary alarm condition. Other smart alarm designs may suggest either a diagnosis or an operator intervention to tell the user more about how to handle the situation, or may offer a context-sensitive information display with specific clinical suggestions.

For instance, imagine a clinical monitoring system that was aware that the patient being monitored had severe coronary artery disease. Knowing that high heart rates are likely to produce coronary ischemia in such individuals, the monitor might offer a default high-heart-rate alarm of 85 beats per minute in such cases instead of a higher default heart-rate alarm (say, 120 beats per minute) that it might offer for patients with normal hearts. Similarly, alarms can be annunciated according to the urgency of the required response. Thus, a high-priority alarm requiring immediate response by a clinician might use a red indicator with a flashing frequency of 2 Hz, while a medium-priority alarm requiring prompt response to deal with a condition might use a yellow indicator with a flashing frequency of 1 Hz, and a low-priority alarm, one simply requiring awareness of a condition or indicating a change of status, might use a constant yellow indicator.

Consider also the following hypothetical example. Imagine a system in which if a patient's heart rate goes too low, say, under 30 beats per minute, it would suggest the administration of intravenous atropine, calling for the crash cart, and checking for low oxygen levels in the patient (using a pulse oximeter). It could even alert the responsible physician or operating-room coordinator by pager to inform him or her that one of the patients is in trouble.

A more mundane aspect of alarm design concerns which alarms can be disabled and for what period of time. As an example, a clinician may want to be able to silence or disable a high-heart-rate alarm for 30 seconds or a minute in order to concentrate on treating the patient. Thus, an alarm policy engine may exist within the software to ensure that the alarm limits chosen are sensible and that important alarms are not disabled or silenced for too long a time. In fact, some alarms should arguably not be disabled under any circumstances. A good example is an alarm signaling a low concentration of oxygen in the gas mixture with which the patient's lungs are being ventilated. This would be an appropriate alarm policy since false alarms are vary rare for the oxygen-concentration signal and low oxygen levels can quickly lead to brain damage. Similarly, an alarm policy engine might indicate what alarms are to be escalated to higher levels (or de-escalated to lower levels) as clinical circumstances evolve.

Another aspect of alarm design involves alarm integration. Until recent years, separate monitors existed for tracking blood pressure, the electrocardiogram, arterial oxygen levels, and so forth, and each monitor had its own alarm system with its own default alarm conventions. Furthermore, all alarms tended to sound the same as manufacturers all used

similar piezoelectric devices to provide audio warning signals. The result was an unintegrated, awkward system of monitors often designed such that when an alarm sounded, the user had to visually scan all the monitors to establish the source of the alarm. Aware of these issues, engineers, manufactures, and standards bodies set about to design integrated alarm systems in which all alarms are routed through a common operator interface in order to facilitate alarm recognition and management. In particular, the International Standards Organization (ISO) has developed ISO standard ISO/IEC 60601-1-8 to specify in detail how medical equipment alarms should be implemented. Such developments offer considerable potential to improve patient safety.

A final aspect of this topic concerns the eventual interconnection and computer control of medical devices in the OR or ICU, such as the anesthesia workstation, patient cardiac monitors, and even drug-infusion pumps. Some of these efforts center on the medical information bus (IEEE Standard 1073, http://www.ieee1073.org). The ability to regulate drug-infusion pumps from a central control point offers obvious advantages when many infusion pumps are used, as is common during cardiac surgery. A less appreciated benefit of such an arrangement is that in principle it allows for the automatic initial management of certain hazardous clinical conditions. For example, it is commonplace to use infusions of dopamine (a drug that raises blood pressure) and sodium nitroprusside (a drug that lowers blood pressure) for cardiac surgery.

However, a clinician may sometimes momentarily forget that a drug infusion is running and forget to turn off an existing nitroprusside infusion as the first response to the management of a hypotensive (low blood pressure) episode, or forget to discontinue an existing dopamine infusion in order to treat an episode of hypertension (excessive blood pressure). The ability to control infusion pumps from a central controlling station offers the potential to provide early warning about such mishaps. It would even be possible to automatically discontinue the offending infusion if no manual response were detected within a given time period. Indeed, the concept of smart alarm systems can even be extended to provide for automatic-initiation drugs to support blood pressure should the crisis not be resolved in a timely manner. Finally, as suggested above, smart alarms can even be designed to automatically call for help should certain clinical crises not be resolved in an acceptable time period.

CLINICAL REALITIES

Despite all these developments, however, many physicians working in the clinical trenches have become quite cynical about many of the developments in medical alarm technology, regarding them as more nuisances to deal with rather than as contributions to patient care. For example, many anesthesiologists note that because they are usually more or less permanently situated near the patient, they are able to keep an eye on the patient on a moment-to-moment basis so that they are usually aware of any clinical deterioration before an alarm sounds. When the alarm does sound, dealing with the alarm (e.g., silencing it, etc.) may distract the anesthesiologist from his or her efforts to treat the patient (e.g., administering drugs to restore the patient's blood pressure into the normal range). (Of course, an important counterargument is that clinicians do not always maintain 100% vigilance, especially when fatigued or distracted, so alarms may notify them of any life-threatening conditions that may have escaped their notice. This argument may be especially true in the ICU setting, where a physician will be caring for many patients.)

The potential value of alarms not withstanding, a high level of frustration exists among healthcare workers about clinical alarm designs. Of all the complaints presented by clinicians about current alarm technology, unquestionably the high rate of false alarms would be first on their list. For example, even small amounts of patient movement can introduce artifacts into the patient's electrocardiogram, pulse-oximeter signal, blood-pressure signal, and other monitored variables. Quite often the artifact is not recognized to be garbage by the alarm-management software, resulting in the false annunciation of some alarm condition. So common and so frustrating is this situation that many clinicians globally disable all alarms to allow them to focus on caring for the patient rather than dealing with false alarms.

Edworthy and Meredith (1994) reviewed many of the issues of alarm design from the perspective of cognitive psychology, with an emphasis on the construction of effective alarm sounds. They point out that there may be circumstances where the excessive use of auditory warnings may be counterproductive, while the principle of urgency mapping (involving a graded series of alarms with increasing perceived urgency levels) may be helpful to produce ergonomically sensible alarm systems.

In a study by Kestin, Miller, and Lockhart (1988), 50 patients undergoing anesthesia were monitored to determine the frequency of false alarms. They found that 75% of all the alarms overall were spurious and 22% represented a change above the upper alarm limits, but only 3% corresponded to patient risk situations. With electrocardiogram alarms the situation was worse, with 81% of the alarms being spurious, 19% representing a change above the upper alarm limits, and 0% representing a patient risk situation. Similar results were obtained with blood-pressure alarms and heart-rate alarms from pulse oximeters.

A similar study by Lawless (1994) reviewed the false-alarm problem in a pediatric ICU. During a 7-day period, ICU staff recorded the type and number of alarms, categorizing them as false, significant, or due to staff manipulations. Of 2,176 alarm soundings, 68% were false and 26.5% were due to staff manipulations, while only 5.5% were significant. Of interest, the pulse oximeter was the largest alarm source (44%), with ventilators (31%) and electrocardiograms (24%) being other common alarm sources. In contrast, only 1% of alarms were from the capnometer, a device that measures expired carbon-dioxide levels from the lung.

As already noted, not infrequently, anesthesiologists disable alarms at the beginning of a case to avoid false alarms and other alarm-related difficulties. McIntyre (1985) conducted a retrospective study in which he asked the question, "Have you ever deliberately deactivated an audible alarm device at the start of a case?" A majority (57%) of respondents replied, "Yes."

These and other studies tend to support two points. First, most alarms (fortunately) do not signify a potentially critical medical event. Second, poorly performing alarm systems may hinder, rather than help, the delivery of clinical care, especially in environments where noise pollution may be problematic (Kam, Kam, & Thompson, 1994).

REFERENCES

Edworthy, J., & Meredith, C. S. (1994). Cognitive psychology and the design of alarm sounds. *Medical Engineering and Physics, 16*, 445-449.

Kam, P. C. A., Kam, A. C., & Thompson, J. F. (1994). Noise pollution in the anaesthetic and intensive care environment. *Anaesthesia, 49*, 982-986.

Kestin, I. G., Miller, B. R., & Lockhart, C. H. (1988). Auditory alarms during anesthesia monitoring. *Anesthesiology, 69*, 106-109.

Koski, E. M., Sukuvaara, T., Makivirta, A., & Kari, A. (1994). A knowledge-based alarm system for monitoring cardiac operated patients: Assessment of clinical performance. *International Journal of Clinical Monitoring and Computing, 11*, 79-83.

Lawless, S. T. (1994). Crying wolf: False alarms in pediatric intensive care unit. *Critical Care Medicine, 22*, 981-985.

McIntyre, J. W. (1985). Ergonomics: Anaesthetist's use of auditory alarms in the operating room. *International Journal of Clinical Monitoring and Computing, 2*, 47-55.

Quinn, M. L. (1989). Semipractical alarms: A parable. *Journal of Clinical Monitoring, 5*, 196-200.

Schreiber, P. J., & Schreiber, J. (1989). Structured alarm systems for the operating room. *Journal of Clinical Monitoring, 5*, 201-204.

Westenskow, D. R., Orr, J. A., Simon, F. H., Bender, H. J., & Frankenberger, H. (1992). Intelligent alarms reduce anesthesiologist's response time to critical faults. *Anesthesiology, 77*, 1074-1079.

KEY TERMS

Alarm Integration: A design approach in which all alarms are routed through a common operator interface in order to facilitate alarm recognition and management.

Alarm Policy Engine: Software structures to ensure that the alarm limits chosen are clinically sensible and that important alarms are not disabled or silenced for an excessive period of time.

Cascading Alarms: Alarm systems that have the ability to change alarm priority with elapsed time, such as a medium-priority apnea alarm changing to a high-priority alarm when no breaths are detected for an additional 30 seconds.

Intelligent Alarms: An alarm design that combines expert-system techniques with conventional alarm technology either to provide more informative alarms, to reduce the frequency of false alarms, or to provide initial suggestions about how to deal with the problem that triggered the alarm. They are also known as smart alarms or knowledge-based alarms.

Sensor Fusion: Employing data from multiple sensors with the aim of improving system reliability.

Threshold Alarm: An alarm that is activated when a monitored parameter exceeds or goes below set thresholds.

Section XIII
Health Economics and Health Services Research

The growth of sciences and technologies during the last decades of the 20th century has resulted in the rapid development of medical science, its benefits, and also models of demand for services of health. A completely organized system of health will aim to combine human, technological, and natural resources so that it is feasible to exercise modern medical practice. It is exceptionally critical for professionals, and future professionals, to comprehend not only the sectors of their professions, but also the nature, organisation, and operation of the systems that make their professions. It is also important for citizens to judge and evaluate the health sector and its economic output in general. This section contains selected articles related to health economic issues.

Chapter LII
Organizational Factors in Health Informatics

Michelle Brear
University of New South Wales, Australia

ABSTRACT

There is a general recognition that numerous organizational factors will influence the success of an informatics intervention. This is supported by a body of evidence from multi-disciplinary and health-specific research. Organizational factors are highly interrelated and the exact nature and contribution of each to the success of an intervention is not clear. A health-specific understanding and recognition of these factors is necessary if informatics applications are to reach their potential in healthcare settings.

INTRODUCTION

The influence of organizational factors on the success of informatics interventions in healthcare has been clearly demonstrated. This health-specific research, informed by a larger body of evidence emerging from interdisciplinary organizational, psychological, and sociological research, has confirmed the view that organizational factors can be the decisive factor in the success of an intervention (Lorenzi, Riley, Blythe, Southon, & Dixon, 1997).

However, it remains rare for organizational factors to be explicitly addressed in the implementation process. As such, their contribution to the success or failure of informatics applications is not properly understood. This has implications for future interventions. Applications that were not utilized or did not perform adequately in a particular setting may be dismissed, while other less appropriate systems may be adopted because organizational factors influenced their success. Explicit study of the role of organizational factors on the implementation of health-informatics interventions is necessary to develop an understanding of their influence in the healthcare context.

Healthcare organizations tend to be highly task oriented, labor intensive, and dependent on interdisciplinary teamwork, so the influence of organizational factors within them may differ considerably from the business settings in which they have traditionally been studied (Chau, 2001). Health organizations are also increasingly underresourced due to the global downturn in government social spending, to health-sector privatization, and to aging populations. It is these characteristics that necessitate the rapid uptake of informatics applications, capable of automating aspects of healthcare provision and reducing labor intensity (Coiera, 2004).

From a technical perspective, rapid and fundamental transformation of the healthcare sector through informatics is achievable. However, without a clear understanding of, and ability to, manage organizational factors, it is unlikely that informatics applications will realize their potential in the health sector. This short review provides an overview of the key organizational factors influencing the success of informatics interventions. It begins by positioning informatics interventions in the broader context of organizational change before discussing the current understanding of selected factors.

INFORMATICS IMPLEMENTATION AS ORGANIZATIONAL CHANGE

Implementing informatics applications is essentially "a politically textured process of organizational change" (Berg, 1999, p. 87), aimed at achieving user acceptance and the utilization of informatics applications. Organizational change requires people to be aware of a need for change, to identify a particular course through which the change can occur, and to take actions to make it happen (Lorenzi, 2004). Resistance to change occurs if users are not aware of the need for change, are not convinced of the course of action set out, or are unable to carry out the necessary action. It is the users, not the technology, that should be the centre of the change process as the decision to utilize the system is ultimately theirs (Berg).

Even the best designed and well-intentioned informatics interventions are likely to lead to productivity losses in the early stages and create major changes (Lorenzi, 2004). The timely and effective training of users can reduce the disruption; however, it is not enough to ensure success as even a correctly used system can have far-reaching effects. Informaticians taking a sociotechnical approach view the application as one component of a complex system (the health organization) whose introduction will disrupt other components of the system (e.g., patients and clinicians). They advocate design approaches that aim to create technology that fits within the complex system (Kaplan, 2001).

The multidisciplinary nature of health-sector organizations makes finding the correct fit challenging (Kaplan, 2001). A range of professionals with different needs, expectations, and work norms are likely to use an application, and each will expect it to fit with his or her work practice. When an application does not fit, resistance will increase. This is often due to valid concerns about increased workload or the ability to care for patients (Timmons, 2003). When systems do not fit, the best way to overcome resistance is to change them. However, when they are essentially effective, resistance can be overcome by changing people's opinions or work norms. Organizational culture and social networks, from which many of these norms and opinions arise, need to be understood and managed.

ORGANIZATIONAL CULTURE

Organizational culture is the set of shared norms, values, and tacit rules within which members of an organization function (Lorenzi & Riley, 2000). "Every culture supports a political and social values system" (Lorenzi et al., 1997, p. 85) that will influence the reaction to an informatics application. Healthcare settings often involve a professional hierarchy between doctors and nurses, are characterized by high levels of informal and disruptive communication, and place value on clinician-patient relationships and patient care.

It is necessary to identify and target the aspects of organizational culture presenting opportunities for and barriers to success when changing the organization through an informatics intervention. Managing change requires mediating the influence of culture on events rather than necessarily aiming to change it (Demeester, 1999). Where organizational culture and informatics applications appear incompatible, adaptation of the application should be considered.

If it is not possible to modify the system, success is dependent on changing the organizational culture to make it compatible. Cultural change directly targeted at the strongly held values of users may only increase resistance. If the organizational culture supports a belief that informatics applications undermine good clinician-patient relationships, attempting to convince clinicians that good relationships with their patients are not important is unlikely to be a successful strategy for winning acceptance of the application. However, it may be possible, through an educational process, to convince clinicians that informatics applications do not necessarily undermine good relationships and in the right conditions can even enhance them. Users may already be convinced of the need to change some aspects of organizational culture

that do not threaten the values they are most passionate about. The structure of an organization, and work patterns and roles of individuals within it are influential and may be appropriate areas to encourage change.

Organizational Structure

The structure of an organization will affect the way in which decisions are made, the type of leadership that emerges, and the way resistance is dealt with in the implementation process. Flatter organizational structures tend to encourage the sharing of ideas, the emergence of innovation, and broader involvement in decision making (Leonard, Graham, & Bonacum, 2004). In these types of organizations, management tends to adopt a collaborative approach, working alongside, listening to, and involving those working on the ground rather than making decisions on their behalf and communicating orders. Management is supportive, approachable, and accountable, and shows dedication to continuous learning (Zimmerman et al., 1993). These types of organizations are more likely to include practicing clinicians in formal decision-making bodies such as management committees. They are also more likely to recognize, encourage, and legitimize the role of grassroots leaders with clinical credibility and presence, and have a commitment to involving informatics users in the implementation process.

User involvement throughout the process "leads to increased user acceptance and use by encouraging realistic expectations, facilitating the user's system ownership, decreasing resistance to change, and committing users to the system" (Lorenzi et al., 1997, p. 86). It also allows a better definition of problems and solutions from the user's perspective, and develops a better understanding amongst users of the application (Lorenzi et al.). Involving users in the design and implementation of a system is more likely to result in applications suited to the current work patterns of the intended users.

Work Patterns and Roles of Clinicians

Any informatics application must be compatible with the current work practices and values of the organization (Greenhalgh, Robert, MacFarlane, Bate, & Kyriakidou, 2004; Kaplan, 2001; Lorenzi & Riley, 2000). Compatibility will differ between organizations and cultures, so applications require the capacity to be tailored to the needs of individual organizations. Take an electronic prescribing system, for example. In one hospital, it may be used to enter prescription orders during ward rounds via a laptop computer; however, a different hospital (or even another ward within that hospital) may find it more appropriate to install the system on a computer terminal at the nurses' stations so that orders can be entered retrospectively. Bearing in mind the necessity to consider the unique context of individual organizations, it is possible to make some generalizations regarding the work patterns and roles of clinicians to broadly inform the design of informatics interventions.

Doctors have traditionally worked with a high degree of professional autonomy and status (Gagnon et al., 2003). Applications perceived to undermine their autonomy and status as professionals or "subvert the art of medical practice" (Kaplan, 2001, p. 4) are more likely to meet with resistance. In a qualitative study examining factors influencing the adoption of a CDSS (clinical decision-support system) involving automatic clinical reminders, Rousseau, McColl, Newton, Grimshaw, and Eccles (2004) found clinicians favored on-demand evidence systems to automatically generated reminders. The latter were perceived to be intrusive, often inapplicable, and not particularly useful for making patient-management decisions.

Clinicians tend to be patient focused, require an ability to maintain control of patient care, and make decisions specific to individuals, which computers are not capable of. They must be convinced that applications will not jeopardize their ability to care for patients (Timmons, 2003). Overly prescriptive systems, or those that attempt to take on the uniquely human quality of thinking, are unlikely to be successful. Rouseau et al. (2004) noted inapplicable reminders were a barrier to effective use and found that practitioners formed a habit of ignoring all reminders. In a study of adherence to electronic HIV treatment reminders, Patterson, Nguyen, Halloran, and Asch (2004) found that the inapplicability of reminders to many patients' specific situations and the time taken to document why the reminders were not adhered to were significant barriers to effective system use.

All applications will create some change to normal work patterns and roles. That is essentially what their implementation is intended to do (Berg & Toussaint, 2003). Users need to be realistically informed of and prepared for changes to normal work practice. It is inevitable that users will expect some future benefit from adapting their behaviors, and realistic communication of the likely benefits, particularly if they are indirect or not clearly visible, should form an integral part of the communication strategy.

Communication

Communication binds individuals together and is integral to the implementation process. Without effective communication, it is impossible to lead, learn, make decisions, prepare individuals for an intervention, or use the intervention effectively (Zimmerman et al., 1993). The lack of communication, or ineffective communication that lacks trust, can negatively influence the uptake of a technology (Ash, 1997). There is no magic formula for effective communication; however, there are some key principles that should be applied to enhance the effectiveness of communication.

Communication must be timely. People require time to digest information and prepare for changes (Tilley & Chambers, 2004). However, they also forget. Users who are trained to use a system months before its implementation may not remember how to use it when it finally arrives. Information must also be communicated at an appropriate time in the day. Disrupting a lunch break or patient care may not be the most appropriate way to inform users about a new application.

Communication must be sincere and truthful. Users must be offered an honest and realistic assessment of the potential negative consequences and expected benefits of an application. For example, if an electronic medical-record application is introduced, it may be realistic to expect its use to be more time consuming in the initial stages while users master the system. However, in time, its ability to provide comprehensive patient information at the click of a button may save time and provide better quality information. It is also important to acknowledge unexpected benefits and problems if they occur.

Sources of communication have an immense impact on the perceived message, its credibility, and its influence (Kaplan, 2001). A manufacturer's leaflet declaring the new system as easy to use is unlikely to carry much weight with users; however, a respected clinical peer conveying this information may be quite influential.

It is essential that the communication be recognized as multidimensional rather than a one-way channel from management to users. Mechanisms for receiving feedback must be created, and where it is not forthcoming, it should be actively elicited from users. Magrabi, Westbrook, Coiera, and Gosling (2004) incorporated two mechanisms for feedback into an online DSS. Users could volunteer feedback at any time; however, it was also actively elicited by randomly prompting users. Once received, feedback should be acted upon to adapt the application to meet user needs (Greenhalgh et al., 2004). For example, in response to clinician feedback, the patterns of automatically generated reminders in a CDSS were altered to limit the number of reminders perceived by clinicians to be inapplicable. Communication through informal structures (e.g., gossiping in the tea room) is inevitable, and the ability to manage it directly is limited. However, the less effective formal communication mechanisms are, the more likely it is that communication will take place through informal channels in the social network.

SOCIAL NETWORKS

A social network consists of the individuals, groups, and organizations with whom, and patterns of communication by which, individuals in an organization interact. It is through social networks that organizational culture and behaviors are reinforced and adapted (Lorenzi et al., 1997). The culture represented within a social network can be influential. For example, Gagnon et al. (2003) found that physicians who perceived social and professional responsibility from others in their social network to adopt telemedicine applications had a stronger intention to do so. The culture represented in each individual's social network will differ, and each individual within will interact and be influenced differently.

To properly understand a social network, it is necessary to examine the interactions, not the individuals. The frequency of interaction is important but should not be viewed in isolation from the style of communication (e.g., formal or informal), the type of communication (e.g., synchronous or asynchronous), the strength of ties between the participants in an interaction, and the power relations involved (Katz, Lazer, Arrow, Contractor, 2004). When implementing an informatics application, interactions that occur in clinical teams and with respected opinion leaders are particularly influential in relation to individuals' decisions to utilize applications.

Effective Teamwork

The clinical team has been identified as the organizational unit most influential in the diffusion of innovation (Gosling, Westbrook, & Braithwaite, 2003). Well-functioning teams facilitate effective communication, encourage continuous learning, and offer a trusting environment in which ideas and issues can be raised. Through these interactions, teams develop shared visions and common goals that support the introduction of new innovations to fulfill these goals. As work in health organizations is highly dependent on teamwork, and it is teams, not individuals, that must adopt informatics applications, well-functioning teams are a prerequisite for successful informatics implementation (Goldstein et al., 2004).

In organizations where well-functioning teams do not exist, an informatics intervention may be an opportunity to develop teams by uniting individuals around a shared vision and common goals that the application can fulfill. Doctors and nurses take on different roles and responsibilities in the process of caring for patients, so a shared vision may not be immediately apparent. However, both groups ultimately work toward the goal of providing optimal patient care, so incorporating an application into a vision of improved patient care may be a way to unite users.

Consideration should also be given to the size and composition of teams. Teams of more than 15 tend to fragment into subteams, while very small teams have a tendency to become cliquish, so ideally they should consist of 10 to 15 members (Gosling et al., 2003). The work environment may largely dictate a team's composition. In healthcare settings, teams are usually multidisciplinary. Individuals, however, are more likely to create ties with those they perceive to be similar, so identifying similarities amongst multidisciplinary teams is pertinent (Katz et al., 2004). Identifying and utilizing the influence of respected clinicians within the team can also be useful.

Clinical Champions and Opinion Leaders

Respected clinicians with influence amongst their peers and who support the intervention play an important role in convincing others of an application's worth, as do those who oppose the intervention. They are commonly referred to as clinical champions or opinion leaders. As the name champion tends to imply a positive influence and does not necessarily imply influence amongst peers (Lolock, Dopson, Chambers, & Gabbay, 2001), opinion leader will be used in this article.

Opinion leaders are individuals with the ability to influence others in the social network and who make a major personal commitment to diffusing information about an informatics application (Lorenzi & Riley, 2000). Such diffusion may have a negative or positive influence and can discourage or encourage the adoption of the application. For example, Ash (1997) identified the presence of champions as a significant factor in the diffusion of e-mail in academic health-science centres. Conversely, Timmons (2003) discusses a "strong and articulate" ward sister whose resistance to using an electronic system in the ward was successful in preventing its implementation. It is not unusual to have both negative and positive opinion leaders within a network.

Whatever their persuasion, they tend to be charismatic individuals with good interpersonal relationships based on trust and understanding. They act through clinical conviction, generally outside of the formal structures, and give applications credibility at a local level. Their role is essentially informal, and, on the proviso their colleagues respect them, they tend to be self-appointed (Lolock et al., 2001). The role is largely dependent on personal motivation and conviction, and therefore it is difficult to formalize. The potential alienating effect of being an opinion leader means that those without sufficient commitment are likely to be reluctant to take on such a role (Lolock et al.)

Despite a general consensus that successful interventions are more likely when champions are present, there is a lack of understanding about exactly what it is they do, the circumstances in which they will be influential, and how best to describe them. As with each of the factors mentioned here, opinion leaders are one small component of a large and complex system (the health organization), and it is difficult to isolate their effect. There is also considerable evidence to suggest that other factors, in particular the suitability of the application, influence the emergence of opinion leaders. Further research is needed to identify how opinion leaders influence, and how the champions amongst them can be encouraged.

CONCLUSION

There is a general recognition that numerous organizational factors will influence the success of an informatics intervention. This is supported by a body of evidence from multidisciplinary and health-specific research.

In particular, research has noted the influence of organizational culture and social networks. Organizational culture, the shared norms and values within which members of an organization function, influences the organization's structure and patterns of communication. Social networks, the individuals and groups with whom one interacts and the interactions that occur between them, are the social space in which teams are formed and work, and in which individuals are influenced, particularly by those individuals known as opinion leaders or clinical champions. Organizational factors are highly interrelated, and the exact nature and contribution of each to the success of an intervention is not clear. A health-specific understanding and recognition of these factors is necessary if informatics applications are to reach their potential in healthcare settings.

REFERENCES

Berg, M. (1999). Patient care information systems and healthcare work: A sociotechnical approach. *International Journal of Medical Informatics, 55*, 87-101.

Berg, M., & Toussaint, P. (2003). The mantra of modeling and the forgotten powers of paper: A sociotechnical view on the development of process-oriented ICT in health care. *International Journal of Medical Informatics, 69*, 223-234.

Chau, P. Y. K., & Hu, P. J.-H. (2002). Investigating healthcare professionals' decisions to accept telemedicine technology: An empirical test of competing theories. *Information and Management, 39*, 297-311.

Coiera, E. (2004). Four rules for the reinvention of healthcare. *British Medical Journal, 328*, 1197-1199.

Demeester, M. (1999). Cultural aspects of information technology implementation. *International Journal of Medical Informatics, 56*, 25-41.

Gagnon, M.-P., Godin, G., Gagne, C., Fortin, J.-P., Lamothe, L., Reinharz, D., et al. (2003). An adaption of the theory of interpersonal behaviour to the study of telemedicine adoption by physicians. *International Journal of Medical Informatics, 71*, 103-115.

Goldstein, M. K., Coleman, R. W., Tu, S. W., Shankar, R. D., O'Connor, M. J., Musen, M. A., et al. (2004). Translating research into practice: Organisational issues in implementing automated decision support for hypertension in three medical centers. *Journal of the American Medical Informatics Association, 11*(5), 368-376.

Gosling, A. S., Westbrook, J. I., & Braithwaite, J. (2003). Clinical team functioning and IT innovation: A study of the diffusion of a point-of care online evidence system. *Journal of the American Medical Informatics Association, 10*(3), 244-251.

Greenhalgh, T., Robert, G., MacFarlane, F., Bate, P., & Kyriakidou, O. (2004). Diffusion of innovations in service organisations: Systematic review and recommendations. *The Millbank Quarterly, 82*(4), 581-629.

Kaplan, B. (2001). Evaluating informatics applications. Some alternative approaches: Theory, social interactionism, and call for methodological pluralism. *International Journal of Medical Informatics, 64*, 39-56.

Katz, N., Lazer, D., Arrow, H., & Contractor, N. (2004). Network theory and small groups. *Small Group Research, 35*(3), 307-332.

Leonard, M., Graham, S., & Bonacum, D. (2004). The human factor: The critical importance of effective teamwork and communication in providing safe care, quality and safety in health care, *13*(Suppl. 1), i85-i90.

Lolock, L., Dopson, S., Chambers, D., & Gabbay, J. (2001). Understanding the role of opinion leaders in improving clinical effectiveness. *Social Science and Medicine, 53*, 745-757.

Lorenzi, N. M. (2004). Beyond the gadgets: Non-technological barriers to information systems need to be overcome. *British Medical Journal, 328*, 1146-1147.

Lorenzi, N. M., & Riley, R. T. (2000). Managing change: An overview. *Journal of the American Medical Informatics Association, 7*(2), 116-124.

Lorenzi, N. M., Riley, R. T., Blythe, A. J. C., Southon, G., & Dixon, B. J. (1997). Antecedents of the people and organizational aspects of medical informatics: Review of the literature. *Journal of the American Medical Informatics Association, 4*(2), 79-93.

Magrabi, F., Westbrook, J. I., Coiera, E. W., & Gosling, A. S. (2004). Clinicians' assessments of the usefulness of online evidence to answer clinical questions. *Proceedings of the 11th World Congress on Medical Informatics* (pp. 297-300).

Patterson, E. S., Nguyen, A. D., Halloran, J. P., & Asch, S. M. (2004). Human factors barriers to the effective use of ten HIV clinical reminders. *Journal of the American Informatics Association, 11*(1), 50-59.

Rousseau, N., McColl, E., Newton, J., Grimshaw, J., & Eccles, M. (2003). Practice-based, longitudinal, qualitative interview study of computerised evidence based guidelines in primary care. *British Medical Journal, 326*, 314-321.

Tilley, S., & Chambers, M. (2004). The process of implementing evidence-based practice: The curates egg. *Journal of Psychiatric and Mental Health Nursing, 11*, 117-119.

Timmons, S. (2003). Nurses resisting information technology. *Nursing Inquiry, 10*(4), 257-269.

Zimmerman, J. E., Shortell, S. M., Rousseau, D. M., Duffy, J., Gillies, R. R., Knaus, W. A., et al. (1993). Improving intensive care. Observations based on organisational case studies in nine intensive care units: A prospective multicenter study. *Critical Care Medicine, 21*(10), 1143-1451.

KEY TERMS

Clinical Champion: Clinical champions are opinion leaders who champion or encourage the uptake of an application.

Opinion Leader: An opinion leader is an individual, respected amongst his or her peers, who acts out of clinical conviction to influence the opinions of others vis-à-vis an informatics application.

Organizational Culture: Organizational culture is the set of shared norms, values, and tacit rules within which members of an organization function.

Organizational Factors: In an informatics context, organizational factors are factors relating to the culture and functioning of an organization that, negatively or positively, influence its ability to adapt to an informatics intervention.

Social Network: A social network consists of the individuals, groups, and organizations with whom an individual interacts, and the interactions that take place between the individual and other components of his or her social network.

Sociotechnical Approach: A sociotechnical approach is one that views informatics applications as part of the broader social and political context within which they are implemented.

Teamwork: The cooperative effort of a small group to achieve a specified outcome.

Chapter LIII
Measurement of Cost and Economic Efficiency in Healthcare

Panagiotis Danilakis
National and Kapodistrian University of Athens, Greece

Pericles Robolas
National and Kapodistrian University of Athens, Greece

ABSTRACT

The developments in new sectors, as in medical physics and biomedical technology, contributed a lot to the progress and especially to the medical practice. However, these developments created a complicated and costly environment in which health services have to take place. This chapter reports on the sensitive sector of finances of health and particularly the ways of cost assessment. Furthermore, it presents the significance of efficiency and effectiveness of technology that is used in the area of health.

INTRODUCTION

During the last 30 years, the financial situation of the health industry has known swift growth. However, the limited resources that are being disposed internationally for the sector of health point out the need of some concern for the cost of provided services. This was the main reason that turned the interest of economists of health from very early to the investigation of factors that influence the growth of expenses for hospital care.

In the economic bibliography, there is a wealth of theoretical and econometric approaches that aim to analyze the cost of hospital care. Naturally, the factors that determine the operation of hospital systems differ from country to country, as well as the structure and the organization of the private sector of care. Constants, functions, means, and the marginal cost exist as the objects of study, and it is supported that not only the objectives but also the more general system of the market and operation of the hospital unit is taken into consideration and is analyzed. One of the sectors that affects considerably the increase or the reduction of cost in the care of health is biomedical technology (biomedical engineering), which constitutes a very important tool for hospital organizations. Biomedical technology is developed continuously, encouraging the creation of new sectors of medical specialization, influencing decisively hospital structures, and simultaneously puzzling its right use with particular accent in the economic dimension.

COST ESTIMATION

The operation of each hospital unit aims at the offering of services of hospital care. Medical, nursing, administrative, and auxiliary personnel as well as certain diagnostic and therapeutic means are used for the offering of these services. The personnel and the means, depending on the way and degree of utilization, have a certain cost. This cost is constant or variable.

- **Constant Cost:** Remains immutable and includes various aspects such as rents and the cost of buildings and instruments. It is independent, therefore, of the number of patients or beds in the hospital. A constant cost is considered a datum and is presented diagrammatically as a horizontal line.
- **Variable Cost:** Influenced by the level of the operation of a hospital and increases proportionally with the number of patients in the hospital, with the duration of their hospitalization, and with the more general use of pharmaceutical products and diagnostic examinations. Sanitary material,

medicines, and diagnostic examinations constitute variable costs.

- **Total Cost:** The total cost of a hospital unit, which can the total monthly or annually, is composed of these two main components. This relation in simple form is expressed as:

Total Cost = Constant Cost + Variable Cost.

Many times in economic analysis, because the total costs do not provide enough information, we seek the determination of average or marginal costs.

- **Average Cost:** With the term this we mean his reason total cost to the number of patients. The average (or medium) cost shows the cost per unit, and in a hospital it can be expressed by a lot of indicators, such as (a) the cost per patient, (b) the cost per day of hospitalization, (c) the cost bed, and (d) the cost per doctor. The significance of the medium cost is important for the exercise of rational economic policy because it provides useful information on the change of costs concerning the productive activity of the hospital.
- **Marginal Cost:** With this term, we mean the change that befalls the costs of the hospital from a small change in patient number. The marginal cost constitutes a useful significance in the economic analysis because it shows how much an increase in the number of patients will affect the medium cost.

EVALUATION OF BIOMEDICAL TECHNOLOGY

As we reported previously, one of the more important sectors that present particular interest in analysis and more generally in the investigation of the relation of cost and effectiveness is the evaluation of biomedical technology. It was built in the '70s by the intense efforts in the search of evaluation methodologies of technologies, and was shaped by the incorporation of the special analyses of cost and effectiveness, and cost and utility. The evaluation of biomedical technology constitutes a sector of the social evaluation of technologies (or social technology assessment, STA), for which the following definition was in effect in the '70s.

- The (social) evaluation of technologies is the dynamic process of the multidimensional analysis, forecast, and estimate of all the short-term and long-term effects of technology in the individual, in society, and in the environment.
- The objective of the evaluation of technologies is the support of decision making (in government, in the hospital, in the industry, and so forth) for the wider comprehension of activities. Society produces, influences, and uses technologies so that they achieve its objectives in the best possible way.
- The aim of the evaluation of technologies is toward the preparation of policies and plans of action that will be useful as points of departure for decision making, via which the negative social repercussions of technologies will be minimized.

The methods of the evaluation of technologies are the following:

- **Heuristic Methods:** Historical retrospections, consensus conferences, hearings, questionnaires, Delphi-analysis scripts
- **Concise Methods:** Analyses of systems, morphological method (Zwicky), analyses of surge flows (Leontieff), dy-

namic models of systems (Forrester), analyses of cost and utilities, analyses of cost and effectiveness, meta-analyses

According to the initial objective of the evaluation of biomedical technology, the collection and treatment of data so that the essential information is produced is required in decision making with regard to investments in new mainly medical technologies. For this aim, a mesh of points of evaluation is proposed that is shaped by considered dimensions and levels, and that fixes the systematic structure of information and also criteria for evaluation. For the confrontation of each question, a particular mesh of criteria is used that is determined by considered dimensions, the levels, and the time horizon.

- **Dimensions:** The evaluation of biomedical technology is not only carried out in the medicine and economic dimensions, but also in the technique dimension. For the indirect cost of medical technology, various technical criteria are proposed in regard to the level of the development of the technology, the type used, safety, the effects of the way of work, the level of the development and support of software, and so forth. Depending on the examined problem of evaluation, additional dimensions are also selected such as further training.
- **Organization Levels:** The evaluation of the social, ethics, law, and education dimensions is carried out on the following levels: (a) the patient (the individual patient and his or her family), (b) the population of the service, (c) the hospital because the technology will alter its structure and way of work according to the population of the service (point of departure for the measurement needs and the demand), and (d) the system of hospitals

that serves the population of the prefecture or sanitary region.

- **Time Horizon:** The time horizon of the evaluation should harmonize itself with the practical requirements: the budget (1 year), the plan for investments (e.g., 5 years), and medium duration of the efficient operation of medical instruments (5 to 10 years).

- **Evaluation Steps:** In each point of evaluation (section of dimensions and levels of evaluation), the following correspond: (a) the placed questions, (b) the methods of collection and treatment essential for the evaluation of data, and (c) the criteria, according to which the data are evaluated so that the information that is required for decision making is produced. Most questions that are placed (or should be placed) to be answered for the evaluation of biomedical technology at the staff level in a hospital, that is to say, at the processes of the syntax of the budget for biomedical technology, belong to one of the following categories.

- **Optimization of the Relation of Cost and Effectiveness:** For the achievement of different (and desirable) medical objectives, to whom does medical technology present the better relation of cost and effectiveness? This question is placed when, for example, it should be decided if investments should be made for the creation of a new radiological clinic or for the automation of a biochemical laboratory, or when deciding on the disposal of existing economic resources for equipment for either a (new) unit for artificial kidneys or for a unit for the intensive hospitalization of nurslings. Still, for the decision-making if is in my interest the supply of chirurgical instrument Laser opposite of some other. Basically, such types of questions are faced with analyses of cost and utilities,

which, however, in practice, are proved inapplicable (or at least applicable with difficulty). It is presupposed that the comparison concerns therapeutic medical instruments and groups as far as for diagnostics should they be taken into consideration as other criteria of evaluation.

- **Optimization of Effectiveness:** For whom will the medical method (or instrument) be more effective so that some predetermined objective is achieved within the given amount of investment? This question is placed for the choice of medical instruments for the achievement of concrete aims when there are limited economic resources. Examples are the choice of equipment for arthroscopy and arthroscopy interventions.

- **Minimization of Cost:** For whom is a medical instrument more economical when given the achievement objective? The effectiveness under examination for medical instruments can be given or even nonexistent. This question is usually examined for the choice of diagnostic instruments. The answer should promote the choice of the more economically acceptable and widespread instrument. Often, the choice of the medical instrument should correspond with a better way to meet needs. Examples are the choice of appliances for the automation of biochemical laboratories, diagnostic technology and appliances for the provision of physiotherapy, and electrocardiographs, monitors, and automated systems for the examination of neurology or ophthalmology.

CONCLUSION

The big growth of science and technology during the last decades of the 20th century resulted in the rapid development of medical science and its benefits, but also of the models of the demand for services of health. These developments, which influenced all the professions of health, helped so that the benefits of services are carried out henceforth in the frames of a completely organized system. Such a system, therefore, will be aim to combine human, technological, and natural resources so that the exercise of modern medical practice is feasible. It is exceptionally critical for professionals and future professionals of health to comprehend not only the sectors of their professions, but also the nature, organzation, and operation of the systems inside that make their professions, as well how important it is to evaluate the sector of health and its economic output generally.

REFERENCES

Abel-Smith, B. (1976). *Value for money in health services*. London: Heinmann.

Abel-Smith, B. (1986). The world economic crisis, part 2: Health manpower out of balance. *Health Policy and Planning*, 309-316.

Butler, J. R. (1995). *Hospital cost analysis*. Dordrecht, The Netherlands: Kluwer Academic Publishers.

Evans, R. G. (1971). Behavioural cost functions for hospitals. *Canadian Journal of Economics*, 198-215.

Evans, R. G. (1972). Information theory and the analysis of hospital cost structure. *Canadian Journal of Economics*, 398-418.

Feeny, D. (1986). New health technologies: Their effect on health and cost of health care. In *Health care technology: Effectiveness, efficiency and pubic policy* (pp. 5-24). Institute for Research and Public Policy.

Lovel, C. (1995). Econometric efficiency analysis: A policy oriented review. *European Journal of Operational Research*, 452-461.

KEY TERMS

Biomedical Technology: The sector that, with the application of scientific and technological methods, aims toward the manufacture of medical technological equipment, for example, monitors and many other appliances. In a lot of ways, this sector is the same as medical information technology. The two sectors use the PC (personal computer), which also has a secondary role in the two sectors. Thus, medical biotechnology focuses on the appliances, and medical information technology focuses on the knowledge and information, and on the management of these with a PC.

Delphi Analysis: A method of the achievement of consent between scientists of prestige on some difficult question.

Effectiveness: A metre that estimates how much a product, service, or program achieves its objectives under real conditions. As the effectiveness of medical equipment is improved, this contribution is in the treating of illness.

Efficiency: The achievement of concrete results with the minimal possible cost of the occasion, or the maximization of results with a given cost for the occasion.

Evaluation of Technology: The evaluation of technology is a dynamic process that examines short-term and long-term social, economic, and legal repercussions from the use of this technology.

Medical Information Technology: It is the way that medical personnel collect, organize, and use data, information, and knowledge in decision making, and the export of conclusions contributing to the quality care of the patient.

Meta-Analysis: A method of evaluating many clashing studies around some question, and the export of useful conclusions.

Reliability of Technical Equipment: It is the faculty of an element, appliance, or technological system to satisfy those requirements that are dictated from the aim for which it was manufactured.

Chapter LIV
Understanding Telemedicine with Innovative Systems

Irene Berikou
Athens University of Economics and Business, Greece

Athina A. Lazakidou
University of Piraeus, Greece

ABSTRACT

A system of innovation (SI) is a new approach for the study of innovations as an endogenous part of the economy. An SI can be defined as encompassing all the important factors that influence the development, diffusion, and use of innovations as well as the relations between these factors. For example, the SI approach is also used as a framework for designing innovation policy at the national level in some EU (European Union) member countries such as Finland and Ireland. It is simply at the center of modern thinking about innovation and its relation to economic growth, competitiveness, and employment. In this chapter, the adaptation of this framework for telemedicine applications is simply presented.

INTRODUCTION

The healthcare sector is in need for innovation during the process of delivering services, and ICT has the potential to change the organization and delivery of health and social services in Europe. The slow rate of telemedicine adoption in a country's healthcare system is not only caused by technology factors related to the speed, security, and capacity of the national infrastructure or by inferior technological arti-

facts. The successful implementation of telemedicine services requires its underlying technologies to be configured in a way that meets the particular needs of the healthcare and social care providers, the individuals receiving care, and all other stakeholders. Technical success alone will not result in the widespread diffusion of telecare technologies (Barlow, Bayer, & Curry, 2003).

Academic researchers have clarified little in understanding the phenomenon of telemedicine in its wider economic and social performance. The complexity of ICT in healthcare has also confused the definition of telemedicine. Many terms have been used by academics, researchers, healthcare professionals, informaticians, the ICT industry, and governmental and nongovernmental organizations to describe the phenomenon.

This chapter is an attempt to use a rather new economic framework in order to define the value and the placement of ICT within the healthcare sector: the way that it transforms previous healthcare delivery into a coproduced activity. Therefore, this effort might prove to be helpful to facilitate implementation issues and to diffuse telemedicine in each healthcare system, no matter if we see it from either a micro or macro perspective.

DEFINITION OF TELEMEDICINE

Telemedicine is an information technology-driven application that provides the means of delivering healthcare services at a distance. The term telemedicine is constituted by two words, *tele* and *medicine*. The first component is the Greek word τηλε that means from far away or at a distance, and the second component is of Latin origin from the word *mederi*, which means healing. It involves not only medical activities for ill patients, but also public-health activities involving well people. In other words, telehealth is a process and not a technology, including many different healthcare activities carried out at a distance (Riva, 2000).

Origins of Systems-of-Innovation Approach in Economist Cycles

Joseph Schumpeter, a classical economist who wrote his famous theory for entrepreneurship, in 1939 was the first to conceive innovation in a much broader way than technical orientation. He specifically mentions new forms of organization and new combinations.

Innovation is the new creation of economic significance of either a material or intangible kind (Edquist, 2001). Innovations may be brand new, but often they are new combinations of existing elements. A useful taxonomy is to divide innovations into new products and new processes. Product innovations may be goods or services. It is a matter of what is being produced. Process innovations may be technological or organizational. They concern how goods and services are produced.

Today, it is widely recognized that technological change is the primary engine for economic development. Innovation, at the heart of technological change, is essentially the innovation process that depends upon the accumulation and development of relevant knowledge of a wide variety. Certainly, individual firms play a crucial role in the development of specific innovations, but the process that nurtures and disseminates technological change involves a complex web of interactions among a range of other firms, organizations, and institutions (Fisher, 2001).

A system of innovation (SI) is a new approach for the study of innovations as an endogenous part of the economy. The SI has emerged only during the last decade or so. An SI can be defined as encompassing all the important factors that influence the development, diffusion, and use of innovations as well as the relations between these factors. These factors can be studied in a national, regional, or sectoral context; therefore, national, regional, and sectoral systems of innovation coexist and complement each other. The SI has diffused surprisingly fast in the academic world as well as in the realms of public innovation making and firm innovation strategy formulation. That is, SI provides a framework, not a theory, of analysis for identifying specific policy issues to understand differences between national and regional economies and various ways to support technological change. For example, the SI approach is also used as a framework for designing innovation policy at the national level in some EU (European Union) member countries such as Finland and Ireland. It is simply at the center of modern thinking about innovation and its relation to economic growth, competitiveness, and employment. In an SI approach, there are at least three main categories of system failure (Edquist, 2001), which are different from market failures as system failures are identified through comparisons between existing systems.

- Organizations in the system of innovation may be inappropriate or missing.
- Institutions or codification may be inappropriate or missing.
- Interactions or links of the knowledge flow between these elements in the SI might be inappropriate or missing.

The development of SI approaches has been influenced by different theories of innovation such as interactive learning theories and evolutionary theories. The first two books exclusively devoted to the analysis of national systems of innovation were Lundvall (1992) and Nelson (1993). However, Chris Freeman (1987) first used the expression in published form. Regional systems of innovation have been addressed, for example, in Braczyk, Cooke, and Heidenreich (1998). Sectoral SIs have been analysed in Carlsson (1995), Breschi and Malerba (1997), and Nelson and Mowery (1999). All these books and others are reviewed in the introduction to Edquist and McKelvey (2000), which is a collection of 43 central articles on systems of innovation.

Tether and Metcalfe (2001) made a major contribution recently to develop the framework for services, shifting the interest from the manufacturer. The adaptation of this framework for telemedicine applications is the following.

TELEMEDICINE AS A SYSTEM OF INNOVATION IN SERVICES

It is known that the sector of healthcare is a service sector. Usually, the definition of a service is embedded with intangibility as it lacks an autonomous physical existence contrary to products.

This sense has reason as the service of healthcare can change our physical being, and in order to offer health services, the process is often indistinguishable from the product, while in the long term the outcome is intangible. All transformation processes transform combinations of material, energy, and information into new, more highly valued combinations of these elements (Tether & Metcalfe, 2001). The differentiated nature of services and the multiple ways that service activities can be defined, or the way telemedicine is defined in the healthcare sphere, are central to an understanding of the complexities of innovation systems of services. The nature of services and the transformations they provide also tend to have a significant bearing on their organizational form. We consider that telemedicine offers an innovation process into the chain of healthcare delivery (Berikou, 2004).

Another characteristic of services is that they are coproduced, involving simultaneous relationships between producers-physicians and consumers-patients. With telemedicine, we have one more new relationship to consider: that between back office experts and front-office physicians in remote areas. The service of healthcare with telemedicine brings to the fore the interactive aspects of a dual character. These complex interactions constitute multiple systems of innovation (den Hertog, in press). As telemedicine may transform previous engagement with healthcare, we may consider that the core function of services in health today is the service delivery of better quality and equity faster than before, and the peripheral form of the service can vary enormously from teleconsulting to telemonitoring at home (Berikou, 2004).

As information technologies and networks have developed, so have new forms of coordination and delivery. Technological developments have reduced the power of location for the service of healthcare. Where traditionally most services were provided locally, with consumers often coming to the service provider, now many services are provided at arm's length, for example, through the Internet. Arm's-length provision typically allows the exploitation of economies of scale, which provide advantages over traditional, local provision (Tether & Metcalfe, 2004). This encourages the development of cooperation between the front office (which deals directly with patients) and the back office that carries out the service processes. It can bring a significant impact on the organization in terms of the size of the healthcare unit, the number of sites, and the location of functions.

As Gallouij and Weinstein mention, the analysis of innovation is difficult because of the "fuzzy" nature of service outputs, in which it can be difficult to distinguish the service product from the background process or the organization of provision. Miozo and Soete have done some attempts at the taxonomy of innovation in services in order to adapt the Pavitt taxonomy into services.

From a system's perspective on the service innovation of Tether and Metcalfe (2001), and

making adjustments for telemedicine, the following apply.

- Services are not normally engaged in the production of tangible products, but cover a huge range of diverse activities associated with various types of transformation, that is, the transformation of people (physically and mentally), things, and information. There are important connections between service innovation (rearrangement in the delivery of healthcare) and artifact innovation (telemedicine applications) as normally defined.

- The study of services brings to the fore to a greater extent the interrelationships between business models, organizational forms, technology, and outputs. The significance of market knowledge and procedural knowledge is highlighted.

- Healthcare with telemedicine shows high degrees of interaction and interdependency between the service provider (physician) and the service user (patient), between the service provider (back-office expert) and the service user (physician in remote areas, front office), as well as between the provider (front office or back office) and equipment suppliers. Such interaction and interdependency is a central feature of systems of innovation. The system involves a wide range of agents from many different sectors (IT suppliers, university researchers, research and development companies and institutes, public sector, healthcare levels, physicians). An interesting feature of these systems is that the agents involved and the interrelationships between these agents can change over time; thus, the boundaries of the system are not fixed but are dynamic and evolve.

- We consider that systems of innovation often develop around identifiable sequences of problems and opportunities, which are themselves framed by a number of contingencies including the regulatory, cultural, and technological context. In this way, the problem or opportunity (telemedicine in remote areas) at the heart of the system of innovation becomes the focusing device around which it is developed. As the problem or opportunity changes or is redefined, so the system of telemedicine can change, changing the agents involved and the relations between these agents: It is a dynamic, distributed process (Coombs, Harvey, & Tether, 2001). One important aspect of this view is that, individually and collectively, firms and communities of practitioners (providers and users) take a leading role in assembling innovation systems in the pursuit of a competitive advantage.

CONCLUSION

Such a framework may help us describe the context of innovation in services for ICT in the healthcare sector, but the field is still fragmented (den Hertog, in press). The problem or opportunity framework must be seen as a context-specific policy tool and not be restricted into a solution for all patterns.

Generalizations under the influence of this framework in telemedicine practice can be given as such: There must be greater capacity and broadband development in between hospitals, and between hospitals and primary health services in order to enable the use of telemedical and IT applications. The clarification of responsibility, rules, guidelines, and rates in connection with telemedical consultations must be a prerequisite. Papers must be removed when electronic applications are implemented. Electronic cooperation with all partners in the sector and with other areas such as pharmacies, relatives, and patients is required. The boundaries of the system are changing as new agents are included, including common standards, the free flow of information between different applications, and the national implementation of important applications. More institutions playing by the rules of the game can constrain, coordinate, and enable activity. ICT development must follow organizational development, changes in work processes, and new forms of cooperation and divisions of labour. This means that learning processes and knowledge bases are going to be established.

REFERENCES

Barlow, J., Bayer, S., & Curry, D. (2003). Integrating telecare into mainstream care delivery. *The IPTS Report.*

Berikou, E. (2004). *Telemedicine systems: A comparison with Norway for innovation and implementation in Greece.* Unpublished master's thesis, Linkoping University, Tema-T Department, Sweden.

Braczyk, H.-J., Cooke, P., & Heidenreich, M. (1998). *Regional innovation systems: The role of governances in a globalized world.* London: UCL Press.

Breschi, S., & Malerba, F. (1997). Sectoral innovation systems: Technological regimes, Scumpeterian dynamics and spatial boundaries. In C. Edquist (Ed.), *Systems of innovation: Technologies, institutions and organizations.* London: Pinter/Cassel Academic.

Coombs, R., Harvey, M., & Tether, B. S. (2001). *Analysing distributed innovation-*

processes: A CRIC position paper. UK: CRIC, University of Manchester, & UMIST.

Den Hertog, F. (in press). Mapping health care innovation: Tracing walls & ceilings. *MERIT.*

Edquist, C. (2001). Innovation policy: A systemic approach. In B. A. Lundvall & Archingi (Eds.), *The globalizing learning economy.* Oxford University Press.

Edquist, C., & McKelvey, M. (Eds.). (2000). *Systems of innovation: Growth, competitiveness and employment.* Gheltenham: Edward Elgar.

Fischer, M. M. (2001). Innovation, knowledge creation and systems of innovation. *Annals of Regional Science, 35,* 199-216.

Freeman, C. (1987). *Technology policy and economic performance: Lessons from Japan.* London: Pinter.

Lundvall, B.-A. (1992). *National systems of innovation: Towards a theory of innovation and interactive learning.* London: Pinter.

Nelson, R. R. (1993). *National innovation systems: A comparative study.* Oxford: Oxford University Press.

Nonaka, I. (1994). A dynamic theory of organizational knowledge creation. *Organization Science, 5*(1).

Riva, G. (2000). From telehealth to e-health: Internet and distributed virtual reality in health care. *Cyberpsychology & Behavior, 3*(6).

Rogers, E. M. (2003). *Diffusion of innovations* (5th ed.). New York: Free Press.

Tether, B. S., & Metcalfe, J. S. (2001). *Services and systems of innovation.* Paper presented at the DRUID Academy Winter 2002 PHP Conference.

KEY TERMS

Adoption: Rogers (2003) differentiates the adoption process from the diffusion process in that the diffusion process occurs within society as a group process, whereas the adoption process pertains to an individual. Rogers defines the adoption process as "the mental process through which an individual passes from first hearing about an innovation to final adoption."

Codification: A process of knowledge conversion between the two forms: tacit and explicit.

Diffusion: The process in which an innovation is communicated through certain channels over time among the members of a social system (Rogers, 2003).

Evolutionary Economics: This science describes the unleashing of a process of technological and institutional innovation that discovers more survival value for the costs incurred than competing alternatives. It explains the evidence and suggests that economies grow faster when there is diverse participation, competitive survival, and the replication of success.

Implementation: The process of putting all program functions and activities into place; it is part of the innovation-decision process quoted by Rogers (2003).

Interactive Learning Theories: Learning by interacting between users and producers, embodying knowledge in new services and products.

Knowledge Flow: The way knowledge travels and grows within an organization.

Chapter LV
A Capacity Building Approach to Health Literacy through ICTs

Lyn Simpson
Queensland University of Technology, Australia

Melinda Stockwell
Queensland University of Technology, Australia

Susan Leggett
Queensland University of Technology, Australia

Leanne Wood
Queensland University of Technology, Australia

Danielle Penn
Queensland University of Technology, Australia

ABSTRACT

There has been substantial interest in delivering ICT training options to rural and remote areas of Queensland, Australia, in order to bridge the rural-urban divide. But there is more than just education and training going on: Participants are being empowered to gain new skills and confidence, form new networks, become active in the community, and be proactive in addressing their own health and well-being needs.

THE RURAL AND REMOTE CONTEXT

Rural and remote populations often experience poor access to services (Simpson, Wood, Daws, & Seinen, 2001; Wagenfeld, Murray, Mohatt, & DeBruyn, 1997). This applies to essential health services, to services that enable individuals and communities to gain the skills necessary to participate in the social changes affecting the population, and to the peer-support services needed by isolated professionals. In Australia, long-standing factors in service delivery to rural communities, such as sparse population, distance, and limited availability of public transport, are being exacerbated by the reduction in and withdrawal of existing face-to-face services. In terms of health services, access constitutes a significant issue for rural communities. At the same time, the traditional jobs base for these communities in primary production is shrinking, resulting in psychological pressures and the need for the re-skilling of many of those people formerly employed in such industries.

Health literacy, understood in its broadest sense, is a key issue for these communities. Parker (2000, p. 280) notes, "... for those with limited health literacy, as health care is becoming increasingly complex and health information is becoming more diffuse in the public domain, there is more reliance on written materials to educate and inform people about their health." As governments at all levels seek ways to simplify, and reduce the costs of, the task of meeting health-service needs, the attractions of e-government for service delivery to a receptive "wired" community are strong (and ICT vendors have encouraged that attraction). However, for those community members used to the supportive environment of face-to-face service delivery and unfamiliar with ICTs, the focus on service provision via the Internet creates new challenges. The incentive for computer literacy (Hamm as cited in Loader & Keeble, 2004) is strengthening.

The problems associated with negotiating the changed rural social and service environment impact particularly those people who have characteristics that may intensify their isolation and lack of access to information, including people of cultural and linguistic diversity (CALD), disabled people, and people with low literacy skills. A socially inclusive society requires informed communities that have the means, skills, and opportunities to communicate (IBM, 1997). For those unable to meet these criteria because of age, ethnicity, disability, income, or circumstance, difficulties associated with the acquisition of everyday information via the Internet can potentially create considerable frustration and distress, increasing the degree to which these people are marginalized within their community, and impacting their health and well-being.

THE CASE-STUDY PROJECTS

The projects build on earlier work that identified the difficulty in accessing accurate current information and in obtaining appropriate health and well-being support for these populations. Interviewees in fieldwork for *Creating Rural Connections* (Simpson et al., 2001) reported a variety of information needs, including more timely access to a wider range of information, and the desire for specific information in response to an identified need (such as to address a health problem), to locate employment, or to improve the family business.

Community members identified two levels of specific need. First is the need for access to specialist services, including medical services and counseling; ongoing access to help, companionship, and mentoring; community-service databases to facilitate better networking and referral services; improved access to services for disability groups, particularly services that have the potential to overcome the effects of communication limitations and personal isolation; and opportunities to identify and reinforce existing support networks. They also identified the need for re-skilling regarding computing skills as a necessary tool in the changing work and social environment. The projects developed to help address these needs have provided an inclusive and supportive learning environment for individuals who had experienced marginalization in their communities. The focus in each project has been on Bella and Bishop's (2004) "building on" community capacity: "helping people believe in their own skills" (p. 13).

HOW THE PROJECTS OPERATE

The projects are built on the recognition that social isolation and access to information are significant issues for marginalized people in far-north Queensland and, in particular, for people who speak little or no English, for indigenous peoples, and for disabled people. Drawing on research that has shown the Internet to be an effective, appropriate means of meeting such needs for a diverse range of people (Communication Centre, 2001; Simpson et al., 2001), the projects sought to:

- enhance the skills base in small communities;
- help create a more informed community and a more equitable society in part via access to information by marginalized groups;
- facilitate the sharing of skills through the development and creation of online and face-to-face social networks;
- develop an innovative and transferable process that will be relevant to other groups and other communities;
- increase awareness of the potential of online technologies for contributing to the social connectedness and overall well-being of potentially marginalized groups, particularly but not exclusively in rural and remote areas; and
- provide "train the trainer" instruction for volunteer community members from

marginalized groups that will assist them in conducting training that is appropriate for their client base, taking into account the specific needs arising from age, gender, rurality, ethnicity, literacy, and/or disability.

While these aims focus on the technical and training needs of people in rural and remote communities, it is how these goals are enacted that creates the powerful social and health outcomes. Projects intended to deliver ICT training to marginalized groups have often failed. When asked what the problems were with computer training programs they had attempted, participants identified the following:

- Modules not relevant to their needs
- Training moved too quickly for them to keep up with the group
- Could not understand the trainer
- Class sizes too big
- Felt alienated from the other students
- Felt alienated from the teacher
- Too old
- Left it too late

As Feinstein, Hammond, Woods, Preston, and Bynner (2003) found, for those who have been away from learning for some time, there are particular qualities in the learning environment that enable the wider benefits to flow. Such programs need to "ensure engagement ... [C]lasses that are not sensitive to learners' needs are not necessarily going to generate the wider benefits. The provision of facilities and encouragement for interaction would also appear to be essential components" (p. 74). The projects described emphasize the need to surmount these issues, and the need for building a supporting and sustaining social infrastructure. The e-life cycle is the methodology common to all these projects,[1] revolving around a five-

Figure 1. Inclusion, connectedness, and information sharing: Making connections face-to-face and online

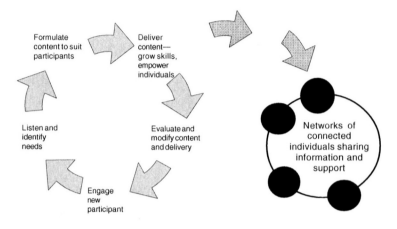

stage approach (illustrated in Figure 1): Engage the marginalized, listen to the learner, identify the need(s), formulate effective programs, and evaluate and modify.

Engage the Marginalized

Engaging the community and ascertaining their training needs is the crucial first step. Tutors publicize their programs through community places like hotels, community centers, and shops, as well as through recruiting clients via other community organizations, which refer people with literacy and/or numeracy needs to the program, and also offer services to learners taking part in the program.

Listen

Developing effective strategies for access and participation that take differences in community needs and the whole range of local social, economic, cultural, and technological factors into account can provide more equitable access to ICTs while increasing the overall success of community informatics initiatives (Rural Women and ICTs Research Team, 1999; Simpson, 2004;

Simpson et al., 2001). Providing an environment in which participants feel they are valued and are treated as capable equals is crucial to the e-life cycle's listening stage; participants here voice their needs explicitly, and those needs are addressed. Empowerment is also important for, as Feinstein (2002, p. 9) found, "Psychological well being, which encompasses a sense of personal control, and freedom from stress and hostility, in turn appears to lead to better health outcomes."

Identify

In this environment, specific training needs can be accurately identified since participants gain a sense that they are valued, that their needs are unlikely to be "way out" or in some way unacceptable, and that their contributions and concerns will be treated with respect. Tutors encourage participants to use the technology to follow their own interests in the belief that something that has direct relevance to their own lives will be more enjoyable and more relevant, and will enhance the internalization of the learning process.

Formulate

Formulating effective programs, then, draws on the expressed interests of the participants. For example, participants might express a desire to be able to e-mail a friend or relative overseas, or to access a particular Web site or support group via the Internet. The learning is structured around this need while following a series of specified guidelines, and it is intended to provide all participants with skills in basic computing and connectivity.

There are both accredited and nonaccredited schemes in operation. In the nonaccredited training programs, material is taught in a flexible, self-paced delivery mode. Participants are encouraged to attend each session but are not penalized for not doing so. Emphasis is on meeting the learner's needs. Feinstein et al. (2003) found that the particular value of unaccredited courses is that they "may equip adults with the personal and social confidence as well as other necessary skills to progress to more challenging accredited courses, especially if appropriate guidance is available" (pp. 76-77).

Evaluate

In the projects in north Queensland, opportunities are provided for trying out new skills, sometimes in real-world situations, enabling the teacher to evaluate and modify the training. Is it working? Are participants moving toward confidence and facility? What adjustments can be made?

PRINCIPLES FOR COMMUNITY WORKERS

These projects have demonstrated a clear link between increased social cohesion and connectedness, health literacy, and health out-

comes. Four crucial aspects of the e-life-cycle approach are the following.

Participation and Inclusion

The equitable and inclusive participation of people in planning, evaluation, and decision making is vital to sustainable community and economic development. The programs are specifically targeted at marginalized individuals, with the trainer taking a proactive approach to inclusion. The existing capacities and experiences of participants are overtly valued and celebrated, with trainers and other class members supporting and empowering one another in an encouraging, inclusive environment.

Content

It is crucial that content is individually tailored in a group setting to the needs and interests of the clients, is culturally sensitive and gender inclusive, and is made accessible by attention to the language and literacy needs of specific groups within the community. Hence, courses are designed around what participants want, using real-life learning needs or desires to shape learning delivery.

Delivery

Delivery must be flexible and responsive to learners' needs, incorporate design features that capitalise on the tools made available by evolving communication technologies, and support access by people with varying levels of ability, including those with mobility, vision, hearing, and cognitive difficulties. In designing training-delivery projects, differences between people therefore need to be taken into account, including gender, age, ethnicity, occupation, and level of knowledge of new technologies.

Time

Allowing sufficient time for the development of the positive attitudes and skills necessary for the effective adoption and utilization of online technology is important. For example, the need for "hastening slowly" is evident in each of the human factors affecting the acceptance and value of Web-based services (Communication Centre, 2001). Taking this into consideration, some courses are self-paced, allowing participants to work through individual modules at their own pace and with the support of peers, tutors, family, or friends. This flexibility allows for work and family commitments, and allows participants to work around farm and seasonal commitments.

FUTURE TRENDS AND CONCLUSION

Advances in information technology and telecommunications may offer many potential benefits to Australia's underserved communities by reducing the barriers of distance and space that disadvantage rural areas; this can only happen where projects enable the participation of all groups in the community. Improvements in the knowledge and use of such technologies have been identified as being beneficial in improving health literacy in rural communities, and they will continue to be an area of attention to reduce health inequities in Australia.

REFERENCES

Bella, L., & Bishop, R. (2004, October 17-19). *Community capacity development: A framework for understanding the contribution of community access computers at MacMorran Community Centre to community capacity, literacy and health.* Paper presented at the Canadian Conference on Literacy and Health, CPHA, Ottawa, Ontario.

Communication Centre. (2001). *Developing indicators to determine the effectiveness of Web-based service delivery: An holistic approach.* Brisbane, Australia: Author, QUT.

Feinstein, L. (2002). *Wider benefits of learning research report no. 6: Quantitative estimates of the social benefits of learning, 2: Health (depression and obesity).* London: Centre for Research on the Wider Benefits of Learning.

Feinstein, L., Hammond, C., Woods, L., Preston, J., & Bynner, J. (2003). *Wider benefits of learning research report no. 8: The contribution of adult learning to health and social capital.* London: Centre for Research on the Wider Benefits of Learning.

IBM. (1997). *The net result: Social inclusion in the information society. Report of the National Working Party on Social Inclusion.* London: IBM UK.

Loader, B., & Keeble, L. (2004). *Challenging the digital divide? A literature review of community informatics initiatives.* York, UK: Joseph Rowntree Foundation & York Publishing Services.

Parker, R. (2000). Health literacy: A challenge for American patients and their health care providers. *Health Promotion International, 15*(4), 277-283.

Rural Women and ICTs Research Team. (1999). *The new pioneers: Women in rural Queensland collaboratively exploring the potential of communication and information technologies for personal, business and community development.* Brisbane, Australia: The Communications Centre, QUT.

Simpson, L. (2004). *Community informatics and sustainability: Why social capital matters.* Paper presented at the Community Informatics Research Networks Conference, Prato, Italy.

Simpson, L., Wood, L., Daws, L., & Seinen, A. (2001). *Creating rural connections.* Brisbane, Australia: The Communication Centre, QUT.

Wagenfeld, M. O., Murray, J. D., Mohatt, D. F., & DeBruyn, J. C. (1997). Mental health service delivery in rural areas: Organizational and clinical issues. *NIDA Research Monograph, 168,* 418-437.

KEY TERMS

Capacity Building: The development of sustainable skills, organizational structures, resources, and commitment to health improvement in health and other sectors.

Health Literacy: The capacity of an individual to obtain, interpret, and understand basic health information and services, and the competence to use such information and services in ways that are health enhancing.

Social Connectedness: The relationships people have with others and the benefits these bring to individuals and society.

ENDNOTE

[1] Workers delivering training refer to the process as "normal mode," a label that downplays its exceptional and innovative qualities.

Index